PREHOSPITAL NURSING

A Collaborative Approach

PREHOSPITAL NURSING

A Collaborative Approach

RENEÉ SEMONIN HOLLERAN
RN, PhD, CEN, CCRN, CFRN

Chief Flight Nurse
University Air Care
University of Cincinnati
Cincinnati, Ohio

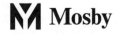 **Mosby**

St. Louis Baltimore Berlin Boston Carlsbad Chicago London Madrid
Naples New York Philadelphia Sydney Tokyo Toronto

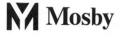
Mosby

Dedicated to Publishing Excellence

Publisher: Alison Miller
Editor-in-Chief: Nancy Coon
Editor: Robin Carter
Developmental Editor: Jeanne Allison
Project Manager: Patricia Tannian
Senior Production Editor: John P. Casey
Senior Book Designer: Gail Morey Hudson
Manufacturing Supervisor: Karen Lewis
Cover Designer: Teresa Breckwoldt

Printed in the United States of America
Composition by Graphic World, Inc.
Printing/Binding by Maple-Vail Book Mfg. Group

Mosby—Year Book, Inc.
11830 Westline Industrial Drive, St. Louis, Missouri 63146

Library of Congress Cataloging in Publication Data

Prehospital nursing: a collaborative approach / [edited by] Reneé
    Semonin Holleran.—1st ed.
        p.   cm.
    Includes bibliographical references and index.
    ISBN 0-8016-7894-3
  I. Holleran, Reneé Semonin.
    [DNLM: 1. Emergency nursing.   2. Transportation of patients.   WY
154 P923 1994]
    RT120.E4P746   1994
    610.73′61—dc20
    DNLM/DLC—dc20
    for Library of Congress   494-16136
                                                                                  CIP

94 95 96 97 98 / 9 8 7 6 5 4 3 2 1

Contributors

LISA MARIE BERNARDO, RN, PhD

Clinical Nurse Specialist
Emergency Department
Children's Hospital of Pittsburgh
Pittsburgh, Pennsylvania

DIANA JAYNES DEIMLING, RN, BSN, CEN, CCRN, NEMT-P

Flight Nurse, University Air Care
University of Cincinnati Hospital
Cincinnati, Ohio

JANICE EVANS, RN, MSN

EMT-A Program Coordinator
Center for Prehospital Education
Department of Emergency Medicine
University of Cincinnati Medical Center
Cincinnati, Ohio

BONNIE L. HOGUE, RN, BSN

Professional Nurse III, Emergency Department
Children's Hospital of Pittsburgh
Pittsburgh, Pennsylvania

ANTHONY T. KRAMER, RN, BSN, NREMT-P

Clinical Coordinator
Center for Prehospital Education
Department of Emergency Medicine
University of Cincinnati Medical Center
Cincinnati, Ohio

ALAN F. MISTLER, RN

Program Director
Center for Prehospital Education
Department of Emergency Medicine
University of Cincinnati Medical Center
Cincinnati, Ohio

MARY ANN NIEHAUS-O'TOOLE, RN, MSN, CEN

Critical Care Nurse
University of Cincinnati
Cincinnati, Ohio

EDWARD J. OTTEN, MD

Professor, Medical Director, Toxicology
Department of Emergency Medicine
University of Cincinnati Medical Center
Cincinnati, Ohio

MIKE ROUSE, RN, CEN, CFRN

Flight Nurse, University Air Care
University of Cincinnati Hospital
Cincinnati, Ohio

MICHAEL SAYRE, MD

Assistant Professor, Medical Director
Center for Prehospital Education
Department of Emergency Medicine
University of Cincinnati Medical Center
Cincinnati, Ohio

T. JANE SWAIM, RN

Patient Care Services Administrator
Nursing Administration
University of Cincinnati Medical Center
Cincinnati, Ohio

JANET M. WILLHITE, RN, BSN, CCRN

Flight Nurse, University Air Care
University of Cincinnati Hospital
Cincinnati, Ohio

CHERYL WRAA, RN, CFRN

Chief Flight Nurse, LIFEFLIGHT
University of California–Davis Medical Center
Sacramento, California

Consultants

JEAN BENING, RN

Program Director, Heartflight
Sacred Heart Medical Center
Spokane, Washington

NANCY L. FOWLER, RN, CEN

Flight Nurse, Heartflight
Sacred Heart Medical Center
Spokane, Washington

PAMELA FRANKEL, RN, MS

Trauma Coordinator
Oregon Health Sciences University
Portland, Oregon

JUDY STONER HALPERN, RN, MS, CEN

Trauma Clinical Nurse Specialist
Bronson Methodist Hospital
Kalamazoo, Michigan

GAIL HANDYSIDES, RN, MS

Instructor, School of Nursing
San Diego University
San Diego, California

LINDA K. MANLEY, RN, MSN, EMT-P

EMS Coordinator
Children's Hospital
Columbus, Ohio

WAYNE McLEOD, RN, BA, REMT-P, CFRN

Flight Nurse, University AIRCARE
University Medical Center
Tucson, Arizona

SUSAN MOORE, RN, MS, CCRN, CEN

Manager, Emergency Department
Washoe Medical Center
Reno, Nevada

CLAIRE RAYMOND, PharmD

Clinical Pharmacist
Washington University Medical Center
St. Louis, Missouri

ANNE RUSSELL, RN, MSN, CCRN

Trauma Clinical Associate
Miami Valley Hospital
Dayton, Ohio

DARLENE T. SCHELPER, RN, MSN, CEN

Clinical Nurse Educator
Hershey Medical Center
Hershey, Pennsylvania

MARIAN STASI, RN, MS, CCRN

Cardiac Clinical Nurse Specialist
Cardiology and Cardiac Electrophysiology
Oak Lawn, Illinois

LORI D. TAYLOR, RN, BSN, EMT-P

Trauma Program Manager
Sacred Heart Medical Center
Spokane, Washington

DONNA YORK, RN, MS, CCRN

Chief Flight Nurse, Stanford LIFEFLIGHT
Stanford University Hospital
Stanford, California

*This book is dedicated to the
patience of my family*

Micke, Erin, and Sara
as well as my
mother

It is also dedicated to all of my colleagues
who practice collaboratively in the "field."

Preface

Prehospital Nursing: A Collaborative Approach was written to describe the practice of nursing in the prehospital care environment. Nursing has been practiced outside of hospital walls for centuries: in homes, communities, and on the battlefield. During the past 30 years the care of the patient before and during transport has developed into both an art and a science. No longer is anyone "too sick" to be moved. Nursing has played and continues to play a significant role in the delivery of care in the prehospital environment.

ORGANIZATION

Prehospital Nursing is organized to present the roles of nursing in the prehospital care environment and to address the nursing and collaborative care that patients require. The book is divided into three parts. The first part discusses the roles of nursing in the prehospital care environment. The second part addresses specific patient populations and the care they require before and during transport. The final part considers the challenges and future of prehospital nursing.

Unlike other areas of nursing practice, there is not a national standard that guides the practice of prehospital nursing. Two texts contributed to the outline of this book: the *National Standard Guidelines for Prehospital Nursing* from the Emergency Nurses Association and the *Air Medical Crew National Curriculum* from the United States Department of Transportation. In addition, the joint position statement from the Emergency Nurses Association and the National Flight Nurses Association provided further direction for this book.

Throughout the text multiple sources are cited to provide information related to the practice of prehospital nursing. These sources come not only from nursing but also from medicine and prehospital care educators and practitioners. Many of the chapters also include additional sources of information that readers may find useful.

Chapters 1, 2, and 3 specifically address the roles of those who practice in prehospital care including nurses, paramedics, emergency medical technicians, and physicians. The specific role each individual plays, as well as the vehicles and equipment used in the prehospital care environment, are addressed throughout these chapters.

Chapter 5 discusses the safety issues related to prehospital nursing practice and includes a section on personal survival.

Chapters 6 through 13 describe patient assessment and preparation in general and with regard to particular patient populations such as the trauma patient (Chapter 7), the cardiac, respiratory, and neurological patient (Chapter 9), the intoxicated patient (Chapter 10), patients with infectious diseases (Chapter 11), and the pediatric patient (Chapter 12). Each of these chapters examines the care of these patient populations before and during transport. Equipment, medications, and potential problems are highlighted by the authors of these chapters. Case studies, tables, and boxes provide the reader with other sources of information and ideas for problem solving.

The final section of the book, Chapters 14 and 15, relates some of the challenges faced by nurses practicing in the prehospital environment and speculates on the future of prehospital nursing practice. Challenges include application of continuous quality improvement (CQI) to prehospital nursing practice, ethical and legal issues such as ceasing futile resuscitation, and the management of stress.

SPECIAL FEATURES

This book was written by nurses and physicians who practice in the prehospital care environment. The nurses who contributed to this book practice in a variety of settings, including ground and air transport, and serve as EMS coordinators and educators. They have been educated and trained for their roles at diverse programs across the country and have practiced in the prehospital care environment for a number of years.

Each chapter begins with objectives, and in the clinical chapters competencies are listed. Nursing care is incorporated in the clinical chapters with the use of nursing diagnosis, collaborative interventions, and evaluative criteria.

Information for the book was contributed from programs and individuals who live and work all over the United States. Chapters contain tables, boxes, illustrations, and examples that enhance the written material. Appendixes include additional information that will be of help to those practicing in prehospital care.

CONCLUSION

The role of nursing in the prehospital care environment continues to develop. Prehospital nursing includes the assessment and identification of patient problems, anticipation and implementation of collaborative interventions, and evaluation of these interventions. It also entails community involvement including education and prevention. Prehospital nursing encompasses a holistic view of people who are ill or injured, incorporating the body-mind-spirit view of the ill or injured patient.

This is the first book that specifically addresses nursing's role in this area of practice. Because there is no national standard for prehospital nursing practice, there are many ideas, opinions, and beliefs. However, this does not alter the fact that nursing has been "out there" for a long time and has made and continues to make significant contributions to the practice of prehospital care.

We hope that this book provides a foundation for the practice of nursing in the prehospital care environment. We also hope that it stimulates a dialogue among all of us who provide care for patients in this setting. Collaboration is the key to ensuring that patients receive the best care before, during, and after transport whether it be from the scene of the injury or illness or between health-care facilities.

ACKNOWLEDGMENTS

I would like to sincerely thank Don Ladig, who planted the seed for this book, and Robin Carter, who reviewed the proposal and nurtured the growth of this book. I would also like to thank Gina Chan and acknowledge all the work and guidance of Jeanne Allison in the completion of this text. The staff at Mosby have offered us wonderful counsel and direction, and the fruit of this is contained in this book.

Renee Semonin Holleran

Contents in Brief

Contents

PART ONE

Introduction to Prehospital Nursing

CHAPTER 1

Role of Nursing in Prehospital Care

Practicing in the prehospital environment is not new to nursing. Historically, nursing has been practiced outside of the hospital for centuries, providing patient care through community and social services, as well as caring for the casualties of war (Donahue, 1985).

Prehospital care of the ill or injured is based on the collaborative efforts of nurses, prehospital care providers, and physicians. The role of the nurse in the prehospital environment is multifaceted and includes practices, research, education, management, consultation, advocacy, and administration.

The purpose of this chapter is to discuss the historical perspective of nursing in the prehospital care environment and to describe the role of the nurse and the skills and education needed to practice in this setting.

HISTORICAL PERSPECTIVE

One of the derivations of the word *nursing* is from the Latin word *nutrire* or "to nourish" (Donahue, 1985). Donahue (1985, p. 9) points out that "men and women have functioned throughout history as nurses because of a natural tendency of humans to respond to the needs of those who are ill or injured." Initially, nursing care remained within a family or was extended only to immediate members of one's tribe. Nurses not only took care of a person's immediate physical needs, but also worked to prevent disease and injury. They recognized that the social needs of people greatly influenced their health status.

Florence Nightingale has been heralded as one of the creators of modern nursing practice (Donahue, 1985). She has also been credited with bringing about the recognition of what women and nurses could provide for the ill and injured out in the field (Figure 1-1). In 1854 she was placed in charge of the Female Nursing Establishment of the English General Hospitals in Turkey during the Crimean War. Within 6 months the death rate in the military hospitals decreased from 47% to 2.2% under her leadership. She went to the battlefront and visited and cared for the ill and injured until she became ill with Crimean fever and had to return to England. Through her work during the Crimean War, Florence Nightingale laid the foundation for nurses' role outside of the hospital.

Just as war brought women and nursing to the forefront in other parts of the world, it did the same in the United States. The Civil War offered opportunities for nurses to demonstrate the care and skill they possessed. Nurses served in the volunteer corps during the Civil War, providing needed care for both the Union and Confederate armies.

True to the nature of nursing, Clara Barton emerged as a symbol of nursing's ability to meet the needs of humans no matter what side they

3

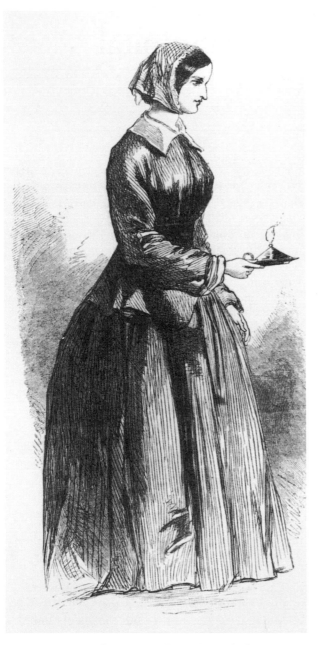

Fig. 1-1   Florence Nightingale. Wood engraving. *Harper's Weekly,* June 6, 1857. (National Library of Medicine, Bethesda, Maryland.)

fought on (Figure 1-2). She was an outspoken advocate against slavery and provided patient care on the battlefield, caring for northerners, southerners, blacks, and whites (Donahue, 1985). She later established the American Red Cross in 1882, which remains one of the major organizations that provides nurses the opportunity to render care in the field.

In the twentieth century nurses have been active participants in World War I, World War II, the Korean and Vietnam Wars, and the action taken in Desert Storm. Hospitals known as mobile army surgical hospitals (MASH) and medical units self-contained and transportable (MUST) have been staffed by nurses, physicians, and corpsmen, many times only miles from the battlefront. The war experience of the twentieth century demonstrated that field stabilization and rapid transport decrease both mortality and morbidity and that nursing played a significant role in the delivery of care (Donahue, 1985) (Figures 1-3 to 1-5).

FLIGHT NURSING

During World War II and the Korean and Vietnam Wars, nurses took on a new role as flight nurses in the prehospital care of patients. The roots of flight nursing emerged a few years before World War II when Laurette M. Schimmoler formed the Emergency Flight Corps in 1933. The name of the group was later changed to the Aerial Nurse Corps of America (Lee, 1987). The nurses were dedicated to defining a role for nursing in flight and patient transport, as well as to evaluating and implementing safety for both patients and crew.

The first public appearance of the Aerial Nurse Corps was at the National Air Races in Los Angeles in 1936. Nurses established and gave care in field hospitals during this event (Lee, 1987).

Through the influence of Ms. Schimmoler, the military opened its first flight nurse training program in 1942 at the 349th Air Evacuation

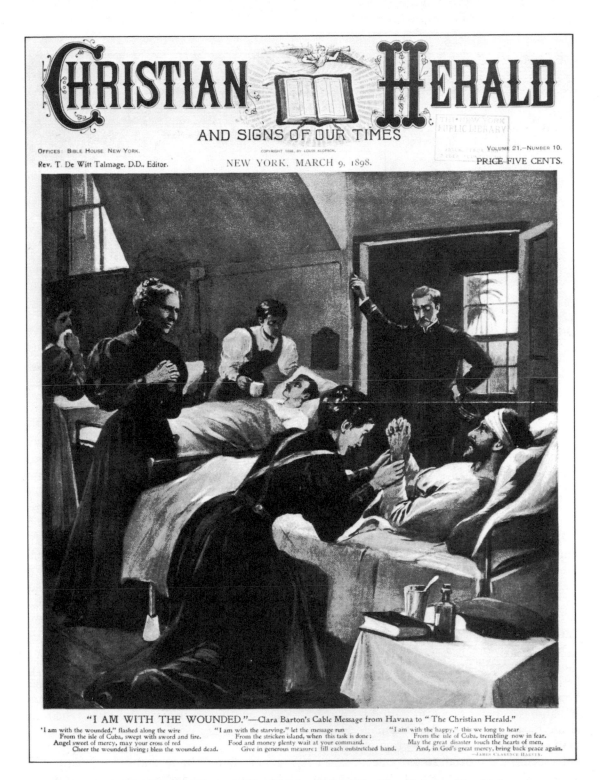

Fig. 1-2   Clara Barton. *Christian Herald*, March 9, 1898. (The Christian Herald Association, Chappaqua, New York.)

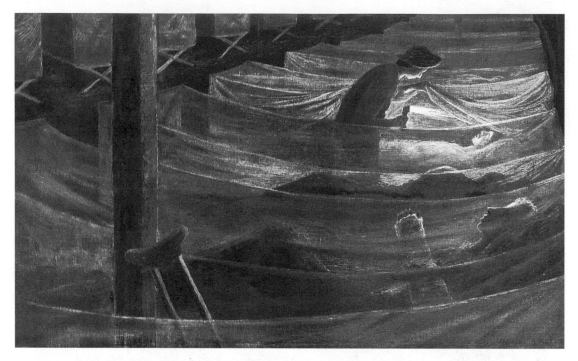

Fig. 1-3   Franklin Boggs, *Night Duty,* 1945.

Group, Bowman Field, Kentucky. The course was moved to Texas in 1944 and required 6 weeks of education that included flight physiology.

During World War II over 1.5 million patients were transported by fixed-wing aircraft with nurses in attendance (Lee, 1987). After the war flight nurse training was conducted by the U.S. Air Force. Flight nurses were reactivated for service during the Korean and Vietnam Wars.

During the Korean and Vietnam Wars, the value of helicopter transport was recognized in the care of the ill and injured. In 1972 St. Anthony's Hospital in Denver established a civilian-based flight program staffed by nurses with critical care experience. Hermann Hospital in Houston began its flight program in 1976 and added the physician to the team.

Since 1972 the number of hospital-based programs blossomed. Flight teams have multiple configurations including nurse/paramedic, nurse/nurse, and nurse/physician. The primary team member is generally a nurse with critical care or emergency experience. In the case of specialty transport, such as neonatal, a professional with experience in that specialty is then included (Figure 1-6).

CRITICAL CARE TRANSPORT

The delivery of critical care before arrival at a hospital was first instituted in Russia in the 1960s. The first mobile coronary care units were used in Belfast and were staffed by physicians and nurses (Colardyn, 1993). Their goal was to identify cardiac problems and to treat the patient at the scene, with the hope of preventing complications and sudden death.

The use of nurses in these units established

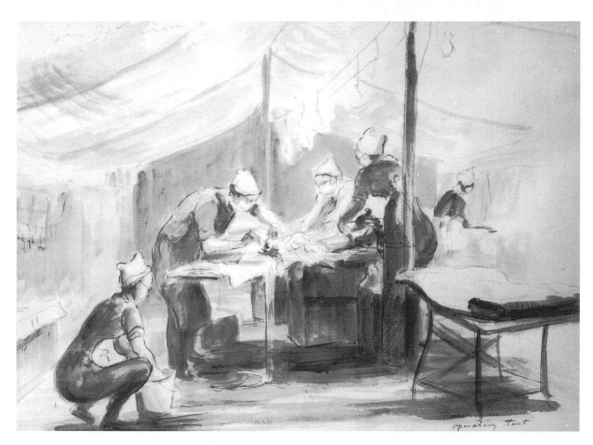

Fig. 1-4 John Groth, *Nurses in the Operating Tent*, Korean War. Watercolor. (Defense Audiovisual Agency, Washington, D.C.)

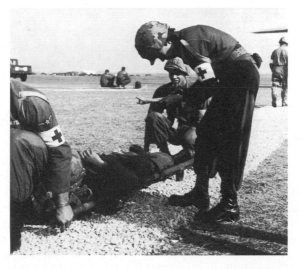

Fig. 1-5 An Air Force nurse checks the identification of an injured man during the Strike Command exercise. (U.S. Air Force Photo.)

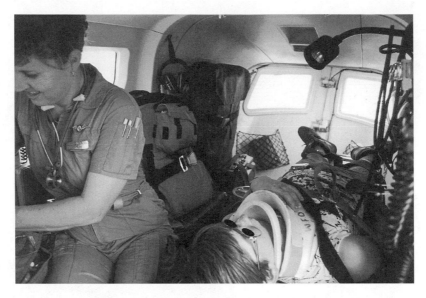

Fig. 1-6   Flight nurse.

their role for the delivery of critical care outside of the hospital intensive care unit. The use of specific critical care equipment (intraaortic balloon pumps), medications (vasoactive drugs, blood), and interpretation of laboratory and X-ray values has shown there is a continued need for nursing to provide this type of care in the prehospital environment (Colardyn, 1993). Critical care transport requires not only highly skilled and experienced nurses to manage the patient, but also the technology necessary to provide care for the critically ill or injured patient.

THE ROLES OF NURSING IN PREHOSPITAL CARE
The Practice Role

According to Robinson (1992, p. 9), "(the) concept of prehospital is to take the expertise of specially trained persons and their equipment to the victim at the scene and maintain that level of care during transport."

Colardyn (1993) enhances this portrait of prehospital care with a description of the following goals of transport:

1. To maintain adequate tissue oxygenation
2. To replace lost fluids, blood, and blood products
3. To immobilize injured parts
4. To deliver early definitive care such as the administration of thrombolytic therapy, methylprednisolone for spinal cord injury, or drugs for cerebral resuscitation.

The education, experience, and skills needed to provide this type of care in the prehospital environment and during transport need to be varied and extensive. Currently there are no national guidelines for the practice of prehospital nursing, although some general guidelines may be used for patient transport, including COBRA law (1984), *Resource Document for Nursing Care of the Trauma Patient* (1992), Emergency Nurses Association's *Interfacility Transport of the Critically Ill or Injured Patient* (1993), and the *Practice Standards for Flight Nursing* (1986). For the critically ill or injured patient who requires transport, a registered nurse, educated, experienced, and skilled in the prehospital care environment, should accompany the patient to achieve the goals of transport, anticipate any additional problems, and provide needed interventions.

In 1987 the Emergency Nurses Association and National Flight Nurses Association released a joint position paper that described the role of the nurse in the prehospital environment. Box 1-1 contains a summary of this position paper.

Three suggested curriculums outline recommended education and skills for nursing practice in the prehospital environment. These are the *National Standard Guidelines for Prehospital Nursing* from the Emergency Nurses Association, the *Flight Nurse Advanced Trauma Course* from the National Flight Nurses Association, and the *Air Medical Crew National Curriculum* from the United States Department of Transportation.

The lack of national standards and a uniform curriculum has caused controversy in some areas of the country as to what type of preparation nurses should have to practice in the prehospital environment. A study conducted by Johnson, Childress, Herron, Boyko, Nowacki, Scanzello, and Lynch (1993) found that 44 of 50 states did not require certification for prehospital nursing. In most of these states, nurses needed both RN and EMT licensure for prehospital practice. Sixty-one percent of the states require nurses to take the entire EMT course, whereas the remaining states allow for some type of challenge examinations and educational courses to meet the EMT requirements. The researchers found that only six states actually had a certification program for prehospital nursing.

At issue is what type of education, training, and licensure nurses should have who practice in the prehospital environment and what type of role they play. Based on the previous historical discussion, nurses have been in the prehospital care environment for a long time. Many of the current issues arose during the 1980s

Box 1-1
SUMMARY OF THE EMERGENCY NURSES ASSOCIATION/NATIONAL FLIGHT NURSES ASSOCIATION POSITION STATEMENT: THE ROLE OF THE NURSE IN THE PREHOSPITAL CARE ENVIRONMENT

1. ENA and NFNA endorse a collaborative role for specially prepared nurses in the delivery of prehospital care.
2. ENA and NFNA believe that a registered nurse who has received the appropriate knowledge and demonstrated skill proficiency related to prehospital care activities need not become certified as an EMT.
3. ENA and NFNA *do* endorse the need for special educational requirements for nurses practicing in the prehospital care environment.
4. ENA and NFNA believe that the practice of the prehospital care nurse should be based on the use of the nursing process which includes assessment; formulation of nursing diagnoses, expected outcomes, and a plan of care; evaluation of interventions rendered; collaboration and coordination with others involved with the patient's care; and communication to the receiving facility.
5. ENA and NFNA believe the role of the nurse in prehospital care includes practice, research, education, management, consultation, advocacy, and administration.
6. ENA and NFNA believe that the practice of prehospital nursing should be regulated by state boards of nursing in which each individual nurse practices.

Note. From *Role of the Registered Nurse in the Prehospital Environment: Emergency Nurses Association Position Statement* (pp. 69-71) by Emergency Nurses Association and National Flight Nursing Association, 1993, Park Ridge, IL: The Author.

when role clarification for both paramedics and nurses was questioned and a nursing shortage resulted in EMTs and paramedics performing traditional nursing roles in such places as the emergency department (Ampolsk, 1989; Ligon, 1993).

As identified in the study by Johnson et al.

(1993), many states have not clearly defined the type of preparation nurses need for prehospital practice. There is no argument that if nurses are functioning as first responders and performing rescue that they should be appropriately prepared to work safely in those environments. Even if nurses are not providing direct care in

---

Box 1-2
COUNTY OF SACRAMENTO DEPARTMENT OF MEDICAL SYSTEMS: REQUIREMENTS FOR MOBILE INTENSIVE CARE NURSE (MICN) CERTIFICATION

All candidates will meet the following certification requirements:
1. Prerequisite criteria (documentation that these criteria have been met must be submitted with the candidates's application for certification.)
   a. Provide evidence of valid and current licensure as a registered nurse in California.
   b. Provide evidence of a valid and current ACLS card according to the standards of the American Heart Association.
   c. Provide evidence of current authorization as a Mobile intensive care nurse (or authorized Registered nurse) in a California county, or
      • Provide evidence of a minimum of 12 months of critical care experience as a registered nurse of which at least 6 months must be within the emergency department of an acute care hospital
      • Provide evidence of successful completion of a basic mobile intensive care nurse course in California approved by the local EMS agency.
2. The candidate will complete an ALS emergency response vehicle observation experience consisting of direct observation of at least eight (8) hours which must include at least two (2) patient contacts in which the patient is assessed. (If two [2] patient contacts are not completed, two [2] ALS patient scenarios will be conducted by the EMT-II/P.)
3. Complete the Sacramento County application form. The completed form must be submitted to the local EMS agency prior to the application deadline for the written MICN examination.
4. Pay all related fees. (Not currently implemented.)
5. Provide proof of employment within the emergency services of a designated base hospital.
6. Successfully complete the Sacramento County Written Examination for MICN Certification with a score of 80% or higher. If unsuccessful, one retest is allowed within 30 days.
7. Successfully complete the Sacramento County Base Hospital MICN Skills Exam.*
8. Attend a County accreditation class to the local EMS system or completion of Sacramento County EMS agency (LEMSA) approved MICN class.
9. Upon successful completion of A-G above, the local EMS agency shall certify the candidate as a base hospital MICN for a period of two (2) years from the last day of the month in which all the certification requirements are met.

Note. From "Mobil Intensive Care Nurse (MICN): Certification" by The County of Sacramento Department of Medical Systems, Office of Emergency Medical Services, 1992.
*Skills would be a test of radio procedure and role-playing scenarios.

these situations, they still need to be aware of the potential hazards of scene work and how to keep themselves and their patients safe.

Some states have prehospital courses that act as bridge courses for nurses to meet the requirements for EMTs and paramedics. An example of this is the prehospital nursing course (PNC) being proposed in Maryland (Miller & Epifanio, 1993). The purpose of the course is to allow nurses to practice in the prehospital care environment without forcing them to train as EMTs or paramedics (Miller & Epifanio, 1993). Many nurses have already mastered parts of the content involved in preparation for paramedic practice. The PNC would contain various modules related to the care of the patient in the prehospital environment, and all but four of the modules could be challenged. The modules that could *not* be challenged include disaster/triage, rescue/extrication, vehicle operation, and orientation/role socialization (Miller & Epifanio, 1993).

The mobile intensive care nurse certification (MICN) is another example of a training course for nurses practicing in the prehospital care environment. The MICN may perform care in the field and also maintain telecommunications between the hospital and EMTs and paramedics. This is generally accomplished through the use of protocols and guidelines. In some states and EMS regions the MICN extends the medical expertise of the physician to prehospital care providers (Selfridge, Sigafoos, & Trunkey, 1987; Cleary, Wilson, & Williams, 1987). MICN functions may include making knowledge-based judgments and providing appropriate direction for field interventions. Box 1-2 contains the requirements for MICN certification in Sacramento, California.

PREHOSPITAL NURSING EDUCATION AND SKILLS
Education Preparation

One of the most important qualifications that has been identified for the nurse practicing in the prehospital environment is clinical experience. Most programs require either emergency or critical care experience, with the number of years required varying from a minimum of 1 to 3.

It has been difficult to develop a course that teaches and enhances clinical decision making for nurses who work in the prehospital care environment. Case studies and direct observation provide two modes of evaluating clinical decision making. The general educational requirements for prehospital nurses are summarized in Box 1-3. The requirements vary throughout the United States.

Box 1-3
SUMMARY OF EDUCATIONAL REQUIREMENTS FOR THE NURSE PRACTICING IN THE PREHOSPITAL ENVIRONMENT

Registered nurse (some programs require multiple licensure when providing care across state lines)
Advanced cardiac life support (ACLS)
Pediatric advanced life support (PALS)
Prehospital care orientation course (determined by state EMS agency)
or
Prehospital registered nurse course
or
EMT/EMT-P certification
Certification in a nursing specialty, for example:
    Certified emergency nurse (CEN)
    Certified critical care nurse (CCRN)
    Certified flight registered nurse (CFRN)
Trauma course, for example:
    Basic trauma life support (BTLS)
    Prehospital trauma life support (PHTLS)
    Advanced trauma life support (ATLS)
    Flight nurse advanced trauma course (FNATC)
    Trauma nursing core course (TNCC)

Box 1-4

SUMMARY OF SKILLS FOR THE PRACTICE OF NURSING IN THE PREHOSPITAL ENVIRONMENT

Airway Management

1. Intubation
   a. Oral
   b. Nasotracheal
   c. Digital/manual
2. Cricothyroidotomy
   a. Needle
   b. Surgical
3. End-tidal CO_2 monitoring
4. Pulse oximetry

Ventilation Management

1. Needle decompression
2. Chest tube insertion
3. Assisting with open thoracotomy
4. Pericardiocentesis
5. Ventilator management

Circulation Management

1. Vascular access
   a. Central line placement
   b. Venous cannulation
   c. Arterial cannulation
   d. Intraosseous line placement
2. Medication administration
   a. Fluids
   b. Blood

   c. Blood products
   d. Vasoactive drugs
   e. Experimental drugs
3. Intraaortic balloon pump management
4. Pacing devices
   a. Internal
   b. External
5. Vital sign monitors
6. Invasive line monitors
   a. Blood pressure
   b. Pulmonary catheters
   c. Intracranial monitors
7. Urinary catheters
8. Nasogastric catheters
9. ECG monitors
10. 12-lead ECG monitors
11. Temperature management
12. Wound care
    a. Control of hemorrhage
    b. Protect from contamination

Additional Skills

1. Pain management during transport
   a. Movement
   b. Motion sickness
2. Emotional care
3. Family care

Prehospital nursing skills also vary depending on service and state and are dependent on state boards of nursing, EMS agencies, and medical direction. In 1990 MacLeod, Seaberg, and Paris pointed out that prehospital interventions included airway management, intravenous access, defibrillation, and drug administration. Today these skills have expanded to include such things as surgical airway establishment, needle thoracentesis and chest tube

insertion, central line insertion, and external pacing (Terhorst & Byrne, 1993). Box 1-4 contains a summary of skills for prehospital nursing practice. Box 1-5 contains a summary of the skills required of nurses who work for the Samaritan Air Evac Services in Phoenix, Arizona.

Learning technical skills can be facilitated through laboratory practice and supervised patient care. Many programs require a specific amount of procedures to be completed quar-

---

Box 1-5
AIR MEDICAL PERSONNEL MINIMUM QUALIFICATIONS IN ARIZONA

Adult/Pediatric Nurse

Arizona RN Licensure

3 years recent ICU/CCU/ER experience

Current ACLS/BLS

CCRN certification within 1 year of hire

Maternal Nurse

Arizona RN licensure

3 years tertiary OB experience

NCC certification within 1 year of hire

Current BLS

Neonatal Nurse

Arizona RN licensure

3 years tertiary NICU experience

NCC certification within 1 year of hire

Current BLS

Note. From "Careful Preparation and State-of-the-Art Procedures," 1993, *Flightlogs*, Spring, pp. 4-5.

---

terly either in the field or laboratory. It has been demonstrated that invasive skills can be safely performed in the field by properly trained nurses (Walls, 1993). As pointed out by Walls (1993, p. 91):

It is rather tragic that we have to focus research efforts on proving what is already known: that invasive procedures can be successfully performed by properly trained field personnel. It is time to put aside the antiquated and totally refuted notion that physicians are somehow intrinsically better than other health care personnel when it comes to technical procedures.

The limits to the type of procedures and the nurse's ability to perform them are directed by state boards of nursing and the medical direction under which they practice.

The educational preparation of the prehospital nurse includes the responsibility to acquire and maintain knowledge and skill levels related to their practice, as well as to provide education for other prehospital care providers, patients, and the community (Emergency Nurses Association [ENA] & National Flight Nurses Association [NFNA], 1993). Developing and participating in safety and injury prevention programs are examples of prehospital nursing education.

PREHOSPITAL NURSING ROLES
Management and Administrative Roles

Initially the education of prehospital care providers was furnished mostly by physicians (Cleary, Wilson, & Williams, 1987). As the number and levels of prehospital care providers grew and state EMS agencies developed, nursing assumed a greater role in the management and administration of prehospital care (EMS Editors, 1991).

Another example of an administrative and management role for nursing in the prehospital care environment is that of the prehospital liaison nurse (PLN). This role has also been described as a prehospital care coordinator (PCC) or an EMS coordinator (Cleary, Wilson, & Williams, 1987). Nurses in this role should have experience in prehospital care practice and EMS policies and procedures. Requirements for this position may be outlined in EMS legislation. The PLN/PCC/EMS coordinator functions as the liaison between the EMS community and the institution or institutions served by the local EMS. In addition, the PLN/PCC/EMS coordinator may also be responsible for coordinating basic and continuing education, clinical skills, and quality management of the EMS provider. In some areas of the country, the PLN/

Box 1-6
CHARACTERISTICS AND RESPONSIBILITIES OF THE PLN/PCC/EMS COORDINATOR

Characteristics	Responsibilities
Effective communication skills	Coordinate advanced life support services
Exceptional interpersonal skills	Assess EMS educational needs
Self-directed and goal directed	Evaluates EMS performance
Leadership ability	Mediates problems
Problem-solving skills	Participates in liaison activities
Emergency department and prehospital care experience	Coordinates EMS quality management
Teaching ability	Maintains data and records
Background in human resources management	
Politically active	Aware of state EMS regulations and requirements

Note. From *Prehospital Care* (p. 38) by V. Cleary, P. Wilson, and G. Super (eds), 1987, Rockville, MD: Aspen Publications.

PCC/EMS coordinator is also responsible for the practice and quality management of nurses working in the prehospital environment. Box 1-6 contains a summary of characteristics and responsibilities of the PLN/PCC/EMS coordinator (Cleary, Wilson, & Williams, 1987, p. 42).

Advocacy and Consultation Roles

The prehospital nurse should advocate for the protection of patient rights, facilitation of patient and family entry into the EMS system, and promotion of recovery and wellness in the community or communities served by the nurse (ENA & NFNA, 1993). Chapter 13 discusses some of the ways that the nurse practicing in the prehospital environment may function in this role.

Since prehospital care requires a collaboration between the nurses, prehospital care providers, physicians, agencies, institutions, and the people served, the consultation role involves enhancing communication between personnel to improve the care provided in the prehospital care environment (ENA & NFNA, 1993). Sometimes this role can be difficult because evaluation can be a painful process. However, when the lines of communication are open and a concerted effort is made to keep them open through case reviews, prehospital care committees, and personal interactions, both the patient and prehospital personnel will benefit.

Research Role

Prehospital nursing involves the investigation of practice, the development of data bases, contribution to the scientific knowledge base of prehospital nursing, application of research findings to practice, and evaluation of their effects on patient care (ENA & NFNA, 1993). Research is needed that describes the role of nursing in the prehospital environment, as well as the patient outcomes related to the care provided by nursing before and during transport. Collaborative research will help demonstrate whether prehospital care interventions make a difference. Research should help to improve current and future patient care (Yealy, 1993).

There are barriers to research in the prehospital care environment including difficulty randomizing patients, controlling for extraneous variables, developing clear inclusion and exclusion criteria, blinding data collectors, patient problems such as the need to perform interventions not on a selected protocol, limited supplies, and lack of enthusiasm related to the project (Menegazzi, 1993). Lack of time and the need to take care of unforeseen problems may also interfere with data collection.

Ethical considerations may make the implementation of research protocols challenging in the prehospital environment. Obtaining consent from patients and their families in life-threatening situations may be difficult as well as potentially disconcerting to patients who may fear not being treated if they do not consent. In addition, some research protocols using new treatment modalities that appear to be working may tempt the nurse to enter and treat a patient who should not be entered into a particular protocol (Davis & Maio, 1993).

Several alternatives have been proposed and used in place of informed consent in the prehospital environment: consent at a distance, consent by proxy, stepped consent, deferred consent, surrogate consent, and consent jury. In consent at a distance, permission is obtained from patients by the person collecting data speaking with them on the radio. Consent by proxy involves the nurse or prehospital care provider obtaining the consent. Stepped consent involves providing the patient with a brief description of the research and the interventions to be performed, obtaining permission, administering the interventions, and obtaining full consent when the patient or the patient's family gets to the hospital. In deferred consent, the therapy is administered, but once the family is present, consent is then obtained. If the family refuses, the treatment is discontinued. This type of consent has been used in resuscitation research, in which delay in treatment

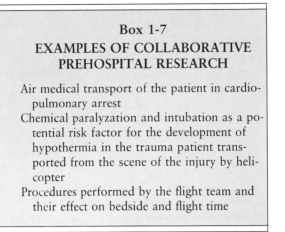

Box 1-7
EXAMPLES OF COLLABORATIVE
PREHOSPITAL RESEARCH

Air medical transport of the patient in cardiopulmonary arrest
Chemical paralyzation and intubation as a potential risk factor for the development of hypothermia in the trauma patient transported from the scene of the injury by helicopter
Procedures performed by the flight team and their effect on bedside and flight time

would only cause further injury. Surrogate consent and consent jury essentially involve the same concepts. A surrogate panel (a group of individuals who have undergone similar treatments) or a group of lay individuals are presented with the experimental protocol and allowed to give input. The internal review boards of the sponsoring institutions and investigators would still be responsible for the study, but this allows others who may benefit from a treatment to give opinions (Davis & Maio, 1993).

Examples of some collaborative research that has been completed and in process in the prehospital environment are listed in Box 1-7. Nurses must develop, design, and participate in the research process to demonstrate that the role they play does make a difference.

Medical Direction

Since EMS has been described as "the practice of medicine in the streets," physicians are also an important part of quality prehospital medical care (Stewart, 1987). Ultimately the Emergency Medical Service's medical director is responsible for the care provided to the patient (Holroyd, Knopp, & Kallsen, 1986). The best prehospital care systems are those with highly visible physicians who make sure that the pre-hospital care provided is equal to that provided in their personal practice (Pepe, 1993). Unfortunately there is only anecdotal evidence that a strong physician medical director improves patient care.

Traditionally the functions of the medical director have been divided arbitrarily into on-line and off-line duties. On-line activities are those that involve direct communication between the paramedics or nurses and the physician at the time patient care is taking place. This type of interaction is sometimes termed direct medical control. Off-line activities are all other functions.

Another classification system defines medical direction as being prospective, immediate, and retrospective (Holroyd, Knopp, & Kallsen, 1986). Prospective functions are those that take place before patient contact, such as training, initial education, and protocol development. Immediate direction is similar to on-line, or direct, medical control. Retrospective functions are those that occur after completion of patient care and include supervision of a quality improvement program, continuing education, and system review.

While all EMS systems, air and ground, should have a medical director, the level of the director's involvement in the system often varies widely. In many systems the medical director does little more than sign papers when asked. However, as Pepe (1993) has pointed out, it is necessary for the medical director to actively participate in the service's activities, including field response.

Personal observation of care delivery provides a perspective that cannot be gained by reading call reports. Field response provides teaching opportunities, as well as demonstrates to the street providers that the physician knows and understands the environment in which they work (Pepe & Stewart, 1986). Without this foundation the medical director will be unable to perform his primary duty, which is patient advocacy (Pepe & Stewart, 1986).

ON-LINE MEDICAL CONTROL

On-line medical control is provided in most but not all EMS systems. The advantages to on-line direction include (Page, Krentz, & Aranosian, 1984):

1. Acceptance of legal responsibility by the physician
2. Close supervision and education of the prehospital provider through prompt feedback and appropriate praise and criticism
3. Transmission of information regarding patient condition, treatment, and progress communicated in a uniform manner
4. If within the scope of the EMS system's authorized capabilities, permission may be obtained to deviate from standing orders or protocols

The disadvantages include the necessity to purchase communication equipment and, most important, to provide the physician time needed. For example, in a system that receives 6000 calls annually and each call requires about 5 minutes of physician time, a total of 500 hours are used yearly. To the extent that this activity occurs when the physician is not otherwise occupied, its marginal cost is negligible. However, when on-line communication takes the physician away from patient care activities, its annual indirect cost may be substantial.

Because of this high cost, some systems, such as California, have used a nurse to fill this role (Pointer, 1985). Unfortunately, this solution adds another layer of bureaucracy to the system, does not make the physician's legal responsibility clear, and does not provide for close physician supervision and education of the prehospital provider. Therefore most busy systems attempt to strike a balance between the demands and benefits of on-line medical control, and they use a physician for their on-line activities.

Research evidence for or against on-line medical direction is quite limited. For example, the use of on-line medical control may increase scene time and delay patient transport (Erder,

Davidson, & Cheney, 1989). However, on-line physician involvement in the decision to request a helicopter for an accident scene may reduce the inappropriate transport of patients (Champion et al., 1988). Notification of the receiving hospital that a patient with a probable myocardial infarction, as determined by a prehospital 12-lead electrocardiogram, is en route has been shown to shorten the time to delivery of therapy, such as administration of thrombolytic agents (Weaver et al., 1993; Kereiakes et al., 1992).

The system's medical director must balance several factors when attempting to determine how much on-line medical control is needed. The first factor is state law and regulations. Some states still have rules requiring base hospital contact for all calls. Second is the amount and type of off-line control present in the system. When off-line control and quality assurance are strong, then less on-line control is needed.

Most of the benefits of on-line control can be achieved by calling whenever possible while the patient is being transported. The benefits of notification of the receiving hospital, as well as education of the providers, are still present. However, the delay at the scene is minimized in such a system.

The medical director must also consider which physicians will provide on-line control. Should a large group of base hospitals provide this service or just one or two core hospitals (Waddington, Neely, Barmache, & Schriver, 1987)? Will emergency medicine residents be used? How will the base station physicians be trained? The answers to these questions will also help to determine the appropriate level of on-line direction in the system.

Another area of controversy in on-line medical direction is the use of telemetry, which is the transmission of an electrocardiographic signal over the radio or telephone (Hitt & Sanders, 1984). These systems are expensive. They require a dedicated base and special transmission units. The limited available evidence sug-

gests that the benefit is small if it is even present at all (Cayton et al., 1985; Stewart, 1985; Erder & Davidson, 1987). Most large EMS systems have found that paramedics are quite good at reading rhythm strips and that little change in patient care results from transmitting a ECG rhythm strip to the base station (McCabe, Adhar, Menegazzi, & Paris, 1992; Peacock, Blackwell, & Wainscott, 1985).

OFF-LINE MEDICAL CONTROL

The EMS system medical director is responsible for a number of activities other than the direct communication between the prehospital provider and physician. These include protocol development, initial and continuing education, provider certification, quality improvement, and risk management.

The medical director should develop protocols that describe how the patient is to be treated. Protocols should address aspects of the EMS system including dispatch, treatment, and triage (Krentz & Wainscott, 1990). Protocols for treatment should be complaint specific, not diagnosis specific (e.g., chest pain, not acute myocardial infarction).

It is important to distinguish between protocols and standing orders. Protocols describe the approach to the particular problem, including assessment and treatment. Standing orders are a subset of the protocol that define specific actions that the prehospital personnel may perform without direct contact with an on-line physician.

The medical director should also be accountable for dispatch decisions. Agencies can purchase medically sound dispatch protocols (Clawson, 1988), but the medical director must be consulted to be sure that the national protocol is appropriate to the local situation. The medical director should also oversee the quality assessment of the dispatch process. Interagency rivalry may interfere with this function, since dispatchers often work for a different governmental entity than the prehospital providers.

The medical director must decide how much autonomy the prehospital providers will have. The decision should be based on the skill level and training of the providers (e.g., registered nurses may generally have greater autonomy than paramedics). The decision should also be based on the components of the local system. For example, in an urban environment with a cadre of highly experienced full-time professionals, paramedics may be permitted greater autonomy than a rural or suburban part-time volunteer.

Education of the prehospital provider is frequently problematic. In many systems there is tension between the time constraints of part-time volunteers and the rapidly changing medical knowledge base. It can be quite challenging to maintain skills with minimal training and experience.

The urban environment provides its own training challenge. Providers in large cities often have a high level of experience. However, many paid paramedics will be reluctant to attend training sessions unless they are compensated. Often the medical director must help convince local government to support training.

Initial training may or may not be under the control of the system's medical director. It is important for the medical director to attempt to ensure that the initial training is effective. There are two techniques that are helpful. The first is to select paramedics who are graduates of programs accredited by the Committee on Allied Health Education and Accreditation (CAHEA). The second is to attempt to recruit paramedics who are nationally registered. To become nationally registered, paramedics must pass a rigorous written and practical examination and then maintain continuing education to remain nationally registered.

Most state governments require that the medical director certify that a paramedic has maintained good clinical standards of care and has kept up to date with continuing education. The rationale for this requirement is that the para-

medic is not an independent practitioner and is therefore only able to deliver medical care with the permission of a physician. Some states are considering allowing paramedics an independent practitioner status.

One of the most important duties of a medical director is to oversee the quality improvement program of an Emergency Medical Service. In many EMS systems, quality is becoming the driving force behind all activities. The medical director is a key player in setting priorities for the system, as well as helping to decide which components to measure. The goal of the quality program must be to improve patient care delivery, not to identify a few "bad apples." Interested readers may wish to refer to R.A. Swor and colleagues' *Quality Management in Prehospital Care* published in 1993 by Mosby, which provides an excellent discussion of the process for designing and implementing a quality improvement program.

The medical director must also ensure that the care provided by on-line physicians is appropriate. Therefore it is helpful if the medical director is also a physician in the major on-line command hospital in the system. This dual role helps to solidify the relationship between on-line and off-line activities. Periodic audits have been suggested as a technique for improving care, although they have not been proven to do so (Pointer, 1987; Wasserberger, Ordog, Donoghue, & Balaserbramanian, 1987; Holleman, Wuerz, & Meador, 1992).

The medical director should have the authority to remove a prehospital provider from active patient care. However, this power should also be used sparingly. First, removal is a poor management technique. Positive training is more effective in most circumstances. Second, use of this power will undoubtedly lead to tension with the street provider, which may negatively affect patient care. If continued poor performance is within the control of the provider and the provider is provided with training and experience and does not make the effort to improve, then suspension may be necessary.

The medical director must also oversee risk management functions of the EMS organization. Problem cases should be brought to the attention of the physician so that appropriate action may be taken to prevent similar occurrences whenever possible. This is important because the medical director is legally and ethically responsible for all patient care provided by the prehospital personnel in the system.

QUALIFICATIONS

Dedication to the task of providing excellent patient care in the streets is the most important qualification for the medical director. Of course, a valid license to practice medicine is also needed. Additional qualifications have been offered, including the following items proposed by Polsky et al. (1993):

Familiarity with the design and operation of prehospital EMS systems, experience or training in the prehospital emergency care of the acutely ill or injured patient, experience or training in medical direction of prehospital emergency units, active participation in the ED management of the acutely ill or injured patient, experience or training in the instruction of prehospital personnel, experience or training in the EMS quality improvement process, knowledge of EMS laws and regulations, knowledge of EMS dispatch and communications, and knowledge of local mass casualty and disaster plans.

Board certification in emergency medicine should ensure that most of the above qualifications are met without additional training.

An effective medical director is a key component of a quality prehospital care system. The medical director must be personally responsible for patient care. Direct field response, overseeing on-line communications, case review, protocol development, and management of a quality improvement program are important parts of the job description. Readers who wish to obtain additional details should obtain a copy of A. Kuehl's *National Association of EMS Physicians: EMS Medical Director's Handbook.* (A new edition of the book is to published by Mosby in 1994.)

Remember, the goal of an EMS system is to save lives (Cummins et al., 1991). With a dedicated, interested medical director, an Emergency Medical Service will find that achieving this goal is enhanced.

References

Cayten, C.G., Oler, J., Walker, K., et al. (1985). The effect of telemetry on urban prehospital cardiac care. *Annals of Emergency Medicine, 14,* 976-981.

Champion, H.R., Sacco, W.J., Gainer, P.S., et al. (1988). The effect of medical direction on trauma triage. *Journal of Trauma, 28,* 235-239.

Clawson, J.J. (1988). *Principles of emergency medical dispatch.* Englewood Cliffs, NJ: Prentice-Hall.

Cummins, R.O., Ornato, J.P., Thies, W.H., et al. (1991). Improving survival from sudden cardiac arrest: The "chain of survival" concept. *Circulation, 83,* 1832-1847.

Erder, M.H., & Davidson, S.J. (1987). Telemetry in prehospital care (letter). *Annals of Emergency Medicine, 16,* 923.

Erder, M.H., Davidson, S.J., & Cheney, R.A. (1989). On-line medical command in theory and practice. *Annals of Emergency Medicine, 18,* 261-268.

Hitt, J.M., & Sanders, A.B. (1984). Prehospital care telemetry: How essential? *Journal of Emergency Medicine, 1,* 417-420.

Holleman, C.J., Wuerz, R.C., & Meador, S.A. (1992). Medical command errors in an urban advanced life support system. *Annals of Emergency Medicine, 21,* 347-350.

Holroyd, B.R., Knopp, R., & Kallsen, G. (1986). Medical control: Quality assurance in prehospital care. *Journal of the American Medical Association, 256,* 1027-1031.

Kereiakes, D.T., Gibler, W.B., Martin, C.H., et al. (1992). Relative importance of emergency medical system transport and the prehospital electrocardiogram on reducing hospital time delay to therapy for acute myocardial infarction: A preliminary report from the Cincinnati Heart Project. *American Heart Journal, 123,* 835-840.

Krentz, M.J., & Wainscott, M.P. (1990). Medical accountability. *Emergency Medical Clinics of North America, 8*(1), 17-32.

McCabe, J.L., Adhar, G.C., Menegazzi, J.J., & Paris, P.M. (1992). Intravenous adenosine in the prehospital treatment of paroxysmal supraventricular tachycardia. *Annals of Emergency Medicine, 21,* 358-361.

Page, J.R., Krentz, M.J., Aranosian, R.D., et al. (1984). *Medical control of emergency medical services: An overview for emergency physicians.* Dallas: American College of Emergency Physicians.

Peacock, J.B., Blackwell, V.H., & Wainscott, M. (1985). Medical reliability of advanced prehospital cardiac life support. *Annals of Emergency Medicine, 14,* 407-409.

Pepe, P.E. (1993). Out-of-hospital resuscitation research: Rationale and strategies for controlled clinical trials. *Annals of Emergency Medicine, 22,* 17-23.

Pepe, P.E., & Stewart, R.D. (1986). The role of the physician in the prehospital setting. *Annals of Emergency Medicine, 15,* 1480-1483.

Pointer, J.E. (1985). The emergency physician and medical control in advanced life support. *Journal of Emergency Medicine, 3,* 31-35.

Pointer, J.E. (1987). The advanced life support base hospital audit for medical control in an emergency medical services system. *Annals of Emergency Medicine, 16,* 557-560.

Polsky, S., Krohmer, J., Maningas, P., et al. (1993). Guidelines for medical direction of prehospital EMS. *Annals of Emergency Medicine, 22,* 742-744.

Stewart, R.D. (1985). When less is more: Teflon and telemetry in the space age (editorial). *Annals of Emergency Medicine, 14,* 992-994.

Stewart, R.O. (1987). Medical direction in Emergency Medical Services: The role of the physician. *Emergency Medical Clinics of North America, 5*(1), 119-132.

Waddington, N., Neely, K., Barmache, M., & Schriver, J. (1987). The effect of on-line medical control on ambulance destination. *Journal of Emergency Medicine, 5,* 299-303.

Wasserberger, J., Ordog, G.J., Donoghue, G., & Balaserbramaniam, S. (1987). Base station prehospital care: Judgment errors and deviations from protocol. *Annals of Emergency Medicine, 16,* 867-871.

Weaver, W.D., Cerqueira, M., Hallstrom, A.P., et al. (1993). Prehospital-initiated versus hospital-initiated thrombolytic therapy: The myocardial infarction triage and intervention trial. *Journal of the American Medical Association, 270,* 1211-1216.

SUMMARY

The role of nursing in the prehospital care environment is not new and continues to develop. Prehospital nursing involves the assessment and identification of patient problems, anticipating and implementing interventions, and evaluating patient outcomes related to these interventions. It encompasses a holistic view of people who are ill or injured and incorporates the "body-mind-spirit" (Guzzetta & Dossey, 1993) of the patient. Nursing involves the experiences that go beyond personal and individual uniqueness, discovering the meaning embedded in life (Guzzetta & Dossey, 1993).

REFERENCES

Ampolsk, A. (1989). Prehospital RNS. *Emergency, 7,* 33-35.

Cleary, V., Wilson, P., & Williams, M. (1987). Base hospital management. In V. Cleary, P. Wilson, and G. Super (Eds.). *Prehospital care.* (pp. 33-63). Rockville, MD: Aspen Publications.

Colardyn, F. (1993). Delivering critical care: A challenge. *Journal of Emergency Medicine, 11*(1), 37-41.

Consolidated Omnibus Budget Reconciliation Act (COBRA) of 1984 (42 USC 13895 dd), as amended by the Omnibus Budget Reconciliation Acts (OBRA) of 1987, 1989, and 1990.

Davis, E., & Maio, R. (1993). Ethical issues in prehospital research. *Prehospital and Disaster Management, 8*(1), S11-S14.

Donahue, P. (1985). *Nursing: The finest art.* St. Louis: Mosby.

Emergency Nurses Association and National Flight Nurses Association (1993). *The role of the registered nurse in the prehospital environment.* Park Ridge, IL: Emergency Nurses Association.

EMS Editors. (1991). Who's on first? *Emergency Medical Services, 20*(6), 29-33.

ENA. (1993). *Interfacility transport of the critically ill or injured patient.* Park Ridge, IL: Emergency Nurses Association.

ENA, NFNA, AORN, AACN, ARN, AANA. (1992). *Resource document for nursing care of the trauma patient.* Denver: American Association of Operating Room Nurses.

Johnson, R., Childress, S., Herron, H., Boyko, S., Nowacki, J., Scanzello, N., & Lynch, M. (1993). Regulation of prehospital nursing practice: A national survey. *Journal of Emergency Nursing, 19*(5), 437-440.

Guzzetta, C., & Dossey, B. (1993). Guiding critical care nurses on the body-mind-spirit journey. *Critical Care Nurse, 8,* 104-111.

Lee, G. (1987). History of flight nursing. *Journal of Emergency Nursing, 13*(4), 212-218.

Ligon, F. (1993). Showdown in Alabama. *Emergency Medical Services, 22*(8), 26-30.

MacLeod, B., Seaberg, D., & Paris, P. (1990). Prehospital therapy: Past, present, and future. *Emergency Medicine Clinics of North America, 8*(1), 57-74.

Menegazzi, J. (1993). Pragmatic problems in prehospital research. *Prehospital and Disaster Medicine, 8*(1), S15-S19.

Miller, P., & Epifanio, P. (1993). Development of a prehospital nursing curriculum in Maryland. *Journal of Emergency Nursing, 19*(3), 206-208.

National Flight Nurses Association. (1986). *Practice standards for flight nursing.* Lincoln, NE: Media Productions.

Robinson, K. (1992). Prehospital care. In S. Budassi Sheehy (Ed.). *Emergency nursing principles and practice.* (pp. 9-17). St. Louis: Mosby.

Selfridge, J., Sigafoos, J., & Trunkey, D. (1987). Training. In R. Cales and R. Heileg (Eds.). *Trauma care systems.* (pp. 65-78). Rockville, MD: Aspen Publications.

Terhorst, M., & Byrne, G. (1993). Survey of flight nursing practice summary report. Unpublished abstract.

Walls, R. (1993). The incredible rightness of being. *Journal of Emergency Nursing, 11*(3), 91-92.

Yealy, D. (1993). Prehospital research. *Prehospital and Disaster Medicine, 8*(1), S5-S10.

CHAPTER 2

Emergency Medical Service Systems and Communications

OBJECTIVES

1. Identify the components of an EMS system
2. Discuss the differences between prehospital and inhospital patient care
3. Describe common EMS provider types
4. Identify the components of an EMS communication system
5. Describe communication equipment used in the field

COMPETENCIES

1. Identify which agency or agencies may govern the nurse's practice in prehospital care
2. Identify the differences between prehospital and inhospital patient care and their effects on prehospital nursing practice
3. Provide patient information from the prehospital care environment using the appropriate communication equipment

OVERVIEW OF EMERGENCY MEDICAL SERVICES

The Emergency Medical Service (EMS) system is a chain of human and physical resources linked together to deliver comprehensive emergency medical care (Grant, Murray, & Bergeron, 1993). The goal of all EMS systems is to stabilize and preserve the life and limb of patients suffering from the effects of an unanticipated illness or injury. This is accomplished by dispatching prehospital emergency personnel to the emergency scene, using on-scene medical intervention, and continuing treatment during transport to a hospital with an adequate staff and the capabilities of caring for acutely injured or ill patients (Norton, Bartkus, & Neely

1992). The concept of extending quality emergency care to the ill or injured outside of the hospital is generally referred to as prehospital emergency care (PEC). In this chapter *EMS* refers to Emergency Medical Service response units including the medical personnel who staff the units, as well as the components and equipment needed for delivering emergency care and transport.

This relatively new and growing medical specialty evolved from public awareness of two major diseases in society: trauma and cardiovascular disease. PEC consists of employing basic life support (BLS) interventions, advanced life support (ALS), or a combination. BLS providers are trained to deliver noninvasive medical care, including basic assessment skills, circulatory support and tissue oxygenation, hemorrhage control, and cardiopulmonary resuscitation (CPR). An ALS provider will have completed extensive training employing both advanced and invasive procedures. These procedures can include intravenous cannulation and pharmacological intervention, advanced airway control techniques (including needle cricothyrotomy and chest decompression) endotracheal intubation, cardiac monitoring, defibrillation, and detailed assessment skills. Traditionally, BLS and ALS have been used to differentiate the two levels of training and services offered in the EMS environment (Hergenroeder & Berk, 1989). Many EMS experts, however, now recognize that there are more than two levels of EMS providers and that the training and practice within these provider levels not only overlap but also are often variable and inconsistent (Dawson, Brown, Chew, Garrison, & O'Keefe, 1993). Revising the methods for EMS response unit classification and standardizing EMS education and practice are important goals of many EMS organizations.

Anyone choosing to work in prehospital and in-hospital emergency settings will find that, in addition to law enforcement, fire suppression, and the EMS system, other components are integral to an EMS organizational structure. Ideally an EMS system provides easy public access, using a well-coordinated telecommunications and dispatch system, dispatches a first responder trained in first aid, followed by a professional EMS response team providing treatment and transportation to a well-staffed and equipped hospital emergency department. In much of the United States public access to the EMS system is now accomplished by dialing 9-1-1 through the public telephone system and reporting the emergency situation to the dispatcher (Bledsoe, Porter, & Shade, 1993). The 9-1-1 system is an easy three-digit number for the public to remember and is designed to quickly alert the EMS response team of a call

for help. Nationwide implementation of this system has been slow, and in spite of federal and state governmental support, 9-1-1 is still not available in many communities.

Historical Review

Providing extended hospital-quality patient care to the sick and injured at the emergency scene is a relatively new development. In fact, only in the last 50 years has emergency care outside the hospital been viewed as a continuum and as an integral link in decreasing morbidity and mortality. The concept of providing care and transport of sick or injured patients can be traced back to biblical times, where litters were used to carry victims to centers of healing (Gazzaniga, Iseri, & Baren 1992). This crude transportation device may be the earliest recorded predecessor to the modern ambulance. The origin of our current EMS system can be traced to the initiatives undertaken by front-line care providers during major military campaigns. These dedicated individuals worked to decrease the high morbidity and mortality rates of soldiers resulting from either disease or trauma. During the Napoleonic wars (1792-1815) ox carts were used to expedite the transport of victims to the medical treatment stations behind the battlefield lines. Although this reduced transport time to a treatment station, mortality remained high, since no care was provided until the patient arrived at the medical treatment area. The concept of using vehicle evacuation, however, was permanently incorporated into military engagement planning.

Significant improvements in medical care for the sick and injured were pioneered by Florence Nightingale (1820-1910) during the Crimean War of 1853-1856. Her innovative methods, emphasis on knowledge, and farsighted approach in setting care standards revolutionized the provision of medical care to wounded or ill soldiers (Yura & Walsh, 1973).

Some of the medical techniques learned in the Crimean and Napoleonic Wars were adopted by nurses and surgeons in the U.S. Civil War, with some success in improving survival rates of battlefield victims. Clara Barton, a nurse, used her experiences in emergency medical care in the Civil War to establish the American Red Cross.

World War I, with the development of the machine gun and devastating explosives, brought a new set of problems to bear on medical care teams. In addition, the unsanitary conditions in the trenches coupled with evacuation times ranging from 8 to 36 hours resulted in shocking mortality rates. World War II forced several important innovations including blood transfusions, infection control practices, improvements in trauma care, and upgrades in ground and air medical transport systems.

The Korean War introduced the helicopter ambulance, and the Vietnam War clearly demonstrated that effective prehospital field care, in conjunction with rapid ground and air medical transport, significantly improved survival rates. From the Vietnam War to the present, the growth of the pharmaceutical and insurance industries, development of computers, major advancements in medical technology, and space-age innovations have had a significant impact on improving emergency care.

Evolution of Current EMS Systems

In 1865 in Cincinnati, Ohio, a specially constructed horse-drawn carriage was designed for carrying the sick (Stewart, 1989). These carriages, which were staffed by interns from the wards of local hospitals, marked the beginning of civilian ambulance services. This practice continued in the United States until the late 1940s and then began to decline. Prehospital care passed into the hands of funeral home directors, and since many ambulance attendants doubled as morticians, this practice clearly involved a conflict of interest. In the mid-1950s emergency services were provided by some fire departments and private ambulance services. Nevertheless, emergency care continued to be

haphazard and consisted mainly of transport only. Before the mid-1960s, it was generally assumed that emergency care began in the hospital emergency department; therefore patients were loaded into an ambulance and transported to the hospital as fast as possible, receiving no treatment en route. Rescue and treatment techniques were unrefined, training for ambulance attendants was nonexistent, medical control standards were lacking, and radio communication was not developed.

Federal Legislation

The lack of prehospital care did not go unnoticed, however, mainly because physicians, nurses, community health officers, and public interest groups began to voice concern over the universal lack of qualified ambulance services. With the development of mouth-to-mouth resuscitation in the 1950s and closed-cardiac massage in the 1960s, the time was ripe for application of these lifesaving interventions by nonphysicians and the lay public (Stewart, 1989).

A 1966 report from the National Academy of Sciences–National Research Council defined the problems of accidental death and disability as "neglected disease." "The White Paper," as the report is now referred, disclosed to the public that there were no standards for ambulance design, medical training of attendants, or equipment requirements. From 1966-1972 a series of federal and private initiatives were enacted, culminating in the Emergency Medical Services Systems Act of 1973, which offered funding for the development of regional EMS systems. Although this immediately raised the national status of EMS, the race for local and state funding was only beginning. The legislation, unfortunately, had failed to address three essential elements: long-term system financing, medical accountability, and quality assurance.

In the 1980s, when the federal government wiped out federal funding for EMS, many systems encountered financially hard times and were forced to turn to their local communities and state government for financial support. The problem of securing operational funds for developing and maintaining EMS services and the state-to-state variance in medical control and accountability have led to major regional differences in the quality of prehospital care (Bledsoe, Porter, & Shade, 1993).

EMS System Personnel and Resources

EMS systems have a number of components, with the prehospital component including the following:
- The public
- Law enforcement officers
- Emergency physicians
- Mobile intensive care nurses (MICNs)
- Flight nurses
- Emergency medical technicians (EMTs)
- EMT-paramedics

The hospital component includes the following:
- Emergency physicians
- Emergency and critical care transport nurses
- Specialty services (e.g., trauma teams and cardiac teams)

In addition, other essential personnel provide support for the preceding components and ensure that the EMS system functions smoothly. Included in the prehospital phase are dispatchers, public safety and fire personnel, and utility workers. The in-hospital phase includes EKG and radiological technicians, respiratory therapists, and a wide array of medical specialists.

The prehospital response team may be composed of the following:

Ground transport, including:
- Emergency medical technicians (EMTs) and paramedics
- Paramedics and nurses
- Combinations of prehospital nurses, EMTs, paramedics, and physicians

Air medical transport, including:
- Two flight nurses
- A flight nurse and a paramedic
- A flight nurse and a physician
- A flight nurse and an allied health professional (e.g., respiratory therapist)
- Combinations of the above

Whichever combination is employed, the emergency team responds to, recognizes, and evaluates the emergency situation. The team provides intervention by using the following systematic approach.

1. *Scene survey:* The emergency scene is evaluated for safety hazards, location of the patient(s), and mechanism of injury if trauma is involved.
2. *Primary survey:* The primary survey is performed to rule out or treat life-threatening conditions. A primary survey quickly assesses the patient's airway and breathing, circulatory status, signs of hemorrhage, and central nervous system function. Upon completion of the primary survey, life-threatening problems should have been discovered and resuscitative interventions initiated by the prehospital care providers. The team should have insight into the seriousness of the patient's condition and be ready to provide either immediate transport with care administered en route or further definitive care at the scene.
3. *Secondary survey:* This survey is part of the overall assessment plan and involves taking a detailed history and performing a head-to-toe physical examination of the patient. It should identify problems that may have not been apparent in the primary survey. This survey is best done en route for patients in hypovolemic shock or for those displaying signs and symptoms of a rapidly deteriorating condition. ALS teams offer the highest level of prehospital care and possess the clinical skills and the technology to provide the following interventions at the scene and during transport:

a. *Advanced airway control techniques:* includes oral or nasotracheal intubation, use of neuromuscular blocking agents to facilitate intubation, end-tidal carbon dioxide detectors, surgical cricothyrotomy, and relief of tension pneumothorax.

b. *Pharmacological agents:* includes advanced cardiac life support medications and thrombolytics and may include additional intravenous solutions or drugs used for treating shock, increased intracranial pressure, labor and delivery problems, or specific medical emergencies such as diabetes mellitus.

c. *High-tech assessment or monitoring devices:* includes 12-lead EKG transmitting machines, infusion rate regulator pumps, and pulse oximetry or glucose assay devices.

EMS and the Chain of Intervention

Usually the first to encounter an EMS emergency is a citizen who activates the system by telephoning a well-publicized emergency number. The first medical person on the scene is termed the *first responder*. A first responder may be a layperson, law enforcement officer, school nurse, firefighter, or anyone who has received medical training in basic first aid, CPR, splinting, and managing basic emergencies. The responsibility of the first responder is to prevent further injury and deterioration of the patient's overall medical condition until more advanced help arrives. The first responder has been identified by the American Heart Association (AHA) as a key link in the chain of survival. The AHA has cited evidence suggesting that early defibrillation in the prehospital setting improves cardiac arrest outcome. The 1992 AHA guidelines recommended that all first responders be trained in the use of automatic external defibrillators (AEDs) for providing early defibrillation. A survey by Cady and Scott (1992) showed that 38% of first responder systems in

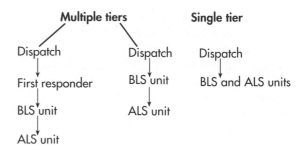

Fig. 2-1 Examples of tiered-response EMS systems.

large metropolitan areas provide early defibrillation.

The next responder may be EMTs in an ambulance or on a fire department vehicle. The EMT may then decide to continue care as being provided, initiate a new care plan, or request an ALS unit. These triage decisions reflect the important role EMTs play in determining both the definitive care a patient will require and which hospital should receive the patient.

The paramedic offers the next line of intervention by providing ALS or, if warranted, calling for a helicopter team. Many EMS systems offer a type of emergency dispatch called *tiered response* (Jackson & Anderson, 1992) (Figure 2-1). A tiered-response system assumes that advanced care is not needed at every emergency scene and sends a BLS unit of basic EMTs who manage the medical care alone, unless the situation requires ALS. In many EMS systems, however, paramedics are dispatched to every call in case ALS is needed. There is some evidence to suggest that a single-tiered system of ALS response is preferred (Wilson, Gratton, Overton, & Watson, 1992). This report examined 6362 calls from January 1989-1990 and showed that 11.7% of all patient calls classified initially as nonemergent unexpectedly received ALS care when they were assessed by ALS personnel. A retrospective study by Lavery, Doran, and Bartholomew (1992) compared hospital-based single-tiered vs. dual-tiered systems using 1989 ALS run reports for cardiac and trauma patients (n = 1024). Results indicate that tiered, dual-response systems are less costly and offer greater flexibility in ambulance assignment.

Response time reliability and the availability of rescue units are essential components in EMS system performance (Cady & Scott, 1993). Variations in the level of services provided by EMS systems across the 50 states are often the result of funding problems, ineffective local or state guidelines, and the perceptions of the citizens and the medical community on the importance of EMS. Even though all states have an EMS agency or board that coordinates EMS education and certification and oversees the state EMS systems, the question of which EMS response configuration is best remains uncertain and requires further research. The future, however, indicates change. Projected changes in health-care reimbursement and financing will continue to affect all EMS systems. With increasing future competition for health-care dollars and the strong possibility of community EMS coverage being contracted out through competitive bids, EMS systems that can offer low-cost, efficient, quick response, and high-quality services will have an advantage over those EMS systems that resist change or restructuring. The most important challenge facing EMS systems in the future is to demonstrate that quality prehospital emergency care makes a difference in improving patient outcome (Cady & Scott, 1993). This can be done only through rigorous data collection and well-constructed research studies.

Differences between Prehospital Emergency Care and In-Hospital Patient Care

PEC differs from in-hospital emergency care in the following ways:

1. PEC is delivered in an uncontrolled environment where the weather, logistical location, on-scene hazards, and an assortment of other circumstances, including family, friends, and onlookers, can interfere with the plan of care; in-hospital care is generally provided in a controlled environment where the weather is irrelevant, lighting is adequate to visualize patient problems or injuries, and interference from family members, friends, or bystanders is minimal.

2. PEC offers only a limited amount of equipment and adjuncts for on-scene intervention; in-hospital care offers a full line of adjunct equipment and services, e.g., X ray, respiratory therapy, laboratory services, and technical support staff.

3. In most cases, especially the county, municipal, and private ambulance services, prehospital emergency care is provided in the physical absence of a physician; in the hospital, physicians and nurses work on parallel tracks and are physically present to direct and manage care of the patient.

4. There are language differences between emergency care providers as exemplified by the following: paramedics operate under written emergency care guidelines termed *standing orders,* or *protocols,* whereas nursing considers established care guidelines and standing orders *standards of care.* Physicians and nurses use the term *diagnosis,* and EMS professionals use *working assessment* in identifying the problem. Both terminologies incorporate treatment guidelines, identification of the problem, and an effective plan of care for managing the situation.

5. Hospital-based air medical services, depending on their situation, can offer first response teams consisting of a physician and a nurse, or two flight nurses, or one flight nurse and one paramedic, and other combinations. These highly trained individuals augment ground ambulance services by providing fast response, a wide level of supportive and invasive skills, and

rapid transport to an appropriate hospital. Although transport times are rapid and the talent and technical "clinical skills" of air medical crews exceptional, the care can be hindered by the terrain, weather, and temperature at the scene, and the range of interventions and equipment at their disposal is still not as complete as that of the appropriate closest hospital.

U.S. DEPARTMENT OF TRANSPORTATION TRAINING CURRICULA
Training of Prehospital Care Providers

Emergency medical technicians (EMTs) make up the majority of certified ambulance personnel in the United States (U.S. Department of Transportation [DOT], 1985). Most rural ambulance services are staffed by volunteer EMTs and EMT-intermediates, and funding is a problem. Although most urban services are usually tax supported, funding is also a problem, but staffing consists of both paid full-time EMTs and paramedics. In an effort to standardize training for all communities in the United States, the U.S. Department of Transportation (U.S. DOT) developed national training curricula for the basic EMT, EMT-intermediate, and the EMT-paramedic programs. The DOT curricula, updated periodically, have been used as guidelines for the past 20 years in training EMTs at all levels of practice.

Training Focus of the EMT

The EMT and paramedic training curriculum was developed as guidelines for training ambulance personnel to manage a variety of emergency situations rapidly and effectively. The didactic sessions focus on the fundamentals of identifying and managing medical and traumatic emergencies; the clinical components, both in-hospital and field rescue unit internships, are structured toward the EMT and paramedic achieving technical proficiency in a number of lifesaving skills. The didactic education gives brief overviews of medical and surgical pathophysiologies but does not delve into any one particular disease or injury. The training emphasis is on speed: rapid assessment, rapid intervention and stabilization, and rapid transport to the closest appropriate hospital. Clinical education focuses on learning skills through repetition. For example, paramedic students practice and repeat a skill such as intravenous catheter placement until proficiency is obtained. The paramedic is also trained to act as a substitute for an on-scene physician.

Prehospital emergency care is organized to be delivered according to preestablished and approved written guidelines and protocols. These protocols serve to guide field care in a standardized fashion and to protect the paramedic in the event that medicolegal questions should arise over the rendered care. EMTs and paramedics are certified according to the state standards in which the educational training was provided. Reciprocity for transferring certification from state to state is neither guaranteed nor easy, since educational and testing standards are not nationally standardized. The lack of national standards has resulted in state to state variations on titles assigned to differing practice levels, even though providers may have the same education and scope of practice (Dawson et al., 1993).

LEVELS OF TRAINING
First Responder

The first responder is the first medical person at the scene of an emergency. This person may or may not have training in first-aid practices. A first responder can be a layperson, firefighter, police officer, school nurse, athletic trainer, lifeguard, or any other public citizen or professional. A first responder in an EMS system should have training in performing initial assessment and first aid, cardiopulmonary resuscitation (CPR), use of airway devices, and knowledge in assisting other medical and rescue personnel. Training involves completion of a 40- to 50-hour course that focuses on stabilizing the patient's condition until advanced care arrives, thus improving patient outcome.

Emergency Medical Technician-Basic (EMT)

The basic EMT curriculum requires 110 hours of instruction, but the number of course hours varies from 100 to 310 hours. EMTs staff ambulances, assess all signs and symptoms, provide interventions, and transport the patient to the hospital. Additional basic EMT responsibilities include the following:
- Thorough patient assessment
- Airway management and oxygenation
- Cardiopulmonary resuscitation
- Spinal and fracture immobilization
- Control of hemorrhage
- Basic vehicle extrication techniques

The recent focus on early defibrillation is prompting the training of EMTs in the additional skill of automatic external defibrillation, referred to as EMT-Ds. This requires 4 to 20 hours of training beyond that of the basic EMT curriculum.

EMT-Intermediate (EMT-I)

Training for EMT-I includes all material in basic EMT training but requires 40 to 80 additional hours. EMT-I training usually includes advanced assessment techniques, intravenous line placement, and administration of some medications, e.g., epinephrine in the event of anaphylaxis. These providers can offer a community a higher level of care than a strictly basic EMT service can provide but with less training and lower cost. Most EMT-Is are trained under U.S. DOT National Standard Curriculum; however, there is great variation between states in both the training and scope of practice for these care providers.

EMT-Paramedic (EMT-P)

The EMT-paramedic is the most extensively trained EMT. Paramedics can provide ALS un-

der written protocols and through a telecommunications device. Most EMT-paramedics are trained in accordance with the U.S. DOT National Standard Curriculum. The training hours range from 700 to 1200+ with a significant portion of the program focusing on clinical assessment and skill repetition.

Interventions a paramedic can perform include the following:
- Dysrhythmia recognition, manual defibrillation, and advanced pharmacology
- Advanced airway control including endotracheal intubation and, in some states, needle cricothyrotomies and decompression of tension pneumothorax
- Insertion of peripheral and central venous lines

A Blueprint for the Education and Training of EMTs at all Levels

Since publication of the first EMT-ambulance course in 1973, prehospital education and training have responded to perceived local needs without a master plan for a comprehensive approach to education and practice (Dawson et al., 1993). To address this issue, a study was commissioned in 1990 by the National Highway Traffic Safety Administration (NHTSA). From this study, a document titled the "National EMS Education and Practice Blueprint" was developed by a task force of experts in EMS and then sent to peer reviewers for comments and clarification. The approved document, which was distributed in September 1993, is endorsed by many major EMS organizations and recommends some significant changes in level of function for prehospital providers. For example, under current training guidelines optimal airway control is limited to oral endotracheal intubation. The "Blueprint" recommends that the EMT-paramedic also be authorized to use nasotracheal intubation, oral intubation with pharmacological sedation, neuromuscular blocking agents, and in some cases, certain types of surgical airways.

Furthermore, the "Blueprint" recommends

that levels of EMS education and practice include knowledge and clinical skills of the preceding certification level. The emphasis is on standardizing prehospital emergency care throughout the country and on bridging the gap between training levels. Throughout the scheme, there are four levels of providers: first responder, EMT-basic, EMT-intermediate, and EMT-paramedic. In most circumstances, the EMT-intermediate will function as current paramedics function. EMT-paramedics will function at a level higher than paramedics currently practice. If these principles are adopted and put into practice, EMS educational curricula and prehospital emergency patient care will change significantly.

Accreditation of EMT and Paramedic Training Programs

All levels of EMT training programs receive accreditation from the state EMS governing agency in which they are located. The accreditation process is not nationally standardized, so there is a wide range of differences between the states on the hours required for EMT, EMT-intermediate, and paramedic training, as well as differences regarding the curricula and scope of practice. An attempt to standardize paramedic education through a national accreditation process is becoming more recognized. National accreditation, however, is currently voluntary and is awarded only to those programs meeting the criteria established by the Joint Review Committee of the Committee on Allied Health and Education and Accreditation (CAHEA), which represents a consortium of health-care providers.

Prehospital Nursing Curricula and Regulation of Practice

In 1988 a committee appointed by the Emergency Nurses Association (ENA) developed the "National Standard Guidelines for Prehospital Nursing Curriculum." This curriculum, published in 1991, was based on surveys of state boards of nursing and state EMS agencies and on guidelines from both nursing and nonnursing-based prehospital education curricula. Also in 1988 the National Flight Nurses Association (NFNA) and ENA released a joint statement recognizing state boards of nursing as the regulatory agencies for prehospital nursing practice and opposing dual-licensure for nurses choosing to practice in the prehospital environment. The NFNA/ENA position paper, however, acknowledged that progress in the area of who should regulate prehospital nursing required a collaborative approach with EMS authorities. The joint statement also recognized the need for nurses to receive additional education and training in specific clinical skill areas of prehospital practice.

The National Association of EMTs (NAEMT) has issued its own statement that supports the viewpoint that nurses should be certified as EMTs by their respective state EMS agency before they are allowed to practice in the prehospital setting. NAEMT's position is based on the concern that if nurses are removed from any accountability to state EMS authorities, then nurses might encroach on EMS employment positions currently held by EMTs and paramedics. The NAEMT also has voiced concern over the development of the prehospital nursing curriculum without input from either EMS professionals or EMS medical directors. They also disagree with some aspects of the lobbying efforts of prehospital nursing organizations, particularly their effort to encourage state legislatures to enact laws designating registered nurses as prehospital professionals regulated solely by the state's nursing practice act.

Other areas of contention revolve around the increased practice of hospitals that employ EMTs and paramedics in emergency departments and other patient care areas. ENA and a number of professional nursing organizations have opposed this practice. Conflict arises over job responsibilities, supervision, and skill levels of the EMTs. The issue is compounded by hospital administrations looking for ways to reduce patient care costs, and employing ancillary personnel is certainly one way to cut costs.

Both nurses and EMTs are trained to provide good patient care. However, differences in historical development, patient care perspectives, and focus of education and training create problems for both in understanding the role of the other. Studies show that problems arise from miscommunication between EMTs, paramedics, and nurses, from misunderstandings of each others' roles, and from different ways of defining a patient care situation (Palmer & Gonsoulin, 1992; Sharp & Sharp, 1985). Clearly, collaboration, compromise, and a team effort from both parties are needed if this issue is to be resolved. There appears to be room for everyone in the practice of emergency care, but professional accountability and job descriptions will continue to be contended until a formal compromise can be negotiated.

EMS and Prehospital Nursing Practice

A 1993 survey of state EMS agencies and the regulation of prehospital nursing was published in the October 1993 issue of the *Journal of Emergency Nursing*. The study was undertaken to gather data concerning prehospital nursing issues and the regulatory practices of prehospital nursing in each state (Johnson, Childress, & Herron, 1993). Essentially the study demonstrated that of the 50 states surveyed, 44 (88%) offered no certification in prehospital nursing. The results indicate also that most state EMS agencies require nurses to become certified at an EMT level to practice on an EMS response unit. Overall the data show that states' adoption of prehospital nursing curriculum recommendations has progressed little since the 1988 NFNA/ENA joint statement.

STATE AND LOCAL REGULATIONS
Nurses in the Prehospital Environment

Nurses have worked both directly and indirectly in prehospital environments since the Crimean War. The mobile army surgical hospital (MASH) units in the Korean and Vietnam Wars served as prehospital care stations. These units were staffed with dedicated physicians, nurses, and medical corpsmen who provided immediate care and stabilization of patients before transfer to better-equipped medical facilities.

Today, however, a nurse who wants to qualify as a BLS or ALS provider with a local EMS response unit may be required to complete additional training to satisfy local or state standards. Some states require basic EMT or paramedic certification as a prerequisite for working in the prehospital environment, whereas other states allow nurses to perform prehospital ALS functions based on the state's nurse practice act. In general, nurse practice acts do not address the role of nurses in the prehospital environment. In a few states the question revolves around whether a nurse ceases to be a nurse when providing treatment in an ambulance. Although most legal opinions indicate the answer to be no, many EMS systems do not accept a nurse as an ambulance member without certification as an EMT or paramedic. Some fire and EMS officers hold the opinion that a nurse without prehospital, emergency, or critical care experience, in spite of having a longer and more extensive educational background, will often not have the specialized ALS skills to manage the life-threatening situations in the prehospital environment. To address this issue, some states have created paramedic training programs to act as a streamlined, or bridge, course for nurses. This bridge course is designed to address only those areas in which the nurse needs more didactic and clinical training and omits those areas in which the nurse demonstrates competency. The respective state EMS agency and state board of nursing should be consulted to determine the EMT, paramedic, and ALS requirements. In states where EMTs and paramedics are in short supply, nurses who are certified in ACLS are often encouraged to be a part of the ALS care team. Currently, 16 states allow RN staffing of EMS services to meet state requirements (Johnson, Childress, &

Herron, 1993). In most states, however, nurses who want to work in a local EMS service need to secure additional certification beyond the requirements of nursing licensure. Certification as a basic EMT is usually considered the minimum state requirement for an ambulance prehospital care provider. If ALS is the community standard, then a nurse may have to obtain paramedic certification to conform with local ordinances or policies. Therefore in most instances nurses who are active members of county-or municipality-based ambulances usually are certified as either basic EMTs or paramedics.

Since many state nurse practice acts do not specifically define the settings in which a nurse can practice, state EMS agencies claim the higher ground in EMS jurisdiction regarding both prehospital certification and the staffing of EMS systems.

Nurses Working in Prehospital Care Roles

In addition to staffing ground and air ambulance services, nurses are also actively involved in prehospital emergency services in the following positions:

- Hospital EMS coordinators
- EMT and paramedic educators
- Mobile critical care nurses (MCCNs) (interfacility transport)
- Mobile intensive care nurses (MICNs) (coordinate field care via a radio-telecommunications device)

Hospital EMS Coordinators

EMS coordinators are registered nurses with training and experience in prehospital emergency care, the emergency department, and critical care unit areas. They are usually employed by the hospital and report to the administrative level. Since there are frequent interactions between patient-bearing EMS services and hospital staff, the hospital EMS coordinator's role involves being the liaison or facilitator between local EMS response units and the hospital. It is

always in the best interests of patient care if the transfer of the patient from the EMS team to the hospital team occurs in a smooth and coordinated fashion. This transfer will go better if each team has an understanding of the other's roles and limitations. This is where the nurse EMS coordinator can help. When a complaint or problem arises, the nurse EMS coordinator is notified; the coordinator then attempts to identify the source of the problem and design and initiate a plan for resolving the issue. Although the roles and responsibilities of these nurses differ between hospitals, they are usually involved in the following activities:

1. Serve as the hospital's EMS contact person for the local prehospital care providers
2. Investigate and monitor state and local legislative activities and attend meetings that affect EMS system issues
3. Initiate and draft hospital EMS interaction policies, review run report information, and update EMS personnel, hospital staff, and administration on evolving policies and procedures
4. Investigate problems and complaints involving EMS, e.g., lost equipment, and offer mitigating solutions
5. Support EMS system continuous quality improvement efforts through continuing education programs and constructive feedback to the local EMS squads

A successful nurse holding this title needs unquestionable clinical competency in both prehospital and in-hospital emergency care, a high degree of political sensitivity in EMS issues, and excellent public relations skills. It is also beneficial if the nurse has training or experience in methods of problem solving and conflict resolution. For example, as a result of different perspectives toward patient care, it is not uncommon for misunderstandings to occur in the emergency department between physicians and EMTs, and nurses and EMTs. If not attended to immediately, these conflicts can create long-term effects of poor cooperation, resentment, and even hostility between emergency and EMS personnel. The EMS coordinator can mitigate the conflict by identifying the source of the problem and having key representatives of the EMS system and the emergency department sit down and discuss both sides of the issue. When conflicts are not addressed and are left to find their own course, they can cause crises requiring intervention by hospital administration and local EMS authorities.

Nurse EMS coordinators are becoming an important link between EMS unit personnel and hospitals. The creation of the EMS coordinator position in hospital emergency departments across the United States demonstrates that hospitals recognize the short- and long-term importance of promoting good working relationships with local EMS units.

Prehospital Educators

Nurses are also involved in paramedic training programs as full-time program directors, clinical coordinators and instructors, and full- and part-time clinical education preceptors. These prehospital nurse educators have an educational background that includes teaching experience and knowledge of EMS systems and the training curricula for EMTs and paramedics. Many also have a 4-year college education, hold ACLS certification, have attended courses in trauma management, and are EMTs, paramedics, or both.

Mobile Critical Care Nurses

Hospital-based mobile transportation units are ground ambulances providing interhospital transfer services and transportation to and from treatment centers for home-care patients who require either BLS or ALS care and monitoring during transit. Mobile critical care nurses (MCCNs) have emergency and critical care experience and are usually employed by the hospital, which serves as their base station. Some are employed as managers of patient transport services. Hospital-based ambulance services are rarely dispatched to emergency scenes as part of the EMS first response, although some do have contracts with counties or municipalities to do so; most act as private carriers and primarily handle interhospital and home-related transport service. There is a difference in the roles of nurses who staff hospital-based ground ambulances providing interfacility transport and those who provide care at the scene of the incident. Responders to the scene environment must have safety and weather-adaptable clothing and have the equipment and clinical skill flexibility and physical endurance to work in extreme weather conditions and rapidly changing patient care situations. MCCNs working with interfacility transport systems, however, rarely respond to the scene of an emergency and usually work in a semicontrolled environment, but many of the patients they care for require extensive critical care nursing experience and in-depth knowledge of pharmacology and technological monitoring devices. Future trends indicate that MCCNs will continue to play an important role in hospital ground emergency transport services.

Mobile Intensive Care Nurses

Mobile intensive care nurses (MICN) are registered nurses with special training in prehospital intervention techniques, protocols, and procedures.

MICNs in California and Indiana issue instructions via a telecommunications device to paramedics regarding assessment of the clinical needs of the patients, implementation of a treatment regimen, and evaluation of the effectiveness of the treatment. MICNs are not recognized to practice in most states. In states where they can practice, the certification training varies from 100 hours to 250 hours and covers all components of telecommunications and emergency medical intervention (see Box 1-2). MICNs must function within the guidelines of state law and the local care standards established within an EMS region (Gazzaniga, Isteri, & Baren, 1982; Pointer, Osur, & Campbell, 1991). In some localities MICNs can issue orders for all approved drugs and medical procedures, whereas in other areas they may do only those activities delegated by a physician. Evidence shows that nurses can independently manage the great majority of the telecommunication calls and, in critical cases, issue stabilization orders until a physician assumes care. An MICN must be an expert in assessing and interpreting incoming information, since it is often necessary to seek clarification of received information and to ask additional questions to get an accurate picture of the patient's condition. MICN responsibilities vary but usually involve on-line telecommunications responsibilities, including medical direction via radio to personnel at the emergency scene.

EMS Systems Configuration

EMS service is provided in a large part because the public recognizes the importance of the service. It is often equated with the public's right and demand for fire and police protection.

The efficient delivery of emergency medical care, therefore, requires both public support and an in-depth analysis of community needs, patient population served, hours of operation, level of services provided, and use of existing resources. Because of these variables, EMS systems are structured according to demographics, geographics and the area to be covered, and the economic and human resources of their respective communities. Although no one best method exists for providing emergency care, some components are considered essential for an EMS system to operate effectively.

Local Administrative Direction

A planning board or operations committee should be established to organize overall EMS system function and to manage resources (Figure 2-2). This organization should include community representatives, local EMS providers, public safety personnel, and members of the emergency medical care community. It is essential that the board develop policies and procedures to ensure that the EMS system functions in accordance with state standards and desig-

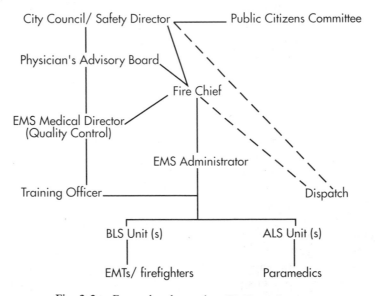

Fig. 2-2 Example of an urban EMS configuration.

nate the level of service (BLS or ALS) and the level of training necessary for serving as a member of the community EMS response team. The board should select a chief administrative officer to oversee and monitor the delivery of emergency care and to attend to the day-to-day administrative duties demanded by the service. Finally, the board should establish a quality control system, in cooperation with a physician medical advisor, for evaluating the efficiency of the service and effectiveness of the provided care.

Medical Control

All EMS systems should retain and be accountable to a medical director who is ultimately responsible for all clinical patient care. The prehospital providers of an ambulance service function on what can be considered the extension of the medical director's license. This makes them designated agents of the medical director and responsible to his or her guidance on compliance with patient care protocols and any other medically related issues. Furthermore the physician should be knowledgeable of emergency medical procedures, take an active interest in EMS training exercises and educational updates, and set up case review and quality assurance sessions for EMS team members.

The process of ensuring accountability of and direction for EMS systems is termed *medical control.* This process should be supported by either a county or municipal medical board that reviews information, approves policies and protocols, and oversees the entire local EMS system. Active involvement and cooperation of the regional medical board provides both guidance and a broad base of support for the EMS medical director who is undertaking medical control responsibilities. Medical control is most consistent and effective when it is mandated by a state EMS agency. In general, medical directors should meet the following requirements:

- Experienced and actively involved in emergency medicine

- Knowledgeable of BLS and ALS prehospital training
- Experience in telecommunications protocol and techniques
- Familiarity with reviewing patient case studies (EMS run reviews)
- Understanding of both local and state legislation
- Knowledge of the political climate of local EMS systems

In addition to physician involvement in EMS training and run review activities, medical control exists in two other ways. The first is direct, or on-line, medical control and occurs when prehospital care providers telecommunicate with a physician or MICN at a base station hospital. The physician, who has ultimate on-line responsibility, or the MICN gives orders based on regionally approved protocols. The best judgments and prehospital medical care occur when physicians and MICNs have established mutual trust and professional working relationships with EMS care providers. Another form of direct control involves the authority of the medical director to set patient care standards and to update and recommend additional training for prehospital staff. In addition to possessing excellent communication skills, it is also essential that physicians and nurses with direct medical control be knowledgeable and experienced in prehospital emergency medical procedures.

The second type of medical direction is indirect, or off-line, medical control. This encompasses medical education, training, personnel development, protocol compliance, patient case study review, and continuous quality improvement goals. With this control the physician can regulate the direction of the EMS system. Effective leadership skills are needed for gaining administrative and squad members' confidence and support. The physician medical director should have disciplinary powers and should have the support of EMS administrative officers with the written backing of the local governing medical board.

Protocols and Standing Orders

The accomplishment of some emergency procedures, such as airway control, is so important, that they should be carried out before direct medical control is established with the hospital physician. These off-line interventions are sanctioned under written standing orders. Voice communication with the hospital base station should always be initiated after the standing orders have been completed. A study by Pointer, Osur, & Campbell (1991) suggests that limited standing orders probably reduce scene time and do not appear to hinder paramedic assessment at the scene or patient outcome. On the other hand, protocols are approved guidelines that designate the step-by-step approach the EMS provider undertakes on all EMS calls and with all patients. A protocol should cover a wide spectrum of emergency complaints, conditions, and signs and symptoms. General headings include treatment for such conditions as coma, seizure, diabetes, chest pain, and a number of other illnesses and injuries. The emphasis of prehospital treatment is not to make a diagnosis but to assess the patient, initiate a plan of care including lifesaving interventions when necessary, stabilize the patient's condition, and continue care en route to the hospital.

Protocols and standing orders should be approved by the local governing medical board, and all life squads, receiving hospitals, and squad medical directors involved should receive copies. A review process should be established to update EMS standing orders and protocols periodically in light of new research reflecting the need to revise emergency care recommendations.

Types of EMS Systems

Public Law 93-154 of 1973 provided funding for EMS systems in a series of grants and encouraged states to set up lead agencies but did not mandate the configuration of EMS systems. The funding was offered to those states

---

Box 2-1
FIFTEEN COMPONENTS SPECIFIED BY THE EMS ACT OF 1973

1. Manpower
2. Training
3. Communications
4. Transportation
5. Emergency care facilities
6. Critical care units
7. Public safety service agencies
8. Consumer input
9. Access to care
10. Patient transfer
11. Standardized record keeping
12. Public education
13. System evaluation and review mechanisms
14. Disaster management
15. Mutual aid practices

---

who incorporated the mandatory 15 components of EMS specified by the law (Box 2-1). This led to a retroactive instead of proactive design of local EMS systems. Thus EMS systems in the United States evolved from historical and geopolitical views of local and state governments rather than from data from scientific evaluation (Wilson, Gratton, Overton, & Watson, 1992). Currently there is a movement for establishment of a national standard for EMS system configuration and for increased scientific research into prehospital care practices (Lavery, Doran, & Bartholomew, 1992).

COMMON EMS PROVIDER TYPES
Municipal-County Services

The majority of EMS systems in the United States are either municipal or county based. The configuration varies, but the design is mainly controlled by economic concerns. A survey of

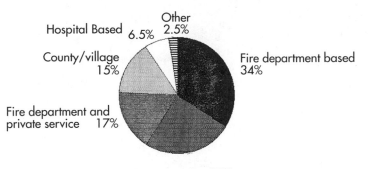

Fig. 2-3   EMS provider types from 1993 survey. (*Note.* From *Journal of Emergency Medical Services*, 1993.)

EMS providers in the top 200 most populous cities is shown in Figure 2-3. Most of these EMS systems are operated through local fire departments. In the early years of EMS development the consensus was that emergency services should become a part of the public safety service system. City and county fire departments seemed to be the most logical choice because they were strategically placed in fixed localities, were available 24 hours a day, and were already oriented toward protecting lives and property (Stewart, 1989). These preexisting delivery capabilities made fire departments the most convenient means for providing prehospital emergency care to local communities. In many cases the responsibility of providing EMS was assigned to the fire departments, which received it with little enthusiasm. The incorporation of EMS within the fire services created funding and logistical dilemmas for fire administrators. In many cases EMS was given little priority, taking second place to fire prevention. Over the years, however, fire codes requiring both old and new buildings to use a number of fire-resistant materials, including sprinkler and alarm systems, significantly reduced the incidence of structural fires in all cities. At the same time, EMS calls have continued to increase annually. According to national statistics maintained by the National Fire Protection Association (NFPA), EMS calls constitute 80% of the total call volume of a fire service, with fire calls making up the additional 20%. These dramatic statistics and the popularity of television programs such as "Rescue 911," "Code 3," and "Emergency Call" are catching the attention of the public and the media and are requiring fire and political officials to fund and provide quality EMS systems in their communities.

Fire department–based EMS units are under the immediate jurisdiction of the local fire chief. The service may be composed of volunteers, who receive either minimal or no compensation, or of full- or part-time paid personnel. The EMS response may be BLS, ALS, or both. The units are supported by a tax base and sometimes by a surcharge for each call. However, funding is an ongoing problem, and the level of care provided is often decided on the basis of fiscal constraints. The fire chief holds an integral position in any fire department–based EMS system, and the chief's cooperation and support are essential for EMS systems to function smoothly and to deliver quality emergency care. Anyone working in this type of system must recognize that the fire chief is also at the head of the administrative power structure; ignoring this fact could shorten the career of anyone working within the service, especially physicians and nurses.

Private Ambulance Services

The private ambulance service is one of the oldest types of EMS systems in the nation. Since it is primarily a for-profit organization or company, the absence of tax support, decreasing federal reimbursement, and spiraling health-care costs strain finances for even the most austere service. These fiscal problems and an increase in mergers may indicate that further consolidation of the private ambulance industry may be necessary for future economic survival.

Some private ambulance providers offer only BLS service, and others provide a combination of ALS and BLS. They must meet the same operational guidelines, however, and provide the same quality of service as any public EMS system, including medical direction and control. Inasmuch as the private services are structured like a business, they must work to maximize efficiency and aggressively market their services to the public. The 1993 annual survey of EMS providers in the 200 most populous cities conducted by the *Journal of Emergency Medical Services* (JEMS) shows that the private sector is responsible for providing EMS to 25% (50 cities) of the cities surveyed. This makes private companies the second most common provider of EMS to major cities, with fire departments providing most services (34%, 68 cities). The collected data also show that 17% of EMS systems use a nontransport, fire department–based ALS first response but employ a private service for transporting patients. These statistics suggest that in major metropolitan cities private ambulance companies play an important role in both the delivery of prehospital emergency care and in the transport of patients.

County or Village EMS System

County or village EMS systems are supported by local taxes but are not fire department based. EMTs and paramedics are employed by the local government, and the service usually operates under the same standards and protocols as authorized by the local physician advisory board. This service type makes up about 15% of EMS services in the 200 most populous cities (Cady & Stout, 1993).

Hospital-Based EMS Systems

Hospital-based EMS systems account for around 6% to 7% of the services (Cady & Stout, 1993). They may be privately owned and operated or they may serve as an extension of the public service areas in providing services to specific geographical localities. Some operate in conjunction with hospital-based air medical services and are administratively managed and financed by the hospital. Direct and indirect medical control is usually excellent because of the close contact and familiarity of the physicians, nurses, and hospital support staff (Stewart, 1989). The possibility of financial changes in private and government health plan reimbursement for this service will restrict the growth of the hospital-based EMS.

Volunteer EMS Systems

Rural EMS could not be maintained if it were not for the commitment of volunteer emergency care providers. The backbone of this system is the volunteer EMT. Most of these individuals have full-time jobs outside of their EMS responsibilities. Furthermore, they are on-call for emergencies, usually for one or two 24-hour periods during the week, and are called out in bad weather and in the middle of the night for accidents and emergencies that sometimes involve friends and neighbors (Garnett, Hall, & Johnson, 1989). Many of these individuals receive little or no compensation for their work and often have to pay for their training and certification expenses. The turnover rate is high, and finding people to staff local EMS squads is becoming increasingly difficult as more families in the community need a double income to pay for living expenses and have less time to give to the local community EMS service.

Summary

EMS systems have evolved from a system that focused on simply racing victims to the hospital to a complex and multidisciplinary system involving cooperation, specialized patient care skills, telecommunications, and a recognition of the various levels of training for all prehospital care professionals. Federal and state laws have established standards for the education and training of prehospital care providers and guidelines for the essential components of EMS systems. The complexity of the system requires the cooperative interaction of many people and organizations for the emergency service process to function smoothly. The contribution of EMTs at all levels of practice, however, has been the main force in elevating EMS response to a level of national prominence.

Medical control is improving as physicians, nurses, and fire and EMS administrators work together in the planning, education and training, patient care process, and development of quality management mechanisms. Nurses are finding new roles in the prehospital setting by becoming training program educators, by providing continuing education for EMTs at all training levels, and by serving as liaisons between the hospital and squad personnel in the hospital EMS coordinator role. When certification is required by either state or local mandate, nurses are becoming EMTs or paramedics and are actively running with their local ambulance service. Flight nursing is becoming a career for many nurses who are interested in prehospital emergency care. Flight nursing provides nurses with excellent opportunities to use advanced assessment techniques, intervention skills, and judgmental abilities to the fullest extent of their training because such employment is offered under the auspices of a medical facility and is not subject to state EMS staffing regulations. Some EMTs are pursuing a nursing education, and the number holding dual certification is increasing. Hospitals are employing the skills of EMTs in emergency service areas, including air medical services, and these practices are under continuous review by nursing, hospital, and EMT organizations.

Funding of EMS systems will continue to be a problem in the immediate future. Budget shortfalls will force states and EMS administrators to find creative ways to finance quality emergency medical services for the public. Fiscal constraints may cause the regionalization of EMS services so that costs can be cut and the expense of funding less well-supported services spread out. The attempts to fund EMS through federal or state legislation could face an uphill battle, since the current mood of many legislators is to balance the budget.

The delivery of prehospital care will be affected in the future by the following:

1. Increasing adaptation of high-tech devices for use by prehospital care providers
2. The continual debate over medical control of EMS systems
3. Funding issues and cost control
4. Politicalization of EMS.

Regardless of these challenges, prehospital emergency care is one of the last frontiers where a medical professional can practice specialized lifesaving skills in an uncontrolled environment.

EMS COMMUNICATIONS
Communication Systems Overview

A reliable and efficient communications network is an essential and fundamental component of prehospital emergency care. The person serving as the integral link in the EMS chain of response is the dispatcher. The dispatcher is pivotal, since citizens accessing the system and requesting help will often have their first contact with a dispatcher. The activities of an EMS communications center are continuously monitored by both computer and a taping process. A modern communications system is equipped with up-to-date technology, is available 24 hours a day, and can be accessed easily and from a wide range of geographical areas. EMS systems must have the capabilities to interface with a variety of groups to provide effective services. This requires coordination between the following:

- Persons accessing the system
- Fire, police, and EMS squads
- Medical facilities
- Base-station medical control
- The media
- Hospital personnel (including medical records)
- Public service administration records
- Disaster networks

All of the above are essential components of a modern communications system. A number of factors, however, influence the type of communications system available in a given area, including funding and resources, geography, and the health and safety needs of the community. Although training of EMS care providers has extensively changed and improved over the past 20 years, it is only recently that attention has been focused on the traditional policies and procedures of the most integral link in the communications system: the dispatcher (Clawson & Dernocoeur, 1988).

In the early 1980s concerned health care and EMS managers began to question long-standing ideas regarding the role of the dispatcher, employment qualifications, organizational structure, and the operational practices of communication centers. According to Suter (1992) the realization of the importance of the dispatcher led to the development of alternative approaches such as emergency medical priority dispatch (EMD) training, computer-aided dispatch (CAD), and systems status management (SSM). These new paradigms recognize the central role of the communications system in controlling overall EMS operations. The efficiency and adaptability offered by these approaches have led to their successful implementation in several cities and counties across the nation. However, because change often runs in the face of both tradition and fiscal restraints, many localities continue to maintain traditional, and somewhat outmoded, EMS communication systems.

Typically an EMS response is initiated by the occurrence of an illness or injury. The incident must then be detected by someone and a call placed to the communications center. Once the information and location of the emergency are obtained, the appropriate EMS provider is dispatched to the scene. At the scene, treatment may include on-line medical control with a base station hospital physician, with periodic radio contact continuing during transport of the patient to a hospital. After delivery of the patient to hospital personnel, the medical run report must be completed, documenting all medical care provided to the patient and recording the dispatch time, on-scene time of arrival, and time of arrival at the hospital. The communications center is alerted when the EMS team has cleaned the vehicle, restocked, and is ready to be put back into service for future emergencies.

Regulations

All radio communications in the United States are controlled and regulated by the Federal Communications Commission (FCC). Currently, EMS communication systems are licensed for operation by the FCC's Emergency Medical Radio Services (EMRS). The FCC allocates radio frequencies, approves equipment, licenses transmitters and repair technicians, monitors frequencies for appropriate usage, and spot-checks communication stations for appropriate licensing and record maintenance (Johnson & Van Cott, 1992).

Radio Frequencies

There are two types of soundwave transmissions: amplitude modulation (AM) and frequency modulation (FM). AM waves follow the shape of the earth and provide a good range of transmission; they are, however, subject to interference that can result in poor reception at the receiving station. FM transmission waves travel in a straight line, are not subject to interference, and are much cleaner and more easily received than AM waves. Therefore most EMS radio communications are conducted on FM frequencies.

Radio frequencies are designated by cycles

per second, called *megahertz* (MHz). Most of EMS communication is conducted in the frequency spectrums termed *very-high frequency* (VHF), which includes low band and high band, and *ultra-high frequency* (UHF). In 1993 the FCC approved a plan to allocate all 800-MHz frequencies for all public safety users, including police, fire, and EMS (Table 2-1). The changes are designed to be phased in over the next several years. Although the FCC does not require public safety service agencies to switch to the 800-MHz band, the advantages offered by the 800-MHz system will probably encourage the change. As agencies and communications centers gradually switch to the 800-MHz system, other UHF and VHF frequencies will be less congested.

Table 2-1   Transmission Frequency Bands

Band	Pros	Cons
800 MHz	Minimal interference Reduced channel noise Numerous channels Requires only a short antenna Excellent for communication in urban areas Can use many 800 frequencies at one time Offers comprehensive frequency coordination Minimal skip, excellent building penetration Not crowded Trunking offers better usage of channels	Expensive equipment Requires repeaters Short range Poor penetration of forests
UHF 450-475 MHz	High-quality and very clear audio Many channels Telemetry and two-way communication available Offers coordination of frequencies Requires short antenna Good penetration of buildings Repeaters already in place in most locales	Range less than VHF Expensive equipment Poor penetration of forests Some channel interference Some degree of skip Few licenses available, since channels are overcrowded
VHF 150-175 MHz High-band	Relatively clear audio Reasonably priced equipment Long-range capabilities Moderate skip and noise characteristics Penetrates forested areas well	Few channels No telemetry capabilities Poor penetration of buildings Many users and no frequency coordination
VHF 32-50 MHz Low-band	Very long range Excellent for forested or open areas	Subject to noise and skip interference Few channels No telemetry capabilities Poor penetration of buildings Many users and no frequency coordination

Cellular Telephones

Many EMS systems are now taking advantages of technological communication networks and are using cellular telephone units to contact medical control. These units are mobile and can both receive and transmit simultaneously using two separate frequencies. They also allow short- or long-distance transmissions without signal distortion. Cellular telephone units can operate only where a functioning telephone system is in place. Cities, counties, and geopolitical areas are divided into "cells," and each has its own receiving units and transmitters. The geographically positioned transmitters are used to interface the portable cellular units with base station control. Calls are then sent to the appropriate destination via preexisting telephone lines. Since low-power transmitters are used, frequencies can be used in adjacent cells without interference. EMS personnel primarily use this field communications system for scene to base station hospital communication. The portability and reasonable cost of cellular telephones may make them the most practical communication device for prehospital personnel. Many hospitals are installing dedicated lines for prehospital personnel to communicate with medical control. Telemetry data can be sent on the same frequency through the use of a demodulator. Technological advances now allow the transmission of facsimiles (faxes) 12-lead EKGs, and computer data to record-keeping computer banks within the communications center.

Biotelemetry

The process of transmitting physiological data, such as an EKG rhythms, over the radio system is termed *biotelemetry,* or *telemetry* for short. A modulator in the EMS unit converts the EKG voltage impulses into audio tones that are transmitted to the local hospital. A demodulator at the hospital converts the audio signal back to voltage impulses to reproduce the EKG. Telemetry interference is often a problem during transmission and can be caused by loose EKG electrodes, muscle tremors, 60-MHz noise, and fluctuations in transmitter power.

Communications Center

The core of all EMS communications systems is the center used for controlling dispatch, using the transmitters and receivers, and coordinating interface between the public, local hospitals, and other public safety agencies. A communications center must have the capability of receiving calls for help from the public and alerting EMS, fire, or police personnel of the emergency. Communications system configuration has three variations: (1) a single facility containing all communication equipment and personnel for coordinating public safety agencies, (2) a center housed within a local fire or police department with EMS integrated into the dispatch process, and (3) police, fire, and EMS personnel functioning separately through their own communications centers. Regardless of the configuration, it is important for prehospital care personnel to be familiar with the operation and protocols of the communications system in their given locale.

Dispatch Procedures

All dispatch and operating procedures must conform to federal, state, and local guidelines. The EMS dispatcher plays a crucial role in EMS function. Recognized courses are available for training dispatchers and are modeled after the "EMS Dispatcher National Standard Curriculum" written by the U.S. Department of Transportation. Responsibilities of the dispatcher include the following:

1. Obtaining, in a rapid manner, as much information about the emergency from the caller as possible
2. Directing the appropriate emergency response unit to the emergency scene
3. Providing first aid or medical instructions for the caller to follow until emergency care arrives

4. Monitoring and overseeing communications between EMS and other public safety personnel

5. Securing and maintaining written records

Dispatchers use questions in the form of algorithms to make quick decisions regarding which vehicles to send to the emergency. This entails knowing which units are available, the location of all vehicles, the various capabilities of each vehicle personnel, i.e., advanced life support (ALS) or basic life support (BLS), and evaluation of whether additional support services are needed. In larger systems computer-aided dispatch (CAD) is used to assist dispatchers in tracking vehicle status, ordering data, receiving calls, identifying the victim's location, and providing codes for describing the acuity of the emergency situation. Some communications systems have mobile data terminals (MDTs) that allow the dispatcher to track on a screen the location of each emergency vehicle. The price of MDTs, however, precludes most centers from purchasing them. These technologies allow the EMS communications dispatcher either to track vehicle location or to follow the movement of dispatched vehicles in real time on a display map.

A dispatcher must gather essential information from the caller before dispatching emergency assistance. This includes the nature and location of the emergency and a call-back number in case of accidental telephone disconnection. The following is an example of the logical order of EMS dispatch:

1. A call is placed and the dispatcher answers.
2. The caller's name and call-back number are obtained.
3. The address and nature of the emergency are confirmed.
4. THE FIRST AMBULANCE IS DISPATCHED.
5. Is the victim unconscious, not breathing, or bleeding severely?

6. Is the victim trapped, or is there a fire or other hazards?
7. AMBULANCE CREW IS UPDATED AND SUPPORT HELP DISPATCHED.
8. The need for immediate emergency care measures is determined, and the caller's capability of performing those measures is ascertained.

Hospital Base Operations

An essential component of prehospital emergency care is the ability of personnel to communicate directly with hospitals via a radio telecommunications device. As previously discussed, the type of communications device must take into consideration the distances the transmissions must travel and the interference caused by the geographics of the area. On-line medical control is best provided by an experienced emergency physician or MICN who is available to answer the radio 24 hours a day in a timely manner. This service appears to work most effectively when medical direction is provided by a single designated base station hospital. Once the information has been received and orders provided to EMS personnel in the field, the physician or nurse notifies the receiving hospital, if different from the base station hospital, of the patient's condition and the care provided. When a system does not have on-line medical control, either because radio communication is not possible or the system is not in place to allow it, the dispatcher can write down the information and relay it to the receiving hospital. This will assist hospital personnel in preparing for the patient's arrival. On-line medical control capabilities do not nullify the need for off-line medical control, such as standing orders, treatment protocols, and policy and procedural guidelines. These also serve as backup systems in the event of communication failure or if the urgency of the situation takes precedence over the early establishment of on-line control. It should be the responsibility of the local EMS governing agency to determine

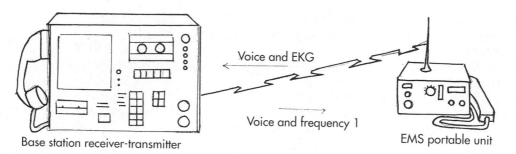

Fig. 2-4   Example of a simplex transmission system.

the appropriate base station hospital and the number of communication channels necessary for ensuring easy access by squad personnel.

Transmission System Characteristics

Radios used for EMS communications use four different systems for coordinating ambulance and rescue dispatch. A prehospital care worker need not have extensive training in the technical aspects of communications systems nor in the aspects of radio etiquette. A general understanding of the various systems and terminology, however, is beneficial for effective operation within the system.

Simplex Transmission

The simplex transmission is the least complicated of the communication systems (Figure 2-4). Communication occurs on one frequency; therefore transmission and reception cannot occur at the same time. The person can send a message but then must release the transmission button for the other person to respond. Simplex is the most common type of communication used by dispatch centers.

Duplex Transmission

A duplex system uses two frequencies and allows simultaneous two-way communication (Figure 2-5). This system operates in the same manner as a telephone conversation. The system can be enhanced by the use of a repeater, which is a device for increasing the power and range of the signal.

Multiplex Transmission

Multiplex transmission allows the simultaneous transmission on one channel of both voice and EKG signals (Figure 2-6). The prehospital caller can provide information about the patient at the same time the EKG rhythm is being sent. The majority of base station hospitals providing on-line medical control for prehospital emergency care providers use multiplex systems.

COMMUNICATIONS EQUIPMENT AND TECHNICAL COMPONENTS
ALS Emergency Vehicles

EMS ground response units offering ALS services must carry a portable battery-powered radio receiver with telemetry capabilities and a battery-powered monitor-defibrillator that can be interfaced with the communications system. The equipment must also be light (no more than 25 pounds), sturdy, dependable, and offer easy-to-use controls. These portable units are used for communicating with either the base station hospital or the local designated communications center. Special equipment is employed by the receiving hospital for receiving both voice information and biotelemetry data.

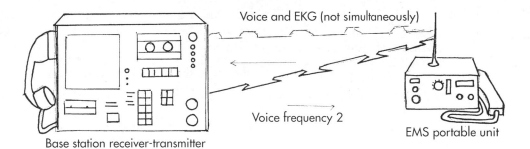

Fig. 2-5   Example of a duplex transmission system.

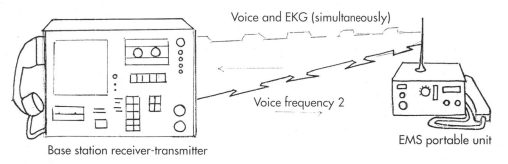

Fig. 2-6   Example of a multiplex transmission system.

Base Station

The base station employs a transmitter and receiver and serves as the primary communications center. Its location should take into consideration the terrain and the service range it is to incorporate. Currently, most base stations offer a power output of 45 to 275 watts and can transmit and receive on only one channel at a time. The maximum allowable base station power is regulated by the FCC and is designated on the base station license.

Mobile Two-Way Radios

A mobile two-way radio suggests a vehicular-mounted transmitter and receiver that operate at a lower output power (usually 20 to 50 watts) than base stations. The range of transmission is usually 10 to 15 miles, providing that

the terrain is of normal configuration and a repeater is not used. Transmissions over flat land or water can increase signal range. Densely forested areas, mountains, and tall buildings, however, can shorten the range of the transmission. A mobile radio may have the capacity to transmit telemetry data and function as either single-channel or multiple-channel units.

Remote Consoles

Sometimes it is not possible or even desirable to have the dispatch center located inside the base station. Control is maintained from a remote control site, which allows the control site to be located anywhere, since it is connected to the base station by dedicated telephone lines and microwave relay.

Satellite Receivers

Since low-power mobile and portable units have a limited range of transmission, additional receivers can be strategically positioned within a large geographical area to ensure that a low-powered signal will be within range of the system. Often, repeaters are used to pick up the signal and relay it to a satellite, which then relays it to a base station via established telephone lines and microwave channels.

Encoders and Decoders

An encoder appears similar to a telephone keypad and, when activated, sends distinct tones over the air. Since many base stations have only one frequency, and because a number of hospitals may be transmitting and receiving on the same frequency, the encoder sends a tone that can be recognized only by another radio's decoder. When a receiving unit with a decoder receives the specific code, or tone, the base station call alarm is activated. Each base station has a unique set of tones that activates their respective receiving system.

Equipment Maintenance

Communications equipment is expensive, but it is an essential component of prehospital ALS units. A few commonsense practices, however, can extend equipment life and prevent breakdowns. Radio equipment should be handled with care and not be taken into harsh environments, if possible. Dusty environments, humid and wet conditions, and dropping the radio are the most common causes of equipment failure. Equipment can be cleaned with a damp cloth and mild detergent or with a cleaner specifically recommended for radio units. Water should be prevented from entering the radio. All radio equipment should be checked on a specific schedule to ensure that it is in working order. Many EMS units check the equipment at the beginning of each shift. Since portable units require battery power, all manufacturer's recommendations for charging, cleaning, and recycling the batteries should be followed. Repairs should be performed only by a certified technician.

Techniques of Communications

Patient assessment incorporates the process of gathering pertinent information, organizing it, and then presenting it in a logical and concise format over the radio to medical control. Proper use of the radio can improve patient care and allow the receiving hospital to prepare effectively for arrival of the patient. Some EMS systems use codes that serve as a system of radio shorthand. The Associated Public Safety Communications Officers (APCO) publishes a 10-code system that is designed for dispatcher use. An example is *10-4,* which signifies "affirmative" or "message received." Codes are best used when the EMS caller wants to protect the privacy of the patient and when air time needs to be shortened. Disadvantages of the code system include the need for everyone in the system to understand the codes and the inadequacy of codes to describe some medical conditions and situations. Many communications specialists believe that plain English works as well and sometimes better than codes.

Radio Communications Techniques

Proper use of the radio results in effective and professional communications. The following are general guidelines regarding the effective use of radio transmission time:

1. Listen to the channel before transmitting to be sure it is not in use.
2. Press down the transmit button for 1 second before speaking.
3. Speak at a close range, around 2 to 3 inches, directly into or across the face of the microphone.
4. Speak slowly and clearly. Pronounce each word clearly while avoiding words that are difficult to hear.
5. Speak in a normal pitch, keeping your voice free of emotion.

6. Be brief. Know what you are going to say before pressing the transmit button.
7. Avoid codes unless they are a part of your EMS communication system.
8. Do not waste air time with excess talking or information.

Transmission Content

1. Always protect the privacy of the patient.
   a. Use codes when necessary.
   b. When possible, use the cellular telephone rather than the radio, since access to an open line is easier.
   c. Turn off the external speaker or radio.
   d. Avoid using the patient's name.
2. Use proper unit numbers, hospital numbers, proper names and titles.
3. Do not use slang or profanity.
4. Use standard formats for transmission.
5. Use the "echo" system when receiving directions from the dispatcher, physician, or MICN. This requires an immediate repeat of the instructions or orders received; this confirms the statements were heard correctly.
6. Use good documentation skills by writing down addresses, orders received, and any other important information.
7. When completing a transmission, obtain confirmation that your message was received.

Written Communications Protocols

The local medical advisory group should develop guidelines (protocols) on prehospital medical care and communicating with medical control. These guidelines should include the following:

1. When a radio call should be placed to a medical control base station
2. How to handle ill patients who refuse treatment or transport
3. Do-not-resuscitate situations
4. Problems with non-EMS physicians or other health-care personnel who interfere at the scene.

Communication of Patient Information

Good radio communication involves securing additional orders for patient care and providing the hospital with enough information to prepare for arrival. The prehospital worker should attempt to paint a picture of the situation for receiving hospital personnel. Although the format varies, it should be concise and include the following:

1. Call unit name and number or name of the caller
2. A scene description
3. The patient's age, sex, and approximate weight
4. The patient's chief complaint
5. Associated signs and symptoms
6. Brief but pertinent history of current complaint
7. Brief past medical history, medications, and allergies
8. Physical examination findings, including:
   a. Level of consciousness
   b. Vital signs
   c. Neurological examination
   d. General appearance and degree of distress
   e. EKG (if applicable)
   f. Trauma or Glasgow coma score
   g. Other pertinent findings
9. Treatment given so far
10. Estimated time of arrival (ETA) at the hospital
11. Name of the patient's private physician
12. Repeat any orders received

Upon arrival at the hospital, a brief synopsis of the patient's history, assessment findings, treatment, and an update on the patient's condition should be provided.

Prehospital Documentation

A properly written patient care record (run report), with documentation including patient assessment and treatment, is an essential component of prehospital care. The value of a well-written medical report serves both clinical and legal requirements. It is important to remember that the written run report of the patient's condition and treatment remains at the hospital long after the prehospital care providers have left. The run report becomes a part of the legal record and a part of the hospital's permanent medical record. Any problems encountered at the scene such as initial refusal of care or transport should be thoroughly documented. The run report serves as a source for medical audits, quality control, data collection, and billing purposes. Run reports must be complete, legible, and signed by prehospital personnel. Documentation formats vary but usually combine *check the box, fill in the space,* and *narrative summary* sections. An accurate and properly completed run report protects the patient, the prehospital emergency service, and the caregivers.

Laptop Computers

Run report records in the future may be typed into a laptop computer by the EMS care provider and then downloaded into an information storage center. Current factors that prevent this innovation include the cost of the portable computers and the poor durability of the digital components of laptops to withstand heat, cold, rain, and the rough treatment they receive in field operation. Nevertheless, computers will continue to evolve into an integral component of both dispatch and EMS function.

Summary

A general knowledge of the overall aspects of EMS communications is important for all prehospital care providers. It is essential to remember, however, that access to the system begins with the citizen and does not end until the patient is delivered to the hospital and the run report is filed and critiqued. Effective and concise communication is required among all involved parties for the system to work, and the larger and more complex the system is, the more technologically advanced must be the equipment and the training of the dispatchers and prehospital care providers.

REFERENCES

Adler, S. (1992). Is EMS communications still at talk? *Journal of Emergency Medical Services, 17*(5):54-64.

Augustine, J.J., Paris, P., & Pappas, G. (1989). Emergency Medical Services communications, In A.E. Kuehl (Ed.). *EMS medical directors' handbook* (pp. 49-58). St. Louis: Mosby.

Bledsoe, B.E., Porter, R.S., & Shade, B.R. (1993). *Paramedic emergency care* (2nd ed.). New York: Brady Publishing.

Cady, G.A., & Scott, T. (1993). EMS providers in the United States: A survey of providers in the 200 most populous cities. *Journal of Emergency Medical Services, 18* (1), 71-83.

Clawson, J.J., & Dernocoeur, K.B. (1988). *Principles of emergency medical dispatch,* (pp. 1-42). Englewood Cliffs, NJ: Prentice Hall.

Dawson, D.E., Brown, W.E., Chew, J., Garrison, H.G., & O'Keefe, M. (1993). National EMS education and practice blueprint: Report from a task force. Paper presented at the Ohio Emergency Medical Services Conference, Columbus, OH.

Editors. (1991). Who's on first? Panel discussion highlights. *Emergency Medial Services, 20*(6), 29-35.

Garnett, G.F., Hall, J.E., & Johnson, M.S. (1989). Rural Emergency Medical Services. In A.E. Kuehl (Ed.). *EMS medical directors' handbook* (pp. 133-140). St. Louis: Mosby.

Gazzaniga, A.B., Isteri, L.T., & Baren, M. (1992). Prehospital emergency care. *Emergency care: principles and practices for the EMT-paramedic* (2nd ed.). (pp. 1-13, 561-575). Philadelphia: W.B. Saunders.

Grant, G.D., Murray, R.H., Bergeron, J.D. (1994 sic). *Emergency care.* (6th ed.). New York: Brady Publishing.

Hergenroeder, P., & Berk, W., (1989). Levels of prehospital care providers. In A.E. Kuehl (Ed.). *EMS medical directors' handbook* (pp 39-48). St. Louis: Mosby.

Jackson, B., & Anderson, C. (1992). ALS intercept and tiered response. *Journal of Emergency Medical Services,* Oct., 65-71.

Johnson, M.S., & Van Cott, C.C. (1992). The FCC may be listening. *Journal of Emergency Medical Services, 17*(5), 19-27.

Johnson, R.I., Childress, S.E., & Herron, H.L. (1993). Regulation of prehospital nursing practice: A national survey. *Journal of Emergency Nursing, 19*(5), 437-440.

Jones, S.A., Weigel, A., White, R.D., McSwain, N.E., & Breiter, M. (1991). *Advanced emergency care for paramedic practice,* (pp. 10-15, 30-39). Englewood Cliffs, NJ: Prentice Hall.

Lavery, B.F., Doran, J., & Bartholomew, J.T. (1992). A survey of advanced life support practices in the United States. *Prehospital and Disaster Medicine, 7*(2), 144-149.

Norton, R.L., Bartkus, E.A., & Neely, K.W. (1992). Compliance with closest hospital transport protocol. *Prehospital and Disaster Medicine, 7*(3), 243-244.

Palmer, E.C., & Gonsoulin, S.M. (1992). Nurse-paramedic interactions: teamwork of turf wars. *Prehospital and Disaster Medicine, 7*(1), 45-50.

Pointer, J.E., Osur, M., & Campbell, C. (1991). The impact of standing orders on medication and skill selection, paramedic assessment, and hospital outcome: A follow-up report. *Prehospital and Disaster Medicine, 6*(3), 303-308.

Sharp, A., & Sharp, B. (1985). Passoff problems. *Journal of Emergency Services, 17*(3), 26-29, 46-47.

Stewart, R. (1989). Historical overview. In A.E. Kuehl (Ed.). *EMS medical directors' handbook* (pp. 3-6). St. Louis: Mosby.

Suter, R.E. (1992). Who calls the shots? EMS operations control and the role of the communications center. *Prehospital and Disaster Medicine, 7*(4), 396-399.

U.S. Department of Transportation, National Highway Traffic Safety Administration. (1983). *Emergency Medical Services dispatcher: National standard curriculum* (2nd ed.). 1-143.

U.S. Department of Transportation, National Highway Traffic Safety Administration. (1985). *National standard curriculum for the EMT-paramedic.* 8-270.

Wilson, B., Gratton, G.C., Overton, J., & Watson, W.A. (1992). Unexpected ALS procedures on non-emergency calls: The value of a single-tier system *Prehospital and Disaster Medicine, 7*(4), 380-386.

Yura H., & Walsh, M.B. (1973). *The nursing process.* (2nd ed.). Englewood Cliffs, NJ: Prentice Hall.

CHAPTER 3

Ambulance Operations and Special Response Situations

OBJECTIVES

1. Describe the components of an EMS vehicle
2. Discuss the equipment needed in an EMS vehicle
3. Describe safe ambulance operations
4. Discuss the components of scene management and the role of the prehospital care nurse in each
5. Describe rescue and extrication procedures

COMPETENCIES

1. Prepare a transport bag stocked with the appropriate patient equipment
2. Identify indications for the use of lights and sirens during patient transport
3. Describe the information needed from dispatch to prepare for patient transport
4. Demonstrate safety practices for a violent patient and scene
5. Name two methods of interaction with the family or crowd at an emergency scene
6. Name two measures to ensure personal safety during extrication

This chapter focuses on two important areas of the prehospital environment: ambulance operations, including scene management, and special response situations. The first section covers the emergency vehicle itself, including vehicle specifications and equipment needed to render patient care in the out-of-hospital setting. It also describes the step-by-step process of an emergency transport, including pre-run preparation, dispatch information, scene arrival, patient transfer to definitive care, and post-run activities. The second section is about special response situations. It describes the simple, single victim rescue and the complex, mass casualty incident using the incident command system. EMS planning is discussed for both a visit from a VIP and for a mass gathering. The section concludes with information on hazardous materials and the impact they can have on the prehospital setting.

VEHICLE OPERATIONS

What is white with orange stripes, weighs 8 tons, and carries five people?

The answer is an emergency transport vehicle, also referred to as an ambulance. The ambulance is an important component of the Emergency Medical Service (EMS). It transports personnel and equipment to the scene and enables patient care to be performed during transport to a medical facility. Several issues regarding emergency transport warrant discussion: emergency vehicle design and engineering, equipment and supplies, ambulance operations, and air medical transport.

Vehicle Design and Engineering

The construction of an ambulance is formulated from a variety of sources. Specifications from the federal government for a "Star-of-Life" ambulance is published in the document "KKK-A-1822C Federal Specifications for Ambulances" (General Services Administration [GSA], 1990). This document establishes minimum specifications and essential criteria for ambulance design, performance, equipment, and appearance. Ambulance manufacturers also consult automobile design engineers, EMS personnel, and fleet mechanics. The object is to make ambulances that will reliably function in the prehospital setting and that are nationally recognized, properly constructed, and easily maintained. There are three components that constitute an emergency vehicle: chassis, driver compartment (cab), and patient compartment (body) (Figure 3-1).

The chassis is the frame of the vehicle. It supports the driver and patient compartments and can be constructed using either a truck or a passenger vehicle frame. The cab is sufficient in size to accommodate a driver and an assistant. It is the mechanical work station for the vehicle, with space to perform driving and vehicle control activities. The instrument panel for the lights, sirens, and radio controls is within reach of the driver and easy to operate. An on-board computer, mounted on the dash, is a recent adjunct in some emergency units. The computer can relay dispatch information, provide street maps, monitor status of vehicle maintenance, and keep a patient database for the emergency care providers.

The body of the vehicle can accommodate two patients and two medical team members.

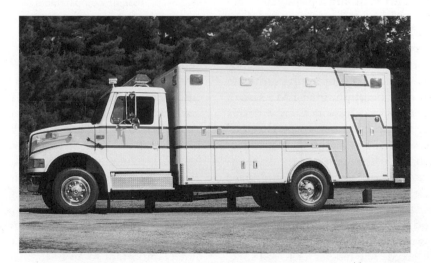

Fig. 3-1   Three components of a type I emergency vehicle: chassis, cab, and body. (Courtesy of Horton Ambulance Company.)

The primary patient is placed on a wheeled elevated cot, and the second patient, if present, is laid on the squad bench. The wheeled cot can be mounted in the center of the compartment floor or against the left wall. The center mount allows for easy access around the entire patient. There is an 18-inch aisle between the wheeled cot and squad bench. A seat with a headrest and seat belt is positioned so that the caregiver can sit facing the patient's upper torso. Storage cabinets and shelf space for medical equipment and supplies are permanently installed and free of protrusions. All equipment and supplies are secured to prevent them from becoming harmful projectiles during an emergency transport. The patient compartment is heated, air conditioned, and ventilated (Figure 3-2).

There are three different models of ambulances: type I, II, and III (GSA, 1990). A type I ambulance is a truck chassis with a modular patient compartment attached to the cab. There is no passageway between the cab and body. A type II ambulance is a standard van with a raised roof and extended patient compartment. There is a passageway between the cab and body. A type III is a van chassis with a modular patient compartment and a passageway between the cab and body (Figures 3-3 and 3-4).

The type of ambulance that is selected by an emergency service is an agency decision. The needs of the organization, type of emergency calls, territory served, and operating costs are all taken into consideration. If an EMS system frequently operates in cities with narrow streets and has short transport times, a type II ambulance may serve their needs best. Patient transport units can be custom designed by the manufacturer. Examples of these special units might include vehicles needed for a wheelchair service, neonatal transport, or mobile cardiac care.

The size and weight specifications of an emergency vehicle can vary according to the model and design selected. The federal KKK-A-1822C dimensions for an emergency vehicle are not to exceed a length of 22 feet, a width of 8 feet,

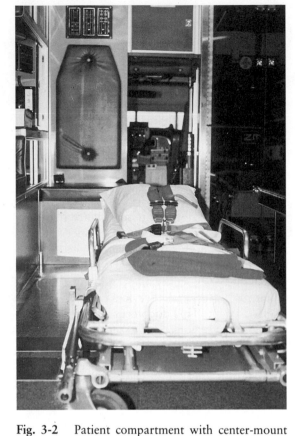

Fig. 3-2 Patient compartment with center-mount cot.

and a height of 9 feet (GSA, 1990). An ambulance is divided into three weight specifications: curb weight, payload, and gross vehicle weight. Curb weight is the weight of the chassis, cab, and body. Payload is the weight allowed for EMS personnel, patients, and rescue equipment (medical, communication, and rescue). The gross vehicle weight is the combined weights of curb and payload. The use of lightweight materials in the construction of the vehicle decreases the curb weight and allows for heavier payloads. The payload a vehicle can accommodate is important to an EMS system, since payload determines the type and amount of equipment and supplies that can be carried safely.

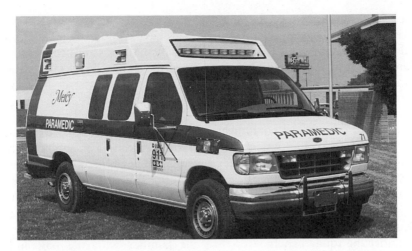

Fig. 3-3   Type II ambulance. (Courtesy of Horton Ambulance Company.)

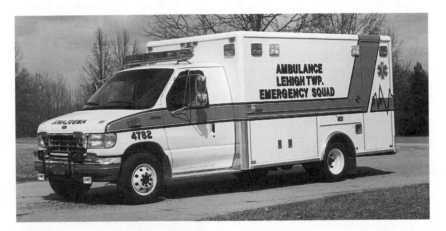

Fig. 3-4   Type III ambulance. (Courtesy of Horton Ambulance Company.)

The exterior color scheme for an ambulance, as suggested by the federal KKK-1-1822C standards, is white with an orange stripe and blue lettering and emblems. The word *AMBULANCE* is mirror-imaged on the front so that the unit can be identified in a rearview mirror. The "Star-of-Life" emblem is usually imprinted on the sides of the vehicle. However, recent studies have shown that a white vehicle, with a stripe of any color, is easily camouflaged in an urban environment. According to these studies, the best color for visibility of an emergency vehicle has been identified as lime-yellow. More than 50% of new fire service vehicles are now being ordered in this color (DeLorenzo, 1992).

Medical Equipment and Supplies

Having the appropriate amount and type of medical equipment and supplies on the emergency vehicle takes planning and preparation.

Equipment specifications are guided by state and regional requirements. Box 3-1 lists suggested essential medical equipment and supplies for an ambulance that provides basic life support (BLS). Box 3-2 lists suggested essential medical equipment and supplies for an advanced life support (ALS) unit.

Inside the ambulance the medical equipment is organized for easy access by the patient care provider. Lifesaving and frequently used items are strategically placed in the cabinets. For example, equipment for airway management and oxygenation is stored near the patient's head. Large bulky equipment, such as vacuum splints, may be stored under the squad bench.

Medical supplies also need to be available for patient care away from the ambulance. Specialized bags or kits are designed to carry portable equipment. The bags are lightweight, durable,

waterproof, and easy to access. The treatment bags have compartments that are organized for specific patient care needs. For example, treatment bags may be specialized for airway management, medication delivery, or pediatric emergencies (Figure 3-5).

A nurse may need to transport a critical patient in a BLS vehicle. Equipment needed for the transport cannot be haphazardly gathered from supplies available in the emergency department or critical care unit minutes before transfer. A transport bag should be organized with ALS equipment to supplement the equipment on the transporting unit. All of the nursing staff should be familiar with the bag and make routine checks of its contents, similar to the daily checks of the unit's crash carts. Under medical direction and protocols, transport nurses must be able to deliver care commensurate with their

---

Box 3-1
MEDICAL EQUIPMENT AND SUPPLIES FOR A BASIC EMS AMBULANCE

Basic Supplies

Stethoscope
Sphygmomanometer
Thermometer
Penlight
Emesis bag
Bedpan/urinal
Cold/heat pack
Sugar packet
Gloves, goggles, mask, gown
Waterless soap
Restraining strap/jacket
Syrup of ipecac
Activated charcoal
Irrigation fluid

Patient Transfer

Wheeled stretcher
Stair chair
Scoop-style stretcher
Reeves-type stretcher
CPR board

Ventilation Equipment

Nasopharyngeal airway
Oropharyngeal airway
Nasal cannula
Simple face mask
Non-rebreathing mask
Bag-valve-mask device
Oxygen delivery system
Demand valve
Suction device
Suction catheter
Pulse oximeter

Childbirth Supplies

Sterile obstetrics pack
Baby blanket/hat
Cord clamp
Rubber bulb aspirator
Sanitary napkin

Immobilization Equipment

Rigid splint
Traction splint
Inflatable splint
Pneumatic antishock garment
Rigid cervical collar
Head immobilizer
Corset-type extrication device
Backboard
Sling and swathe

Dressing Supplies

Cravat
Roller bandage
Sterile gauze pad
Multitrauma dressing
Occlusive dressing
Ace bandage
Eye pad
Sterile burn sheet
Trauma shears

educational preparation and current nurse practice standards.

Ambulance Operation

One goal of prehospital care providers is to deliver the patient to the hospital safely. Good driving skills are essential for an ambulance driver. There are more than 40,000 ambulances and first response vehicles in the United States, and it is estimated that 1 out of every 10 ambulances will be involved in a collision each year. Intersections are the most frequent site for an incident to occur (DeLorenzo, 1992). Emergency vehicles are subject to all state, local, and agency traffic regulations. In about 95% of all emergency calls, transport can be conducted by obeying the regular traffic laws (Hafen & Karren, 1989). Exemption from traffic regulations is given only when responding to an emergency. The U.S. Department of Transportation (DOT) defines a true emergency as a situation in which there is a high probability of death or serious injury to an individual and that the action of the ambulance driver may reduce the seriousness of the situation (U.S. Department of Transportation, National Highway Traffic Safety Administration, 1978). Examples of traffic exemptions include proceeding cautiously past stop signs, exceeding speed limits, passing in a no-passing lane, and traveling against the flow of

---

Box 3-2
MEDICAL EQUIPMENT AND SUPPLIES FOR AN ADVANCED
LIFE SUPPORT AMBULANCE

Ventilation Equipment

Esophageal obturator airway (EOA)
Esophageal gastric tube airway (EGTA)
Laryngoscope
Magill forceps
Macintosh, Miller, Wisconsin, or Flagg blades
Endotracheal tube
Malleable stylet
End-tidal CO_2 detector
Pharyngeotracheal lumen airway (PLT)
Esophageal tracheal combiTube airway (ETL)
Percutaneous transtracheal jet ventilation equipment
Automatic ventilator
Chest decompression equipment

Intravenous Therapy

Intravenous tubing
Intravenous fluid
Angiocath
Armboard
Intravenous start kit (venous constricting band, antibiotic swab, gauze dressing, tape)
Intraosseous needle
Assorted syringes with needles
Blood collection tube
Sharps collection container
Glucose chemstrip

Cardiac Monitoring

12-lead EKG monitor with electrodes
EKG graph paper
External cardiac pacing equipment
Monitor/defibrillator
Conduction medium

Medications

Activated charcoal
Adenosine
Albuterol
Alupent
Aminophylline
Atropine
Bretylium
Dexamethasone
50% dextrose
Diazepam
Diphenhydramine
Dobutamine
Dopamine
Epinephrine
Furosemide
Haloperidol
Hydrocortisone
Isoproterenol
Labetolol
Lidocaine
Magnesium sulfate
Mannitol
Methylprednisone
Morphine sulfate
Narcan
Nitroglycerine
Nitronox
Norepinephrine
Oxytocin
Phenothiazines
Procainamide
Procardia
Propranolol
Sodium bicarbonate
Sodium nitroprusside
Succinylcholine
Syrup of ipecac
Terbutaline
Thiamine
Verapamil

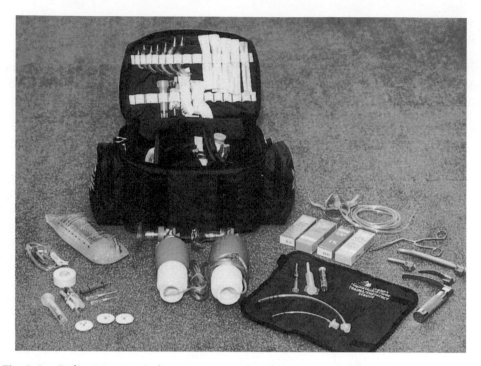

Fig. 3-5 Pediatric transport bag. (Courtesy of Children's Hospital Medical Center, Cincinnati, Ohio.)

traffic. All of these exemptions apply only during an emergency call and must be performed with due regard to the safety of others. If a collision occurs, EMS personnel can be held criminally and/or civilly liable. The incident investigators ask two main questions: Was the situation a true emergency? Was there due regard for the safety of others?

Lights and sirens are the primary warning signals of an ambulance. They are to be used when exercising the exemption from regular traffic laws and to inform traffic of the emergency vehicle's presence. The use of warning devices does not negate the responsibility of the ambulance driver to regard the safety of others.

According to the KKK-A-1822C specifications, each emergency light shall flash on/off 75 to 80 times per minute and illuminate 20 square inches (GSA, 1990). Warning light colors of red or white are the most common. The bright white light of the flashing strobe is a popular emergency warning light. Red warning lights, by themselves, can lose their effectiveness in heavy traffic because of the brake lights from other vehicles. It has been found that a combination of two colors is better than one. Headlights are also part of the emergency lighting system, since they are easily seen in the rearview mirror of other motorists. It has been found that warning lights are least effective at dawn and at dusk (Henry & Stapleton, 1992a).

Audible warning signals should be in a frequency range of 1 kHz to 4 kHz. To be most effective, siren sounds, such as wail, yelp, and hi-lo, are recommended to rise rapidly in pitch with rapid cycling time (DeLorenzo, 1992). In a 1977 U.S. DOT study it was found that the maximum distance a siren can be heard at an urban intersection is 25 to 40 feet. Thus an automobile approaching an intersection at 35 miles per hour can outdrive the siren range, and the siren would not be heard. In addition, sound does not travel around buildings or corners (DeLorenzo, 1992), making urban intersections extremely dangerous. The siren also competes with automobile engine noise, road noise, car radios, and ventilation fans. As demonstrated, the siren has limitations as an effective warning device. Some motorists panic when they hear the siren, making it difficult for the ambulance driver to predict their action; it may be better at times to turn the siren off.

Previously, ambulance driver training was only available on the job. Now, principles of emergency driving are taught in the basic EMT-ambulance program. In addition, special driving programs have been designed, including the emergency vehicle operations course, developed by the U.S. DOT.

An EMS agency can use several programs for evaluating driving techniques. One program is the Allsafe Driving System, which measures the amount of lateral force exerted on a vehicle by the driver's acceleration, braking, and turning. The driver receives feedback from a computer device that measures performance. This program advocates that low-force driving can reduce the risk of collision, vehicle maintenance cost, and fuel consumption (Lucia, 1993).

Other types of vehicles are used for emergency calls. An EMS supervisor in a backup unit may use an all-terrain vehicle to transport additional equipment to the scene. If an EMS agency operates in a territory with a large body of water, a boat may be necessary for transportation. The air ambulance is another form of patient transport that became popular in the 1980s.

Air Medical Transport

In 1972 the first civilian hospital–based EMS flight program began. Today, more than 150 programs are in operation (Jones, Weigel, White, McSwain, & Breiter, 1992). Air medical transport is an integral team player in the EMS system, since patient care of the critically ill or injured is enhanced by the quick response time to the scene with a medical team trained in advanced patient care skills.

The following guidelines for the efficient use of a flight medical team have been established by the Association of Air Medical Services (1990):

1. For transport of seriously ill patients to a tertiary care center
2. For provision of ALS in areas where land-based ALS ambulance units are not available
3. For decreasing transport time for critically injured or ill patients
4. For patients located in an area inaccessible to ground transport
5. For lengthy extrications and when the patient's injury requires delivery of a critical care team to the accident scene.

Fixed-wing aircraft and helicopters are the vehicles used in air medical patient transport. The helicopter is used for response to emergency scenes and for interfacility transports. Its service area is a radius of 100 to 150 miles, and it flies at low altitudes. A fixed-wing aircraft is used for long-distance transfers, usually over a 120-mile radius, and mainly for interhospital transfers. Fixed-wing flight time is longer and flying altitudes are higher in comparison with the helicopter. The air ambulance medical team may include a combination of specially trained physicians, nurses, paramedics, and respiratory therapists.

In the prehospital setting there are three operational issues to consider when a patient is transported by helicopter: (1) establishing a safe landing zone, (2) approaching the helicopter, and (3) patient loading/unloading procedures. An appropriate square foot area free of trees, poles, and loose debris is selected for the landing zone. Flags, lights, or other signaling devices are used to outline the perimeter of the landing zone. Rotor wash winds generated by the main rotor when the aircraft lands can be in excess of 60 miles per hour. EMS personnel need to protect themselves from loose dirt and sand. Nothing should be raised above head level, and all hats and helmets should be secure.

Upon the direction of the pilot, personnel approach the front of the helicopter; approaching from the rear is dangerous because of the tail rotor. When advancing toward the helicopter, emergency responders should crouch down, since the main rotors in some aircraft dip as low as 4 feet (Heckman, 1992b). The terms *hot* (when the helicopter is on the ground and its rotors are spinning) and *cold* (when the helicopter is on the ground and its rotors are not spinning) are used in reference to patient movement to and from a helicopter. One criterion for determining a hot or cold load/unload is based on the condition of the patient. Only under the direction of the flight personnel should the prehospital care nurse (PCN) assist with patient loading and unloading.

Helicopter transport in the prehospital setting is common in most areas of the country and has proven to be a valuable patient care tool. For further information on the subject, refer to the U.S. DOT publication *Air Ambulance Guidelines* (1991) (Heckman, 1992b).

Overview

The involvement of the PCN with emergency vehicles can encompass a wide range of responsibilities. Besides administering patient care en route to a hospital, a PCN may be involved in the selection of an emergency vehicle for a hospital transport unit, may participate in a quality assurance program for ambulance drivers, or may oversee a maintenance program for a fleet of emergency vehicles.

Many hours of planning are spent on selecting an emergency vehicle and the medical equipment and supplies it will carry. The needs of the organization, initial cost, resale value,

and operating expenses are all considered before a final decision is made. Vehicle operations encompass a wide range of issues for EMS personnel. The main objectives are to provide quality patient care and safe transport to a medical facility by the best possible means.

From the initial call for help to patient transport to a medical facility, a unique process takes place that is particular to the prehospital setting. This chapter now examines the management of the emergency scene and the activities of the medical team.

SCENE MANAGEMENT

It is 1400 hours and your ALS crew is dispatched to 115 Howard Street for a "child struck by a car, person unconscious." The address is directly across from an elementary school. Are you prepared to run? Will you have the necessary equipment you need to handle the call? Will you need help? What is the safest, fastest route there?

No matter what role the prehospital care nurse plays, the following factors must be considered before, during, and after call completion (Emergency Nurses Association, 1991):

- Pre-run preparation
- Dispatch information, including information received and factors affecting response
- Use/nonuse of emergency lights and sirens
- Assignment delegation
- Scene response, including safety considerations, patient assessment, and patient packaging
- Transfer of patient to a definitive care facility
- Post-run activities

Pre-Run Preparation

Pre-run preparation begins with inspection of the equipment and vehicle. This is conducted at every shift and after each emergency call, be it an ambulance, helicopter, or fixed-wing aircraft. The medical team systematically checks to make sure the equipment is available and functioning. If an item is found missing or non-functional, a notation is made detailing the problem and its resolution. The inspection is facilitated by a checklist, which ensures a systematic approach and accountability to the process. Lack of preparation for an emergency call could result in the loss of a patient's life, for example, if airway equipment is not functioning properly at the scene, not to mention the legal ramifications that could ensue (Figures 3-6 and 3-7).

The emergency crew also performs a routine and daily vehicle check. The ambulance body, tires, and light systems are inspected. It is also necessary to check the fluid levels, hoses, battery, and fuel.

Stocking the ambulance with medical supplies can be accomplished several ways. One system requires the EMS crew to return to the base station to restock medical supplies. Under this system the EMS agency usually charges the patient for the items used. Another restocking system allows the emergency care providers to restock medical supplies from the hospital

where they have taken the patient. The hospital then charges the patient for the items used by the EMS crew. Whichever system is used, it should be efficient, cost effective, and time saving.

An interfacility transport of a critical patient may involve a nurse accompanying the EMS team. The nurse should be knowledgeable about the equipment available during the transport and confirm that it is functional. A systematic approach to the equipment check is the *ABC* format. *A* is for airway. The equipment necessary to open an airway, such as an oral airway and suction, must be available. *B* is for breathing. Is a resuscitation bag and oxygen available? How much oxygen will be needed? The amount of oxygen available in an oxygen cylinder depends on the pressure in the cylinder and the rate of flow.

Box 3-3 presents a formula that determines a cylinder's duration of oxygen flow in minutes. *C* is for circulation. Equipment needs might include a blood pressure cuff, military antishock trousers, and intravenous fluids. Using the ABC format to check a transport unit allows the PHN to identify and examine the equipment

---

Box 3-3
DURATION OF FLOW FROM AN OXYGEN CYLINDER

$$\frac{\text{Gauge pressure in psi—the safe residual pressure} \times \text{constant}}{\text{Flow rate in liters/minute}} = \text{Duration of flow in minutes}$$

Residual pressure = 200 psi
Cylinder constant   D = 0.16   G = 2.41
               E = 0.28   H = 3.14
               M = 1.56   K = 3.14

Determine the life of an M cylinder that has a pressure of 2000 psi and a flow rate of 10 liters/minute.

$$\frac{(2000 - 200) \times 1.56}{10} = \frac{2808}{10} = 281 \text{ minutes, or 4 hours and 41 minutes}$$

Note. From *Emergency Care* by H.D. Grant, R.H. Murray, & J.D. Bergeron, 1994, Englewood Cliffs, NJ: Prentice Hall/Brady.

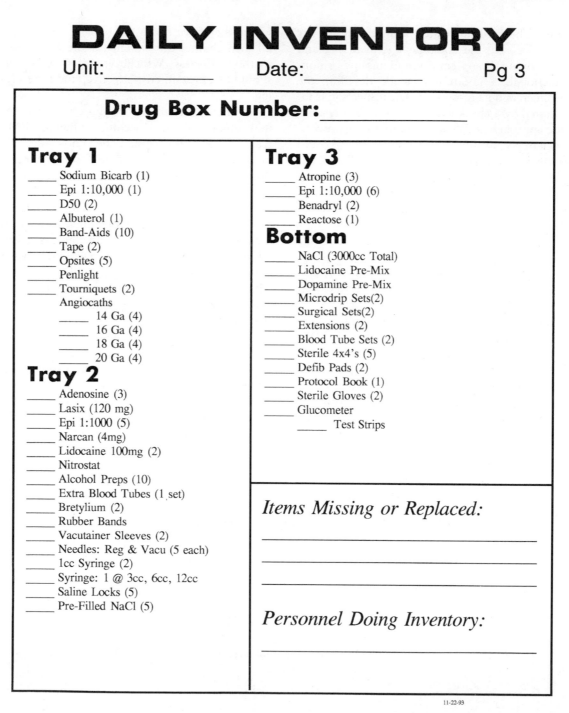

DAILY INVENTORY

Unit:_____ Date:_____ Pg 3

Drug Box Number:_____

Tray 1
- _____ Sodium Bicarb (1)
- _____ Epi 1:10,000 (1)
- _____ D50 (2)
- _____ Albuterol (1)
- _____ Band-Aids (10)
- _____ Tape (2)
- _____ Opsites (5)
- _____ Penlight
- _____ Tourniquets (2)
- Angiocaths
  - _____ 14 Ga (4)
  - _____ 16 Ga (4)
  - _____ 18 Ga (4)
  - _____ 20 Ga (4)

Tray 2
- _____ Adenosine (3)
- _____ Lasix (120 mg)
- _____ Epi 1:1000 (5)
- _____ Narcan (4mg)
- _____ Lidocaine 100mg (2)
- _____ Nitrostat
- _____ Alcohol Preps (10)
- _____ Extra Blood Tubes (1 set)
- _____ Bretylium (2)
- _____ Rubber Bands
- _____ Vacutainer Sleeves (2)
- _____ Needles: Reg & Vacu (5 each)
- _____ 1cc Syringe (2)
- _____ Syringe: 1 @ 3cc, 6cc, 12cc
- _____ Saline Locks (5)
- _____ Pre-Filled NaCl (5)

Tray 3
- _____ Atropine (3)
- _____ Epi 1:10,000 (6)
- _____ Benadryl (2)
- _____ Reactose (1)

Bottom
- _____ NaCl (3000cc Total)
- _____ Lidocaine Pre-Mix
- _____ Dopamine Pre-Mix
- _____ Microdrip Sets(2)
- _____ Surgical Sets(2)
- _____ Extensions (2)
- _____ Blood Tube Sets (2)
- _____ Sterile 4x4's (5)
- _____ Defib Pads (2)
- _____ Protocol Book (1)
- _____ Sterile Gloves (2)
- _____ Glucometer
  - _____ Test Strips

Items Missing or Replaced:

_____

_____

_____

Personnel Doing Inventory:

_____

11-22-93

Fig. 3-6 Daily inventory checklist of EMS drug box. (Courtesy of Milford-Miami Township EMS, Milford, Ohio.)

MAJOR INVENTORY

Units 22, 23, 24   Date:_____

_____ Car Seat	_____ Chux
_____ XP-One	_____ Sterile Pour Solutions (4)
_____ Vacuum, Air, SAM Splints & Triang Bndgs	_____ Baby Wipes
_____ Infection Control Kit #_____	_____ Baby Powder
_____ Reel Splint	_____ Peroxide
	_____ Rubbing Alcohol
_____ Stair Chair	_____ Kleenex
_____ Soft Tool Pouch	
_____ Large Bolt Cutters	_____ PDR
_____ Hard Hats (2)	_____ Rateminder Clips
_____ Flashlight Lanterns Batteries O.K._____	_____ Bio-Hazard Bags
_____ Goggles (2)	_____ Germicidal Cleaner
_____ Safety Vests (2)	
_____ Flares (5)	_____ Syrup of Ipecac (2)
_____ Gloves (2 Pair)	_____ Tauma Shears
_____ Orange Safety Triangle	_____ Ring Cutter
_____ Fire Extinguisher	_____ Tongue Blades
	_____ Rescue Blanket (1)
_____ Backboards w/CID Bases (3)	
_____ Padded Board Splints	_____ Eye Shields (2)
_____ Scoop Stretcher	_____ Tape
_____ Pedi Half-Backboard	_____ Chest Wound Seals
_____ Ropes	_____ Small Exam Gloves (Box)
	_____ Medium Exam Gloves (Box)
_____ OB Kit (Non-Disposable)	_____ Large Exam Gloves (Box)
_____ OB Kit (Disposable)	
_____ Sterile Aluminum Foil (1)	_____ Needle Tray
_____ Sterile Gloves (4)	_____ Syringes: 2 @ 1cc, 3cc, 6cc, 12cc
_____ OB Pads	_____ Extra Blood Tubes (2 Sets)
_____ Bulb Aspirator	_____ Needles (5)
	_____ Vacutainer Needles & Adapters (5 Each)
_____ Sterile Burn Sheets (2)	_____ Vacutainer Sleeves (2)
_____ Multi-Trauma Dressings (6)	_____ Rubber Bands
	_____ Tourniquet
_____ Stiffneck C-Collars	
_____ Pedi No-Neck (1)	_____ Garbage Bags (Reg)
_____ Pedi (1)	_____ Rico Suction Liners
_____ No-Neck (3)	_____ Emesis Hoop
_____ Short (2)	_____ Suction Catheters (3)
_____ Regular (2)	_____ Yankauer w/Tubing (2)
_____ Tall (2)	_____ Evidence Bags (5)
_____ CID Blocks & Straps (3)	
	_____ Blood Tubes w/Syringe (2)
_____ 1200cc Suction Canisters w/Lids (2)	_____ Surgical Sets (4)
_____ EKG Paper (3)	_____ Microdrip Sets (4)
_____ Defib Pads (2)	_____ Extensions (4)
_____ EKG Electrodes (5 Sets)	
_____ Battery Eliminator w/Cord	Pg 1 of 5
_____ Defib Gel	
_____ Backboard Straps (4)	
_____ Leather Restraints (4)	

11-19-93

Fig. 3-7 Equipment/supply checklist. (Courtesy of Milford-Miami Township EMS, Milford, Ohio.)

and supplies necessary for an emergency situation before they are needed. If the equipment and medication needs of the patient exceed what is provided by the transport unit, then usually the transporting facility provides the necessary equipment (e.g., cardiac monitor/defibrillator, pulse oximetry, or infusion pump).

Another piece of valuable equipment that the prehospital nurse does not want to be without is a two-way radio. This allows communication with the base hospital, where medical direction can be obtained, if the patient's condition worsens.

Dispatch

Dispatch information may be the most vital component of any EMS call. Information gathered by the dispatcher sets the tone for the entire call—for example, red lights and siren versus nonemergency response, whether additional units are needed, or whether police response should precede EMS response. Information gathered from the dispatcher includes but is not limited to the following:

- Location and condition of patient
- Number of patients
- Severity of injury(ies)
- Need for additional units
- Scene hazards
- Traffic problems
- Provision of prearrival instructions

It is also necessary to inform the dispatcher of problems encountered en route to the scene. Any delay in response may necessitate the dispatch of additional units. Factors that may affect response and delay arrival include the day of the week and the time of day. A weekday at rush hour will have a significantly higher traffic flow than the same time on a weekend. Special events such as concerts and parades increase traffic volume during a normally quiet time. Weather has an obvious effect on response time with rain, fog, ice, and snow hampering travel time. Detours, railroad tracks, and school zones can cause traffic backups, as well

as other simultaneously occurring incidents. It would be well advised for any EMS provider to take an emergency vehicle driving course.

Use/Nonuse of Emergency Privileges

Before departing from base, the ambulance must decide if the response will be hot (with red lights and sirens activated) or cold (no lights or sirens) (Clawson & Dernocoeur, 1988). Depending on the EMS system, the dispatcher will determine that response or the decision is made based on the dispatcher's information. Either way, five items must be taken into consideration when deciding on a hot or cold response. First, will time make a difference in the final outcome? For example, if the patient is awake with no other complaints except for a possible fractured ankle, will the extra 5 minutes it takes to get to the scene matter? Second, how much time leeway do you have for the problem? A "cardiac arrest situation" or "child choking, turning blue" call leaves no time to waste. Third, how much time can be saved by running hot? The need to run hot to get through traffic at rush hour probably does not exist at 0400 hours. Fourth, what time constraints exist in the system? An EMS volunteer system may have to wait for a crew, but this does not necessitate the use of lights and sirens to make up for lost time. Finally, when the patient gets to the hospital, will the time saved running hot be significant to the time spent awaiting care? This question is relevant when transporting the patient to the emergency department. It's of no benefit to save 3 to 5 minutes running hot if the patient has to wait 20 to 30 minutes before receiving treatment from a physician (Clawson & Dernocoeur, 1988).

If running hot were without risks or ramifications, then the decision would be easy. However, numerous incidents have occurred as a result of direct emergency vehicle collision, but many others are caused by "wake effect," which is when an emergency vehicle causes a collision but is not directly involved. Many of these incidents are not attributed to the emergency vehicles in the accident reports (Clawson, 1991; Clawson & Dernocoeur, 1988). As many as 12,000 emergency vehicle collisions occur each year as a result of running hot (Clawson, 1991).

With the use of a medical priority dispatch system (MPDS), assigning hot or cold response based on defined, written criteria has dramatically decreased the number of accidents involving emergency vehicles. In Salt Lake City a 78% reduction in emergency vehicle accidents occurred after the use of red lights and sirens was reduced by 50% by the implementation of MPDS (Clawson, 1991).

Assignment Delegation

While still en route to a scene (field or hospital) it is necessary for the crew leader (nurse, paramedic, physician) to delegate assignments and anticipate equipment needs. Based on the information received from the dispatcher, a decision must be made as to additional units, police support, air medical response, or the need for fire and rescue personnel. Also, some units may not routinely take pediatric equipment out of the unit to the scene, so knowing the age of the victim is essential.

Assignment of equipment to be taken from the unit on arrival at the scene should be made en route. One person needs to secure the airway equipment, including oxygen. Others may take cervical collars and other immobilization devices if the mechanism of injury is trauma. No matter what the call, equipment needs must be anticipated to prevent the crew from making frequent, unnecessary trips back to the vehicle.

Scene Arrival

The crew leader or driver is responsible for positioning the vehicle on arrival at the scene. Before a decision is made where to park, the following factors must be considered:

1. Is the vehicle and access around it safe? Due to curiosity and diverted traffic flow, the crew is at an increased risk of being hit by a passing vehicle. The driver must position the ambulance in a protected area that still allows safe and quick access to the scene.
2. Does the ambulance placement block traffic? If so, then the crew must be aware that one side of the ambulance will be exposed to passing traffic and that access will be inhibited.
3. Can an easy departure be made from the scene in the direction of the most appropriate hospital? This must be considered before parking the vehicle. If the vehicle cannot be easily parked because of space confinements, then, if crew size permits, the driver can allow the other members to get out of the ambulance with their equipment and begin patient care so that the ambulance can be positioned for rapid egress.
4. Is the ambulance close to the patient? The goal is to provide easy, safe access to the ambulance for the crew and patient (Childs & Ptacnik, 1986).

When deciding where to park, the driver must consider any existing hazards, such as downed electric wires, fire, spilled fuel, hazardous materials, traffic, and incoming or departing emergency vehicles. The ambulance should be upwind, uphill, and at least 100 feet away from the incident. If hazardous materials are involved, that distance may increase a hundredfold. Associated problems, such as these, necessitate the response of other agencies (fire department, hazardous material team, and others) to stabilize the scene.

With scene safety being a primary concern of the EMS team, the ability to identify dangers, such as those already stated and others, is paramount to survival. Whenever dealing with the human element, there is a degree of unpredictability associated with every event. The following rules of thumb should be adhered to for every emergency incident:

1. A scene in which the mechanism of injury or illness involves some form of violence or self-destruction (overdose, suicide, fight, and the like) should *never* be approached without police accompaniment.
2. A means of egress should always be maintained during treatment of a patient. If the family or patient should suddenly become violent, the driver and team should be able to get out immediately.
3. Emergency responders should stand to the side of a door or window when knocking on it or opening it.
4. The paramedic, nurse, and ambulance and life squad staff should always identify themselves.
5. Police always enter first when accompanying an emergency response team.
6. An EMS responder should never remain in a room alone with a potentially violent patient or upset family members.
7. Each patient should be visually inspected for potential weapons.
8. Weapons should be physically searched for as part of the physical examination. For example, weapons are checked for when examining the legs for deformity, pain, and the like.
9. If an EMS member gets close to a weapon or other contraband during the examination, the patient may become defensive; therefore the patient should not be aggravated, and the police or hospital security should be notified as soon as possible.
10. A sternal rub or nipple twist should not be used to try to elicit a response to pain; other, more appropriate methods will accomplish the goal and not upset family members and friends.
11. If a scene is out of control, there is nothing wrong with moving the patient to the

squad. This will remove all EMS personnel and the patient to a more stable environment.
12. The EMS team should make sure that their uniforms do not resemble those of the local police departments. Although some people will not discriminate between EMS and police when trying to do harm, there are still those who consider EMS personnel as the "good guys" and the police otherwise.

On-Scene Physician

The presence of a physician on the scene of an EMS call can be advantageous if there are preestablished, well-defined guidelines dictating the role of the physician. The Academy of Medicine of Cincinnati, which underwrites the paramedic protocol for Hamilton County, Ohio, has developed standing orders for when a physician is present at the scene of a medical emergency. These specific guidelines correspond with the American College of Emergency Physicians Emergency Medical Services Committee position statement "Control of Advanced Life Support at the Scene of Medical Emergencies" (American College of Emergency Medical Services Committee, 1984). A different set of responsibilities exist when the physician knows the patient and has established a previous doctor-patient relationship, as opposed to when no such relationship exists. The service's medical advisor or on-line medical command physician is generally responsible for patient care (American College of Emergency Medical Services Committee, 1984).

When a previous doctor-patient relationship has not been established, it is recommended that the physician present proof of identity along with current licensure to practice in the state. Also, the physician must agree to ride with the EMS unit, abide by the authority of the on-line medical control physician, and sign all orders. The physician can issue orders within the scope of the EMS team's training and practice. Any orders or procedures beyond their scope of practice must be carried out by the on-scene physician. However, the on-line medical control physician has the ultimate authority over all issues (Academy of Medicine of Cincinnati, 1993; Natt, 1989).

If the physician has a previous doctor-patient relationship, as when responding to a doctor's office, and the physician wants to assume control, then all criteria must be met as if the previous relationship did not exist. Patient assessment and management is conducted just as it would be in any other location. The on-scene physician may refuse to ride with the patient, but gives orders to the EMS team that are in contrast to standing orders. For example, the physician may not want the EMS staff to treat a patient with symptomatic bradycardia or may give EMS personnel a medication order that may be lethal. If this happens, EMS personnel should immediately package the patient for transfer to the vehicle, resume communication with on-line medical command, and treat the patient accordingly.

Evidence Preservation

Although patient assessment and treatment take precedence over most EMS activities (other than safety), emergency responders must be cognizant of the necessity for evidence preservation at the scene of a crime or potential crime. Police should be notified as soon as a crime is suspected at the scene. Visual observations should be made and notes taken as is appropriate for the situation. If removal of clothing is necessary, the clothing should be put in a paper bag. Evidence should not be placed in a plastic bag because moisture can cause the evidence to deteriorate (Bledsoe, Porter, & Shade, 1991; Hafen & Frandsen, 1985).

If any call may have legal implications (e.g., a crime scene or a call from a distraught family that did not approve of a responder's actions), all observations of the call should be written down in a chronological format—the sooner

the better. These notes should be filed as an addendum with the patient report. All notes should be written with the understanding they can be reviewed by patients or their attorney if the case should go to litigation. Only facts should be recorded, statements should be quoted accurately, and the notes should be devoid of the responder's opinion. In the attempt to deliver patient care, evidence may be destroyed, and therefore these notes may be law enforcement's only mechanism to re-create the crime scene. If a crime scene is suspected, the number of people entering the patient care area should be kept to the minimum necessary to deliver safe, competent care.

Family and Crowd Control

When entering the scene it is important that the EMS crew take control of the situation, including the crowd. When possible, one person should be dedicated for dealing with family and friends. A rapport must be developed with the bystanders, since they may be able to provide valuable information that may make the difference between life and death for the victims. When engaging in conversation with the family, it is imperative that a clear, calm voice be maintained without raising the voice. If the bystanders are loud or all are talking at once, then a technique called *repetitive persistence* can be used. In this technique the EMS provider, in a calm, nonthreatening voice, repeats a phrase over and over until the attention of the bystanders has been gained. For example, if a child has been hit by a car, and family members are screaming at the EMS crew, a crew member could repeat the phrase, "If you want to help your child, you are going to have to listen to me." In most situations, family members' attention is gained momentarily because they have been offered an opportunity to help (Clawson, 1989). If this seems to be failing, a person who appears to be calm should be selected to discuss the situation. Questions can be addressed to this person, and the others will start paying attention as they overhear the questions and answers.

To gain the confidence of the bystanders, the EMS crew leader must first let them know that EMS team members are working on the patient. After information is obtained it is imperative that some type of communication is maintained between the bystanders and the EMS team.

It can be as simple as telling them what hospital will be receiving the patient or as elaborate as a description of why CPR is being performed. All explanations should be made in simple layman terms; "a tube to breathe for them" is more appropriate and relevant to the family than an "endotracheal tube."

If the bystanders are hindering patient care or communication is lacking, it may be necessary to gather the help of ancillary personnel at the scene. For example, if the crowd has consumed a significant amount of alcoholic beverages or drugs, the police would be able to help protect the EMS crew and the patient. When at the scene of an obvious fatality, when the victim will not be treated or transported, the family or significant others become the patients. Clergy, other family members, or personnel trained in dealing with critical situations, such as social workers or critical incident stress-debriefing teams, can prove invaluable for dealing with the survivors. When the situation is potentially dangerous for the crew or patient, the patient should be quickly packaged and transported.

The Media

Cooperation with other professionals is requisite to the delivery of health care. Prehospital care is no different. Cooperation with fire, police, disaster personnel, and others makes for the smooth, safe delivery of care. One group of professionals that most nurses have not had direct exposure to is the media. Although most prehospital providers read the newspaper and watch the news on television, paying particular attention to EMS-related events, some of these same people consider the media as obtrusive people who are willing to go to any length to get a story or photograph. So how can the "meddlesome media" get their story, which EMS providers may consider as an invasion of the patient's right to privacy, and provide news coverage to the public? The answer is simple, cooperation.

The news media is made up of professionals who are educated and provide a public service. They would rather be considered nursing allies than adversaries. Following are some tips on how to use the media to the best interests of the patient and the EMS team:

1. The media need to be informed, so emergency responders should not be secretive. Without divulging discriminating or confidential information, the EMS team should inform them that the patient is critical or stable.

2. One EMS person should act as a liaison to speak to the media; if reporters have a question, they can be referred to a single EMS representative.

3. As long as they are not hindering patient care, the media should be allowed to take pictures or shoot video footage. Many EMS providers feel uneasy knowing that their actions and words may be on the evening news. This reason alone is insufficient for not allowing the media to do their job. If the patient's body is being exposed and it is feared that the media may videotape exposed breasts or genitalia, this fear should be allayed, since videographers and editors carefully go over the tapes and pictures so as to show only pertinent material to the public.

4. Many news agencies would be happy to copy the unedited news footage for an EMS system if provided with a videocassette tape. Hours of videotape are shot to provide a 10-second segment on the news. This unedited version can be an excellent form for quality improvement.

5. For the media to film an incident effectively, they need sufficient lighting. Most prehospital incidents require the same, so by allowing the videographer to tape the incident up close, emergency responders reap the benefits of their lights. On May 18, 1988, a school bus carrying children and chaperons collided with a car on Interstate 71 in Carrollton, Kentucky. There were multiple fatalities and casualties. Local EMS systems and state police used a Louisville, Kentucky, television station's lighting equipment to supplement their own.

6. If the media must be removed from a scene, they should be given an explanation as to why they are being removed and informed that they will be updated at the earliest opportunity.

Cooperation between all professionals (nursing, paramedic, fire, police, media) allows them to accomplish their primary task, which is to serve the public.

Patient Assessment and Intervention

To assess and treat the patient, access must be gained. While this may be as simple as walking through a door, difficulties arise that deny the provider direct contact. For example, an auto collision with entrapment requires extrication from the vehicle before contact occurs. The scene of a shooting may require that the area be secured by the police first. Scores of issues must be addressed, such as pre-run preparation, dispatch information, safety, scene response, and so forth, before contact with the patient is made and assessment is performed. Patient assessment, interventions, packaging, and transport are discussed in Chapter 6.

Transfer of Patient to Definitive Care

A decision must be made early on during the call as to when transport will take place and where the patient will be transported. If a problem such as airway control arises during the primary assessment that cannot be remedied immediately, then expeditious transport is indicated at once. When a problem such as a "surgical abdomen" or shock is suspected, then early transport is given priority after the ABC system check.

Some of the most frustrating moments for prehospital providers involve the decision as to which hospital the patient should be transported. Many services know that certain hospitals can treat specific patient problems but not all problems. For example, for a trauma victim who has had an episode of hypotension that responded to fluids, a level III trauma center would be inappropriate, but a level I center would require 15 more minutes of transport time. The decision is not easy and must not be made at the scene. Strict medical control with standing orders and protocols that address transport issues must be in place before EMS involvement in the prehospital setting.

After departing the scene and before arrival at the destination, radio or cellular phone contact should be made with the receiving facility alerting them to the estimated time of arrival, patient condition, and the like.

Upon arrival and the safe removal of the patient from the ambulance, a verbal report to the nurse or physician is made. To save time and effort, the person who will be taking care of the patient should be contacted. Once that person is identified, the following information is given:

1. *Chief complaint,* either the patient's verbalized complaint or an estimation of the patient's most serious problem.
2. *Present history,* including the patient's complaints, events leading up to the incident, bystanders' reports, aid before EMS arrival and by whom, and any other subjective history available.
3. *Medications and drug allergies,* if known.
4. *Past medical history,* especially that which may prove relevant in the care of the patient, for example, a patient with paroxysmal supraventricular tachycardia and a

University of Cincinnati Hospital
University Paramedic Services/Mobile Care

Medical Record No. _____

Run No. _____   Date: _____

Name: _____ Sex: M F   SS #: ____ — ____ — ____   Age: _____ DOB: _____

Address: _____ City: _____ State: _____ Zip: _____

Phone: _____ Resident: Y / N   Family Physician: _____ WT: _____

Situation Found: _____

Chief Complaint: _____

Medications: _____

Allergies: _____

	EMS Unit	Call Rec'd	Responding	At Scene
	To Hospital	At Hospital	Returning	At Qtrs

Location of Call: _____

Nature of Call: _____

Responding From: _____

Medic Response: _____ Medic Transport: Y / N

Other Responding Units: _____

Receiving Hospital: _____

Communications: ☐ Phone   ☐ Telemetry   EKG Sent: Y / N

Base: _____ MD: _____

HISTORY

☐ HEART DISEASE _____
☐ RESPIRATORY _____
☐ SEIZURES _____
☐ CANCER _____
☐ OTHER: _____

☐ HYPERTENSION
☐ CVA/TIA
☐ DIABETES
☐ PSYCHOLOGICAL

PHYSICAL FINDINGS

MENTAL STATUS
☐ ALERT & ORIENTED NORMAL
☐ DISORIENTED/CONFUSED
☐ RESPONDS TO VERBAL STIMULI ONLY
☐ RESPONDS TO PAINFUL STIMULI ONLY
☐ UNRESPONSIVE

SKIN COLOR
☐ NORMAL
☐ CYANOTIC
☐ PALE/ASHEN
☐ FLUSHED
☐ JAUNDICED

SKIN CONDITION
☐ NORMAL
☐ WARM/HOT
☐ COOL/COLD
☐ MOIST
☐ DRY

PUPILS

	RT	LT
EQUAL		
REACTIVE		
DILATED		
CONSTRICTED		
UNEQUAL		
NON-REACTIVE		

GLASCOW COMA SCALE

	TIME				
EYE OPENING SPONTANEOUS 4 / TO VERBAL COMMAND 3 / TO PAIN 2 / NO RESPONSE 1					
VERBAL RESPONSE ORIENTED & CONVERSE 5 / DISORIENTED & CONVERSE 4 / INAPPROPRIATE WORDS 3 / INCOMPREHENSIBLE SOUNDS 2 / NO RESPONSE 1					
MOTOR RESPONSE OBEYS COMMANDS 6 / LOCALIZES PAIN 5 / W THDRAWL 4 / FLEXION - DECORTICATE 3 / EXTENSION - DECEREBRATE 2 / NO RESPONSE 1					
TOTAL SCORE					

BREATH SOUNDS

	RT	LT
CLEAR		
RALES		
RHONCHI		
WHEEZES		
DIMINISHED		
ABSENT		

☐ STRIDOR

VITAL SIGNS

TIME	B/P	PULSE	RESP	O₂ SAT	GLUCOMETER

MEDICATIONS / DEFIBRILLATION / IV FLUIDS / EKG

TIME	MED / DEFIB / SOLN / ANGIO	DOSE / JOULES	ROUTE	MONITOR RHYTHM	INIT

BLS TREATMENT

☐ PATIENT ASSESSED
☐ TRANSPORT ONLY
☐ OXYGEN
  ☐ CANNULA @ _____ LPM
  ☐ SIMPLE MASK @ _____ LPM
  ☐ COMPLEX MASK @ _____ LPM
  ☐ OTHER @ _____ LPM
☐ VENTILATION
  ☐ BVM
  ☐ VENT @ RATE: _____
☐ AIRWAY INSERTION
  ☐ ORAL
  ☐ NASAL
  ☐ EOA / PTL BY: _____
☐ PULSE OXIMETER

☐ CPR   TIME
  ☐ BY-STANDER _____
  ☐ SQUAD _____
☐ BLEEDING CONTROL
☐ BANDAGING
☐ BURN CARE
☐ C-SPINE IMMOBILIZATION
  ☐ C-COLLAR
  ☐ CID
  ☐ OTHER: _____
☐ SPINAL IMMOBILIZATION
  ☐ XP-1 / KED
  ☐ LONG BACKBOARD
  ☐ SHORT BACKBOARD
  ☐ SCOOP
  ☐ OTHER:

☐ EXTRICATION   MINUTES: _____
☐ SPLINTING
  ☐ BOARD
  ☐ TRACTION
  ☐ AIR VACUUM
  ☐ OTHER: _____
☐ COLD PACK
☐ PASG/MAST   TIME
  ☐ IN-PLACE ONLY _____
  ☐ LEGS ONLY INFLATED _____
  ☐ FULLY INFLATED _____
☐ OB DELIVERY
☐ RESTRAINTS _____
☐ IPECAC   AMOUNT: _____
☐ CRISIS INTERVENTION

ALS TREATMENT

☐ CARDIAC MONITOR
  ☐ STANDARD   ☐ 12-LEAD
☐ ENDOTRACHEAL INTUBATION
  ATTEMPT # _____
  ET TUBE SIZE: _____
  ☐ ORAL BY: _____
  ☐ NASAL BY: _____
☐ CRICOTHYROTOMY BY: _____
☐ DEFIBRILLATION
☐ SYNCHRONIZED CARDIOVERSION
☐ PACEMAKER
  OUTPUT: _____
☐ CHEST DECOMPRESSION
  ☐ RT   ☐ LT
☐ INTRAOSSEOUS INFUSION
  ATTEMPT # _____
☐ IV ATTEMPT # _____
  IV ATTEMPTS BY _____

PATIENT ASSESSMENT: _____
_____
_____
_____
_____
_____
_____
_____
_____
_____

WRITTEN BY: _____

EMS CREW: _____

Fig. 3-8 A run form is completed at the end of each patient contact. The format allows basic assessment and frequently used skills to be checked off while leaving adequate room for a more specific narrative.

I. D.O.A.

AUTHORITIES NOTIFIED BY _____ TIME _____ A.M. / P.M.

RELEASED BY _____ TIME _____ A.M. / P.M.

PRONOUNCED DEAD BY _____ M.D. TIME _____ A.M. / P.M.

II ALTERNATE HOSPITAL AUTHORIZATION

I _____ HAVE REQUESTED TRANSPORT TO A HOSPITAL OTHER THAN THE CLOSEST HOSPITAL. I AGREE TO RELEASE (DEPARTMENT NAME) AND THE ATTENDING (EMT/PARAMEDICS) FROM ANY ADVERSE CONSEQUENCES THAT MAY RESULT FROM THIS DECISION.

PATIENT'S
SIGNATURE _____

CREW CHIEF   WITNESS
SIGNATURE _____   SIGNATURE _____

III. TREATMENT/TRANSPORT RELEASE

I _____ PREFER NOT TO BE TRANSPORTED TO THE HOSPITAL BY AMBULANCE FOR MEDICAL TREATMENT. THE POSSIBLE ADVERSE CONSEQUENCES OF SUCH A DECISION HAVE BEEN EXPLAINED TO ME.

PATIENT'S
SIGNATURE _____

CREW CHIEF   WITNESS
SIGNATURE _____   SIGNATURE _____

VICTIM WOULD NOT SIGN REFUSAL FORM _____   REASON _____
_____

IV. CALL DELAY REASON _____

STRIP #1	TIME: _____	LEAD: _____	INTERPRETATION: _____

STRIP #2	TIME: _____	LEAD: _____	INTERPRETATION: _____

STRIP #3	TIME: _____	LEAD: _____	INTERPRETATION: _____

Fig. 3-8, cont'd   Depending on the system, some items may be added, such as trauma scores or specifics for neonates and children.

history of asthma, making beta blockers a lethal treatment modality.

5. *Physical assessment* including pertinent negatives.
6. *Treatment* including extrication and immobilization.

When the patient's condition is worsening, a brief, pertinent verbal report can be made and then expanded on when the patient's condition and staff availability permit.

Written documentation should include all of the above but in more detail. Attention should be paid to the time that events occurred and when treatment was rendered. The written report is not an individual effort; the team should be consulted so that a clear, concise report is made that can be recalled years later (Figure 3-8). Also, it is important that another healthcare provider such as a critical care nurse can read the report and understand what happened to the patient in the prehospital setting.

Post-Run Activities

Equipment exchange and restocking should take place after the used equipment and vehicle have been cleaned and decontaminated. All equipment must be inspected before the next call. If a drug equipment box has been opened, it must be inspected to ensure that all drugs and supplies are there. In the haste of a scene, equipment may have fallen out or been displaced; therefore it is imperative to inspect the vehicle and all equipment and supplies. Medical gases, such as oxygen, are checked and must be at least full enough to handle a prolonged, high-flow oxygen incident.

Special incidents may arise that challenge the prehospital nurse, as well as the rest of the EMS team. The remainder of this chapter examines some of those situations and gives the PHN some background on how to deal with them.

RESCUE AND EXTRICATION

The incident is a head-on collision between a van and a passenger car. The car rolled down a hill and over a 10-foot embankment, coming to rest on its roof. After witnessing the collision, a bystander calls the 911 dispatcher and reports that a victim is pinned underneath the car. The Emergency Medical Service system is activated, and the appropriate equipment and personnel are dispatched to the scene.

When confronted with an emergency rescue situation, specialized skills and equipment are required to rescue the victim safely. The term *rescue* applies to the process of gaining access to and then removing the victim without compromising the victim's condition. Extrication goes hand-in-hand with rescue and involves the application of specific tools and techniques for releasing the entrapped victim. Examples of various rescue situations include (1) a laborer's hand caught in an industrial machine, (2) a construction worker buried in a trench cave-in, or (3) multiple victims entrapped by debris from a collapsed building. The most common rescue performed by prehospital care providers involves victims of motor vehicle incidents (Heckman, 1992a). Rescue operations involve combined efforts of fire, police, and EMS personnel.

Roles and Responsibilities in Extrication

The composition of the rescue team and the logistics of its base of operation may vary from one locale to another. In large cities a separate rescue team that specializes in extrication is usually housed and staffed by the fire department. In some locations responders may be trained in both patient care and rescue procedures. Dual-trained responders function according to the needs mandated by the emergency situation. The specific roles of emergency care providers, EMTs, and paramedics during a rescue situation are to provide patient assessment and medical treatment and ensure safe removal of the victim from the vehicle.

Personal Safety Measures of Extrication

The predominant on-scene hazards that emergency providers encounter are fire, debris, sharp objects, traffic, and contamination from toxic agents (Henry & Stapleton, 1992b). Protective clothing is one measure rescuers use to shield against these potential hazards. Rescue personnel wear turnout gear, which consists of fire-resistant clothing and gloves, sturdy boots, and a helmet with a face shield. Protective clothing should also be reflective, weather appropriate, and allow for mobility in a variety of rescue situations.

The victim also requires protection from on-scene hazards. One example is protection from flying debris. Frequently, rescuers must use extrication tools in close proximity to entrapped victims. Using extrication tools, such as center punches and hydraulic power tools, often results in flying glass and pieces of metal. A fire-resistant blanket should be placed over the vic-

tim before such tools are used. Two excellent sources providing standards and guidelines for safety in the prehospital work environment are the Occupational Safety and Health Administration (OSHA) and the National Fire Protection Association (NFPA).

Principles of Extrication

The procedure of extrication at a collision scene follows three basic principles. These principles, identified by Heckman (1992a), are (1) survey and control the scene, (2) gain access to the victim and initiate medical care, and (3) remove the victim from entrapment and transport to an appropriate medical facility. These principles are now discussed, using a rescue and extrication situation involving a motor vehicle accident (Figure 3-9).

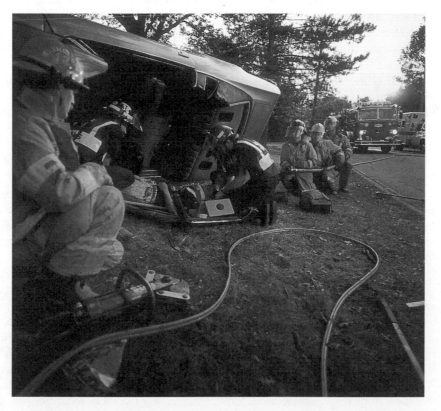

Fig. 3-9   Extrication of a victim involved in a motor vehicle incident.

Survey and Control the Scene

The emergency call starts at the time of dispatch, when the rescue team gets mentally prepared for the emergency scene and develops flexible operational plans. The initial evaluation of the scene is focused around the issue of safety. Work hazards at a collision scene can be significant. A rescuer needs to make personal safety a number one concern. The rescuer cannot be an effective patient care provider if incapacitated by an injury (Grant, Murray, & Bergeron, 1994b).

For protection from environmental hazards, emergency vehicles should be parked uphill, upwind, and at least 100 feet away from the incident to assess the scene initially (Henry & Stapleton, 1992b). Binoculars may be used to look for displayed hazardous material placards, downed wires, fuel leaks, or other dangers. If the scene presents too much risk, the rescue attempt is halted until the scene can be stabilized. The decision to request additional rescue personnel or special extrication equipment is made at this time.

Environmental conditions such as rain, snow, or high winds are noted during the scene assessment. The need to provide the rescue team protection from adverse weather should be considered. For example, to protect the rescuers from frostbite, a designated rescue vehicle may be established as a warming area.

Included in the scene assessment is information provided by bystanders. What did they witness? How many vehicles were involved? What was the speed at impact? Rescuers then inspect the interior and exterior of the vehicle for type of deformity. Is the steering wheel bent? Is the windshield broken? The basic trauma life support program identifies four common types of automobile collisions: (1) head-on, (2) lateral impact, (3) rear-end, and (4) rollover. Each type of collision presents an index of suspicion for particular injuries specific to the mechanism of the injury (Campbell, 1988b). Thus vehicle assessment provides important information for the emergency care team.

Information pertaining to the victims must also be gathered. How many victims are involved? What are their ages? Were any victims thrown from the vehicle? If so, what kind of terrain will need to be searched: a ditch, woods, tall grass? In concordance with the mechanism of injury, what injuries could the patients have sustained?

Scene Access and Initiation of Medical Care

When the scene is considered safe, the vehicle is secured to prevent it from rolling, rocking, or tipping over (Figure 3-10). Stabilization can be accomplished by using extrication equipment, such as air bags or cribbing, to disperse the weight of the vehicle over a large surface area. The medical team then approaches the patient. The initial plan of action is to assess for life-threatening injuries. If the patient is determined to be unstable, lifesaving treatment should be initiated and prompt transport provided to an appropriate medical facility. This usually involves administering treatment while en route. Primary patient care must focus on five assessment steps, as follows:

1. Patency of the airway with cervical spine control
2. Quality of ventilation
3. Quality of the cardiovascular system
4. Hemorrhage control
5. Level of consciousness

The scene time for an extricated critical patient should be less than 10 minutes. Every minute spent in the field takes away from the patient's golden hour (Campbell, 1988a).

A rule of extrication is to immobilize the victim before removal from the wrecked vehicle (Campbell, 1988c). This is done by applying a cervical collar and corset-type extrication device to immobilize the neck and spine while the victim sits in the car. The victim is then rotated out of the automobile and placed on a long backboard with a head immobilizer. When a victim is in critical condition or the scene becomes unstable during the extrication, rapid ex-

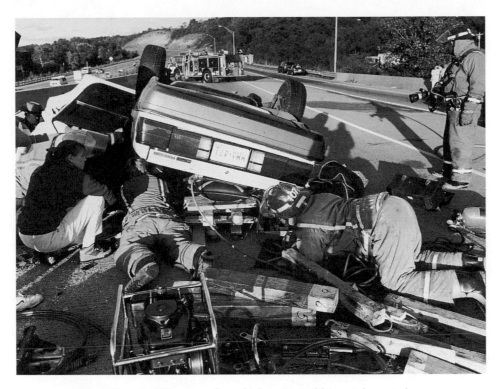

Fig. 3-10   Stabilization of a vehicle using cribbing and an air bag.

trication can be performed, which involves manually removing the victim from the vehicle with limited immobilization devices (Campbell, 1988c). Because of the importance and complexity of rapid extrication, the procedure needs to be practiced regularly by the emergency care team to maintain proficiency.

Removal and Transport to a Medical Facility

Once extrication is complete, emergency care providers continue patient assessment, medical treatment, and patient stabilization. The patient is transported by either ground or air transport, with a full complement of medical personnel, to the closest appropriate medical facility. A detailed report describing the collision scene, vehicle, and extrication is given to the emergency team at the receiving facility. A Polaroid photograph of the scene can enhance the EMS report, since it can be used for both scene documentation and insight into the mechanism of injury (Holmquist, Lee, & Songne, 1989).

Extrication Equipment

Guided by state specifications, ambulances are required to carry basic extrication equipment to enable simple entry or disentanglement. Larger, more specialized rescue equipment is usually transported to the scene by a designated rescue vehicle. Extrication tools are divided into five main categories: (1) hand, (2) cutting, (3) spreading, (4) pulling, and (5) lifting (Heckman, 1992a). They can be generated either manually, pneumatically, or by a gasoline/electric engine.

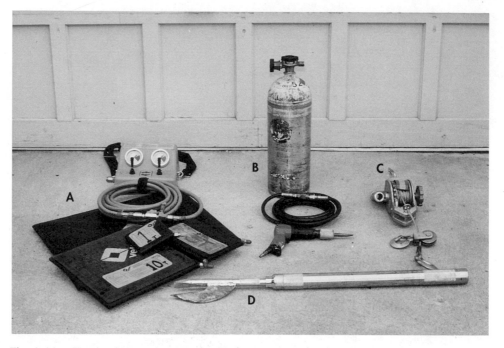

Fig. 3-11 Extrication equipment. **A,** Air bag. **B,** Air chisel with compressed air cylinder. **C,** Come-along. **D,** Can opener.

A hydraulic tool that has gained much recognition for its specific function of opening jammed vehicle doors is called the "jaws of life." Rescue tools can possess hazards of their own. A hydraulic tool can weigh up to 60 pounds, making it very cumbersome to handle. The friction from cutting sheet metal creates sparks and, in the presence of combustibles, produces a potential for fire. Thus at the scene a fire department maintains a charged water hose when the rescue is in progress. Tools containing hydraulic fluid, a corrosive, can leak or spray, even when operated correctly. The noise from the power tools tearing and cutting metal can frighten the victim. Explaining the sounds and vibrations from extrication maneuvers can minimize the victim's anxiety.

The following list is a description of extrication tools frequently used in the prehospital setting (Figures 3-11 and 3-12):

- Cribbing (shoring): stacked blocks of wood used to stabilize a vehicle
- Porta-power: a manually powered hydraulic pump
- Center punch: a spring-loaded hand device that, when pressed against tempered glass, causes the glass to shatter
- Pry axe: used for prying and cutting of sheet metal
- Hacksaw: used to cut through steering wheels, roof posts, and brake pedals
- Knives: used to assist in the removal of windshields
- Air chisel: driven by compressed air to cut sheet metal and support columns
- Can opener: manually powered device used to cut sheet metal
- Handwinch (Come-Along): combination of a cable, pulley, and breakaway handle

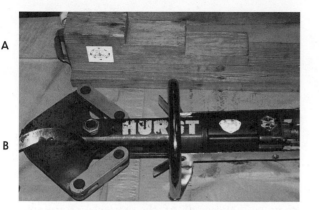

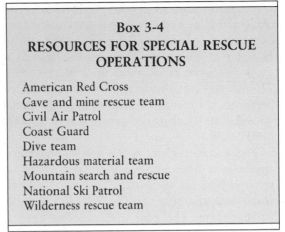

Fig. 3-12   Extraction equipment. **A,** Cribbing. **B,** Hydraulic cutting tool.

Box 3-4
RESOURCES FOR SPECIAL RESCUE OPERATIONS

American Red Cross
Cave and mine rescue team
Civil Air Patrol
Coast Guard
Dive team
Hazardous material team
Mountain search and rescue
National Ski Patrol
Wilderness rescue team

that is used, attached to chains, to pull steering wheels and displace seats
- Hydraulic spreaders (jaws of life): used to spread metal and for lifting
- Hydraulic shears: used to cut support columns
- Hydraulic rams: powered pump to push and spread metal apart
- Air bag: bag filled with compressed air capable of lifting 2000 to 150000 pounds.

Adjunct Resources for Rescue Operations

It is not practical for an EMS/fire department to maintain the equipment or expertise for every rescue situation they could encounter. Rescue personnel should be knowledgeable of local, state, and national organizations able to assist in rescue situations. Obtaining additional help may be as simple as requesting mutual aid from an adjacent fire department or as complex as locating a cave and mine rescue team to supplement a rescue operation. Box 3-4 lists additional rescue and extrication resources.

Role of the Prehospital Nurse in Rescue and Extrication

At the accident scene the PHN is a member of the emergency care team and works along-

side of the EMS and fire personnel. Activities of the PHN are to ensure a safe working environment, perform patient assessment, and provide medical treatment. The patient care and extrication teams coordinate the treatment of the patient. This is illustrated when patient assessment indicates a tension pneumothorax that needs immediate decompression. The rescuers, who are getting ready to pull the steering wheel, are alerted that a medical procedure needs to be performed. The rescuers halt, temporarily, so that the patient can receive the lifesaving procedure.

The entrapped victim is dependent on the rescue team. Good judgment in regard to the patient's safety and treatment is in the hands of the caregiver. The PHN is a patient advocate. The activity around an entrapped victim can be overwhelming. Communicating with the victim, explaining rescue procedures, and informing the victim of medical treatment can make a difficult time more tolerable.

Curious bystanders are a part of the accident scene. As a patient advocate, the PHN can intervene. A blanket screen can be devised to safeguard the victim from the video cameras of nonprofessionals and from onlookers.

Another responsibility of the PHN may include acting as a family liaison, especially if the extrication is lengthy. At a rescue attempt in New Jersey, family members or close friends at the scene were given a red armband to wear. This alerted emergency workers of the family's presence and identified them as needing special consideration during the stressful event (Noose, 1989).

The accident scene is full of challenges and excitement. The rescue mission is focused on what is best for the victim. It is an all-out effort by the rescue team. The PHN is a member of that team. The goal is to expedite extrication and transfer the victim in the best possible condition to the medical facility. There are triumphs and there are losses. Maintaining special knowledge and skill proficiency in rescue and extrication are essential components for prehospital care providers.

MASS CASUALTY INCIDENT AND THE INCIDENT COMMAND SYSTEM

Although nursing has functioned in the out-of-hospital environment for years as public health nurses, home health nurses, and as prehospital care providers in EMS systems, the advent of disaster nursing has necessitated that the nurse have a basic understanding of mass casualty incidents (MCIs). An in-depth examination of multicasualty incidents and disaster nursing is beyond the scope of this text; instead, a general review of MCIs and their structure will be addressed.

Mass Casualty Incident

The registered nurse (RN) typically has had more in-depth education in anatomy, physiology, and pathophysiology than the EMT and paramedic, who have had more extensive training in safety, extrication, and rescue techniques than the RN. Although these differences may come into play during an MCI, the nurse, EMT,

and paramedic may function on an equal level depending on their assignment. Therefore the prehospital nurse must be familiar with all roles involved in response to an MCI.

An MCI exists when (1) the number of patients and the nature of their injuries make the normal level of stabilization and care unachievable; (2) the number of personnel and ambulances that can be brought to the scene within the time allowed is not enough; or (3) the stabilization capabilities of the hospitals that can be reached within the time allowed are insufficient to handle all of the patients (Butman, 1985).

Through retrospective studies, the following common problems were found at most MCIs:

1. Failure to alert responders adequately
2. Lack of rapid primary stabilization of all patients
3. Failure to move, collect, and organize patients rapidly at a suitable place
4. Failure to provide proper triage
5. Use of overly time-consuming and inappropriate care methods
6. Premature commencement of transportation
7. Improper use of personnel in the field
8. Lack of proper distribution of patients, resulting in improper use of medical facilities
9. Lack of recognizable EMS command in the field
10. Lack of proper preplanning and lack of adequate training of all personnel
11. Failure to compensate for malfunction and remedy problems
12. Lack of adequate or proper communication (Butman, 1985)

Keeping in mind these problems and the definition of an MCI, the structure and mechanisms developed to alleviate these problems and to restore the victim and community to a normal state of existence are discussed in the following paragraphs.

Identical incidents may pose different problems based on the area in which they occur. An event that may be easily handled by the EMS system and the local hospitals in one area may be almost catastrophic when it occurs elsewhere. For example, a drive-by shooting injuring five people would be handled with relative ease in the inner city or suburbs. That same shooting in a rural area with the nearest neighboring EMS agency 20 minutes away would be classified as an MCI for that community. If the quantity of personnel and resources needed are not available within a specific, reasonable time frame, then the quality of the personnel and their abilities becomes more important.

Two types of MCIs exist, closed incidents and open incidents. An incident is termed *closed* when patients are confined to a small, undesirable place. It would be necessary then to expeditiously, yet cautiously, remove these patients from the confined area and transport them with stretcher or ambulatory to a designated triage area. An example would be a school bus crash in which many people are injured in a confined space, making extended triage and treatment infeasible. In this incident it is necessary to visually identify the most severe cases quickly and to extricate them from the vehicle. If the incident area leaves the EMS team or the patient in any type of danger, then expedient removal of the patients by any mechanism may be warranted.

An incident is termed *open* when the patients or the scene is spread out over a large area. An example would be a plane crash in which the victims can be found throughout a large geographical area. As planes hit the ground, their debris is spread over a large area. Surviving victims may be found in the wreckage no matter how far from the initial impact. It would then be necessary for the rescuers to bring the victims to a designated location for triage, stabilization, and transport. Also, closed incidents may turn into open incidents. An example of this is the fire that occurred at the Beverly Hills Supper Club in Southgate, Kentucky, on

May 28, 1977. Victims who suffered from smoke inhalation were exiting from various parts of the building. It became extremely difficult for rescuers to find the victims, triage them, treat them, and arrange for their eventual transport from the scene. A preplanned MCI response was not in effect at the time of the incident. An organized MCI response would have addressed the problem by alerting all rescuers to move the injured parties to a predesignated triage area for triage and eventual dispersement.

Incidents may be classified as either contained or continuing. A contained incident is when the cause of the incident has ceased, for example, a motor vehicle collision into a school bus. Additional injuries probably will not occur after the initial impact, unless there is a danger of fire or hazardous material exposure. A continuing incident occurs when the cause of injury continues. Examples include a hazardous materials spill where the spill and its gases have not yet been confined, or a multistory building fire where effective rescue of all occupants has not yet occurred. This must be taken into consideration when evaluating an MCI for personnel and equipment needs.

Although any type of work at an MCI is potentially dangerous, some areas pose a greater threat to the prehospital care nurse. The area surrounding the immediate scene presents the greatest risks and is frequently referred to as the *hot zone*. It is imperative that prehospital nurses be protected with the proper clothing or turnout gear, including shoes, helmets, gloves, pants, and jackets. The area immediately outside of the hot zone may be referred to as the *cold zone*. Most of the contact that prehospital care nurses have with the patient occurs in this area. Triage, treatment, and transportation are set up in this region. The nurse must be educated and cognizant at all times of hazards that may occur. These include but are not limited to fire, explosive material, downed power lines, smoke or other toxic gases, fallen debris, floods, crowd violence, or collapsed buildings (Garcia, 1985).

Incident Command System and the MCI

The prehospital nurse must understand the structured hierarchy referred to as the *incident command system* (ICS), which consists of procedures for controlling personnel, facilities, equipment, and communications. It is designed to begin when an incident occurs and to continue until the requirement for management and operations no longer exists. The ICS is dynamic and continues to evolve until the incident is cleared. *Incident commander* is a title that can apply equally to the chief of a department or to the first EMS personnel arriving at the scene; that person is ultimately responsible for the total operations of the incident. The structure of the ICS can be established and expanded depending on the changing conditions of the incident. It is staffed and operated by qualified personnel from any EMS agency and may involve personnel from a variety of agencies (Federal Emergency Management Agency [FEMA], 1989).

The system can be used for any type or size of emergency, ranging from a minor auto accident to a major MCI. It is designed for application to emergencies caused by various mechanisms, such as floods, earthquakes, fires, tornadoes, civil disturbances, hazardous material incidents, or any other natural or human-caused disasters.

The ICS has five major functional areas: command, operations, planning, logistics, and finance. These tasks are similar to those that business managers perform and include planning, directing, organizing, coordinating, communicating, delegating, and evaluating. The responsibilities of the incident commander also includes gathering and evaluating information for preplanning and size up, as well as development and communication of plans. (*Size up* is the term used for describing the collection and evaluation of initial information received at the beginning of the incident.)

The incident commander must be involved with directing available resources to accomplish incident goals through operational and command responsibilities. To ensure proper incident management by coordination of overall operations of command tactical operations and support functions, a responsive organization must be developed (FEMA, 1989). The overall effectiveness of the incident action plan must be evaluated continually based on the results of previous operational decisions. Using these data, the incident commander modifies the action plan. This type of operation is similar to the nursing process. Both involve preplanning, assessment, plan of action, implementation, reassessment (evaluation), and updated plans based on data collected.

The incident commander may delegate functional authority down line but retains ultimate responsibility for the incident. If choosing not to delegate authority for one or more functions, the incident commander must perform the functions as required by the incident.

Incident priority includes life safety, incident stabilization, and property conservation. Although life safety is always primary, incident stabilization may be necessary before issues of life safety can be pursued. For example, a truck containing hazardous materials collides with a car; the victims must be attended to, but first a hazardous materials team must secure the scene and move the victims to a safe area.

Incident Command System and EMS

The incident commander is in charge and has absolute responsibility for the entire incident. Obviously, no one person can undertake such a task at a large MCI. Therefore the incident commander delegates responsibility down line so that the incident as a whole can be studied. The incident commander delegates to an operations officer, who in turn delegates fire responsibilities to a suppression officer, and EMS responsibilities to an EMS officer. The EMS officer then delegates responsibilities to the triage group, treatment group, and transportation group. Also, under the transportation group is the EMS staging officer.

The following rules pertain to the down line delegation of authority:

1. Each officer is in charge of three to seven people (the average is five).
2. Although individual officers make their decisions about operations and patient care, the up line officer must be kept informed at all times about decisions that affect the incident or group as a whole.
3. Typically the incident commander is the first officer to arrive at the scene of an MCI. The incident command position is then relinquished to a higher ranking officer after a thorough in-depth report has been given.
4. The incident command system is a dynamic structure that must be readily expanded or condensed to meet priority needs.
5. The EMS officer, as well as the triage officer, treatment officer, and transportation officer, must have a system for recording incident events, location of equipment, and location of personnel (Figures 3-13 to 3-15).

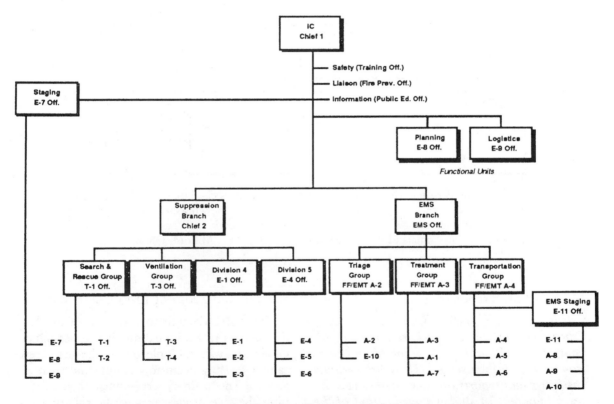

Fig. 3-13   The incident command flowsheet illustrates the chain of command that exists at a mass casualty incident. The incident commander has delegated responsibility for various operations that need to be performed for this event. The EMS branch officer has assigned personnel to the triage group, treatment group, and transportation group. Identification of groups that will staff the triage, treatment and transportation zones is made by apparatus assignment (*A*, ambulance; *E*, fire engine; *T*, ladder company).

FACILITY LOCATIONS
Command Post
Triage Area
Treatment Area/s
Helicopter LZ
Morgue
EOC
Media Center
Other

COMMUNICATIONS
Channel Freq. Use Comments

LEVEL 2 STAGING
Location
Best Route
Staging Officer

TYPE OF UNIT	REQUESTED OR ENROUTE	AT STAGING
Ambulances		
Non Transport Units		
MCI Supply Units		
Buses		
Helicopters		
Other		

EMS TACTICAL COMMAND WORKSHEET
Date: Time: Location:
Type of Incident:
Incident Commander EMS Commander:
Fire Commander: Police Commander:
Rescue Commander: Liaison Officer:
Public Information Officer: Safety Officer
Weather Forecast:

Transport Unit	Hospital	No. of Patients & Conditions	Time		Transport Unit	Hospital	No. of Patients & Conditions	Time		Transport Unit	Hospital	No. of Patients & Conditions	Time	

ESTIMATED TOTAL NUMBER OF PATIENTS:

NUMBER OF PATIENTS IN TREATMENT AREA

RED	YELLOW	GREEN	BLACK

HOSPITAL CAPABILITIES AND UTILIZATION
Name
Specialties
Patient Capabilities:
# of Red:
# of Yellow
# of Green
Number of Patients Sent:
Red
Yellow
Green

COMMAND ASSIGNMENTS COMMAND ASSIGNMENTS

Sector Division Group				TRIAGE OFFICER	TREATMENT OFFICER	TRANSPORTATION OFFICER
Name of Officer						
Radio Channel Freq.						
Units Assigned Location Needs Additional Information						

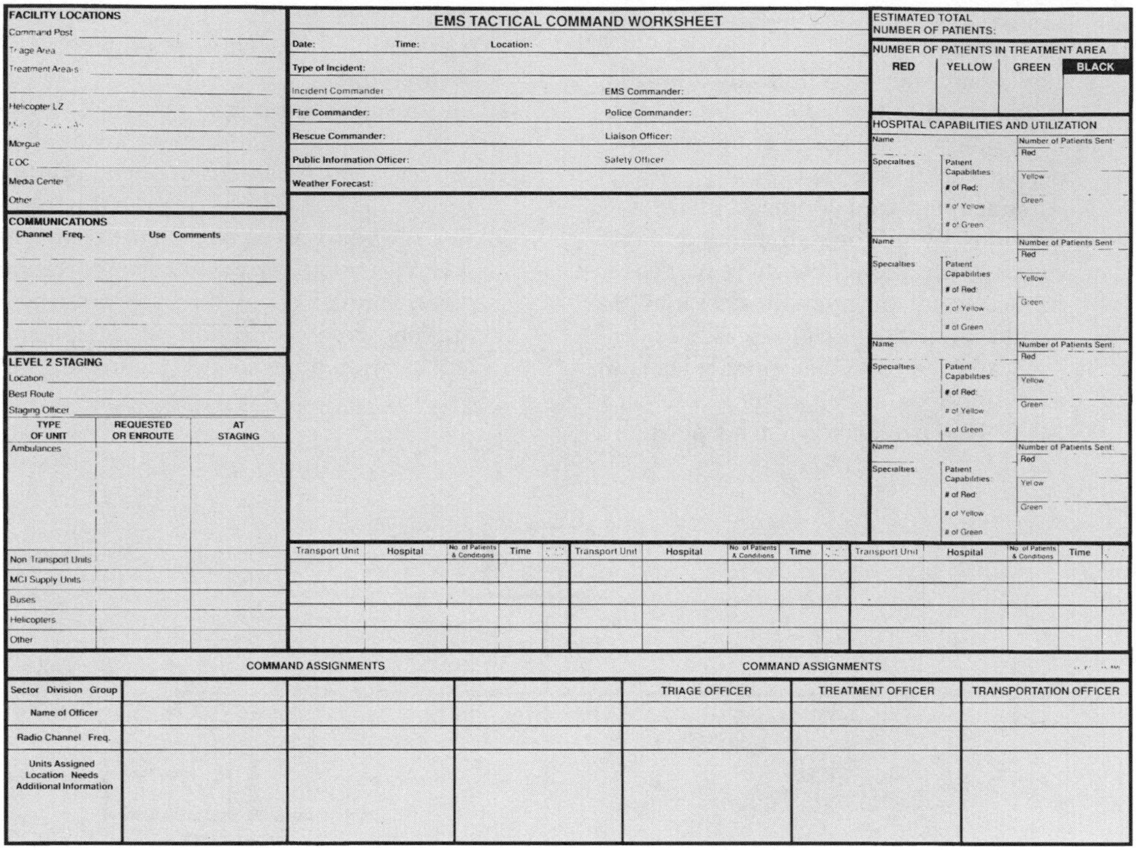

Fig. 3-14 The person in charge of the EMS sector at a mass casualty incident must have a worksheet to keep track of the evolvement of the incident. The worksheet can be either paper or a board that can be written on with an erasable marker. (Worksheet printed with permission of The Command Post, a Division of AMEC, Inc., Milford, Ohio.)

MCI and the Prehospital Nurse in Action

It is Wednesday, 1:00 PM, *on a warm, sunny September afternoon. You are responding with your local EMS unit to the scene of an explosion at a local high school. There are multiple casualties and reports of some deaths. You observe hundreds of students out in front of the school with many of them collapsed on the ground. The incident commander has assigned your crew the task of being medical command. What do you do?*

Size Up and Setup of EMS Command

The first EMS unit to arrive at an incident may consist of a minimal number of personnel. Obviously, with multiple victims the basic crew cannot feasibly begin to examine and treat all people. The primary crew must then switch from the role of caregiver to the role of mass casualty incident managers and begin to take on their preplanned, assigned roles. Treatment should not be started in this phase. The crew must quickly assess the situation, determining

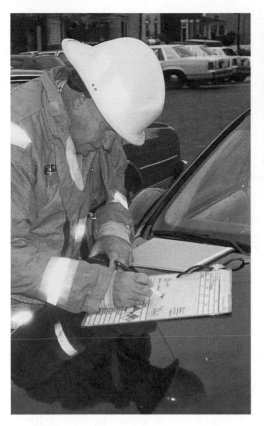

Fig. 3-15   The incident commander keeps track of vital information such as personnel assignments, weather, evacuations, and notifications of ancillary services such as utilities, hospitals, and neighboring emergency services. The board also acts as a reminder to the incident commander in case he or she forgets to perform a task or notify somebody.

the approximate number of patients and the number of EMS units required and assess the need for any special equipment or services.

An EMS commander must be identified at this point. This role is taken by the most qualified member of the first on-scene EMS crew. The commander should set up a command post and remain there throughout the duration of the incident. Realizing that the goal of a mass casualty response is to "strive to achieve the greatest good for the greatest number of potential survivors," a size up must be made and officer assignments given. The commander requests additional EMS units as needed and places others on standby for response as the situation dictates. Evacuation or triage is set up when personnel become available and it is safe

to do so. Hospitals are notified as soon as possible of the potential of multiple victims. At this point, it would be advantageous for the dispatch center to call local hospitals to ascertain their bed availability and number of critical patients that they can take. **Note:** It is at the beginning of a multicasualty incident that EMS providers feel the greatest temptation to start rendering treatment and transportation for the first scene victims. If the EMS team is to do the greatest good for the greatest number of people, it is imperative that they follow preplans and the medical incident command system. Triage, treatment, staging, and transportation officers are then assigned by the EMS commander.

Triage Officer

The triage officer sets the stage for the remainder of the incident. It is an absolute necessity that the triage officer not take on any other roles. This officer has two functions: (1) to assess the patient's condition quickly and to assign the patient to a priority category in the treatment zone and (2) to communicate with the treatment officer to ensure that an adequate number of personnel are assigned to each zone.

Initial field triage takes place as the triage officer quickly scans the incident and makes an assessment of the number of victims. This information is relayed to the EMS commander. The triage personnel then begin at the farthest end of the incident and quickly assess the ABCs of the victims and provide treatment limited to the rapid correction of life-threatening injuries, for example, airway stabilization and bleeding control. Large, bright-colored ribbon (that corresponds with the four basic color categories of triage) is attached to an extremity of the victim. Stretcher bearers (preferably EMTs trained in patient handling) then remove the victims to the treatment area. The patient is retriaged upon entering the treatment/collection area. The patient is then assigned to the designated treatment area according to the patient's condition. Once in the designated colored section, a full primary and secondary survey is then performed. More detailed treatment can then be delivered to the patient. Patients are removed from this area based on their severity of injury and chances of survivability and not on a "first in, first out" system. If a person remains in the treatment area for a significant period of time, retriage should ideally occur every 15 to 20 minutes.

As the triage officer and personnel begin their field triage duties, they will be making decisions that are atypical as to how they were trained. Anybody who is in cardiac arrest, or has deteriorated to such a condition that survivability is improbable, is triaged as such and no treatment rendered. If treatment of these people were initiated, chances are that more lives would be lost that would have had a possibility of survival.

Triage Categories

The four basic triage categories are given the following color categorical assignment:

I. *Red*—Urgent/critical: Injuries or medical problems that are not immediately dealt with will lead to death; the patient is otherwise salvageable.

II. *Yellow*—Delayed: Patient's condition will likely deteriorate without medical intervention, but as such is not yet critical.

III. *Green*—Minor: These patients have sustained minor injuries and with a minimal level of support can wait long periods before reaching a medical facility for definitive treatment. (Try to avoid using the term *walking wounded*. Not all ambulatory patients have injuries that are minor in nature, and not all patients with minor injuries are ambulatory.)

IV. *Black*—Obviously dead or terminal: These patients have suffered mortal injuries that, despite immediate care, will suffer absolute demise. An example would be a traumatic arrest or a patient who has suffered burns to 80% to 90% of the total body surface area.

Any rescuer who goes down during the incident is automatically classified as *red*. It is imperative that rescuers are transported in the next available ambulance because of the psychological impact this has on fellow rescuers.

Different types of triage tag systems have been developed to assist the rescuer in labeling the victims, and the rescuer should be familiar with the tags used in the area. The ideal tag must be waterproof, easily written on with a pen or magic marker, color coded, possess the quality of being both upgraded and downgraded as retriage occurs, and provide a space for a brief initial assessment and treatment rendered.

Treatment Area

The treatment area is usually within short proximity of the disaster or incident site, unless a dangerous environment exists that forces it to be located farther away. In general, it is better to keep it closer to the site so that the stretcher bearers and ambulatory victims will not have a long transit before they reach the treatment area. Equipment used for the triage and treatment of victims is sent to this area and is disseminated as needed by a supply officer who keeps records of what was used and assesses the need for more equipment in consultation with the treatment officer. The treatment area is divided into three main zones that correspond with patient severity and priority for transportation. A red zone (critically injured patients) is set up and may be designated by a red banner or red flag. These patients are transported first. Yellow and green zones are similarly set up with treatment and transportation priority given to the yellow-zone patients first.

Treatment Officer

The treatment officer is more of an administrator than a medical care provider. The officer should not necessarily be an EMS person most qualified in patient care. Personnel who are best qualified in the area of patient care and treatment should be applying themselves to what they do best, treating patients. The treatment officer must establish an area that is capable of accommodating large numbers of patients and equipment and that will have room to grow. When choosing the area, the officer must consider factors that may affect the safety of patients and personnel, such as the weather, security, and hazardous materials. The area must be readily accessible and have clearly designated entrances and exits.

Patients should only leave the treatment area at the direction of the treatment officer. It is the treatment officer's responsibility to make sure that all patients are transported according to their triage designation and treated as such. As more personnel arrive at the scene to assist, the officer will assign the more advanced trained personnel, such as physicians, nurses, and paramedics, to the red and yellow zones, respectively. Basic EMTs may be used to assist the ALS personnel or they can be assigned to the green zone.

Accountability for setting up a morgue area (black zone) is left with the treatment officer. The coroner or medical examiner should be notified as soon as possible. The morgue must be set up away from the treatment areas in a secure spot that is not accessible to the public. Large refrigeration trucks may be commandeered from food transportation agencies to store the bodies if local hospitals are unable to accommodate them. This task should be turned over to the police or coroner's office as soon as possible.

Transportation Officer

One of the most challenging assignments during an MCI is that of the transportation officer. The transportation officer is responsible for the routing of patients from the treatment area to the hospital, while taking into consideration the capabilities of the hospital. As mentioned earlier, bed count and availability to treat patients are ascertained at the beginning of an MCI. The transportation officer must keep track of this count to prevent hospital overloading. Although general overall hospital bed counts may prove useful, emergency department beds and availability of operating room suites are what count the most. Since trauma is basically a surgical disease, dividing the patients up between as many hospitals as geographically possible allows for patients with the most serious conditions to receive surgical intervention in the shortest period of time.

Ambulances arrive at various times during the incident. The first units to arrive at the scene probably will not be used for transport because of the need for additional help and resources in the various areas such as triage and treatment.

Depending on variables, such as traffic and weather conditions, the next ambulances to arrive can be used to transport patients out of the red zone. After that point, a continual flow of ambulances to and from the treatment area can be anticipated. After ambulance personnel turn over patient care to the hospital, they may be called back into service to transport more victims.

The transport officer notifies the hospital as the ambulance leaves the treatment zone. Information included is the name of the unit responding, the number of patients being transported, a brief description of the patients by category or specific injury, and the estimated time of arrival of the transport unit. The individual ambulances should not contact the receiving hospital unless the patient's condition deteriorates and physician consultation is needed.

Information should be recorded on each patient leaving the treatment area. If enough emergency responders are available, a scribe can be assigned to work with the treatment officer to record all information.

The surrounding community not involved in the MCI must be appropriated a level of protection during the incident that meets its EMS needs. Neighboring communities can move their equipment into a staging area to provide protection to the rest of the community and to the MCI, if needed.

Staging Officer

The staging officer is in charge of traffic control. As EMS, fire, and rescue units are dispatched to an MCI, they are to report to a location known as the *staging area*. The staging area should be readily accessible, easy to locate, and big enough to handle large numbers of vehicles. It needs to be far enough away from the scene so as not to cause congestion, yet close enough to make accessibility to the scene rapid and efficient. The staging officer is in charge of making sure enough units are available to pro-

tect the community and are readily available to meet scene needs. No equipment or personnel goes to the scene unless released by the staging officer. The burden of determining which particular unit to send to the scene is lifted from the treatment officer and incident commander and given to the staging officer. For example, all the treatment officer would have to request is a BLS unit and the staging officer would then dispatch one from the staging area. This would also work the same with the fire department. The operations officer would request an engine company, and it would be up to the staging officer to dispatch a particular unit. Fire department and EMS staging is generally combined with one staging area and one staging officer (Figures 3-16 and 3-17).

After the Incident

Postincident events are geared at minimizing the psychological trauma that occurs for all participants of a multicasualty incident. Responders (EMS, fire, American Red Cross, media, and so on) and victims and their families are all at risk after an MCI. The goal of postincident care is to address the feelings and emotional trauma early to prevent long-term manifestations and problems. Responders may have feelings of inadequacy, frustration, powerlessness, fear, guilt, and insecurity (Butman, 1985).

Individuals involved in critical incidents are normal people who have undergone psychological and physiological trauma during an extraordinary event. They will experience grief, guilt, anger, anxiety, vulnerability, depression, isolation, and problems in relationships with emergence of old problems (Hafen & Frandsen, 1985). Relatives of victims may undergo the same type of feelings, such as uncertainty, blaming, guilt that they survived, and separation anxiety.

Treatment for psychological emergencies and emotional trauma begins in the preplanning phase for MCIs. Incorporation of trained social workers, psychiatric nurses, critical incident

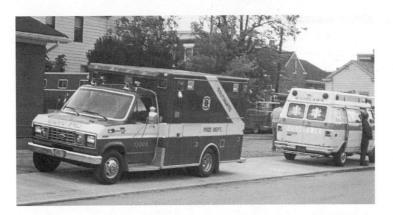

Fig. 3-16   The EMS staging area is where all responding EMS units meet and receive assignments from the staging officer. Units may be dispatched from this area directly to the incident site or to other incidents that may occur.

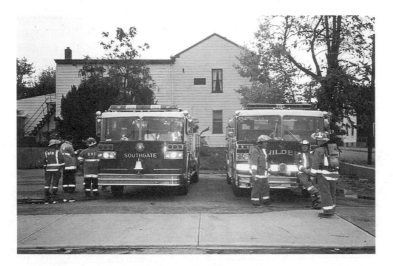

Fig. 3-17   In some mass casualty incidents the fire service may be used to supplement EMS personnel. Fire service personnel are pictured here waiting for their assignments at the EMS staging area.

stress-debriefing teams, and the ministers working with rescue, fire, police, and EMS response enhances a total team concept and addresses the physiological, psychological, and spiritual needs of all participants and victims. Careful documentation of all patient contact, as well as who responded to the scene, allows for health-care professionals to follow-up with all parties involved.

MCI and Disaster Planning

Traditionally, preplanning for disasters and MCIs has been the responsibility of fire and EMS services. Nursing's role has been to preplan for the effect that a disaster would have on hospitals. Nurses' backgrounds, however, make them ideal candidates for initiating disaster and MCI planning in the community. Nursing continually seeks out information, defines a problem or need, plans for it, acts on it, then reevaluates whether the need was met. In light of this, a brief explanation of disaster and MCI preplanning follows.

Each community has different potentials for the occurrence of MCIs and disasters. For example, California must preplan for earthquakes, forest fires, and, most recently in the Los Angeles area, riots. Meteorological disturbances, such as hurricanes, ravage the coastal states, and tornadoes torment the Midwest. Each community must define what its potential problems are and address them with preplans.

Community leaders, including fire, police, EMS, and hospitals, must meet and identify hazards within their communities that could pose threats to the welfare of the people. Schools, hospitals, nursing homes, and neighborhoods near transportation routes that carry hazardous materials must be identified and plans developed to address the potential needs should an incident occur.

All participants must identify what they believe their roles would be if an MCI were to occur. After this is completed, the group as a whole defines what will be needed by each participant. After discovering what each group has to offer in ways of personnel, equipment, and resources, discussion and planning are aimed at specific targets in the community that may be affected by an MCI.

It is advantageous to include in the preplan which group will supply the incident commander for a particular scene. For example, most incidents fall under the reign of the fire service. Some MCIs, however, would be under the direction of law enforcement, such as a sniper or hostage situation. A disaster may go beyond the scope of the fire service or law enforcement and fall under the realm of municipal, state, or federal government. An example of this is Hurricane Andrew, which devastated southern Florida. Since numerous incidents occurred at once over a wide geographical area, municipalities set up local command posts to address the needs of their particular area. On a larger scale the state government became the incident command center with the governor as the incident commander. The governor then solicited the aid of the federal government through the Federal Emergency Management Agency (FEMA).

After much discussion and preplanning, a "tabletop" exercise is planned with representatives from all involved agencies participating. It can be here that problems are discovered and preplans are modified. The representatives from the respective agencies then return to their personnel to review the preplans.

A mock MCI/disaster is then enacted with all participants engaging in their assigned duties. This must be taken seriously and made to be as realistic as possible. Representatives from outside agencies who have had experience in MCI/disaster planning should be invited to critique the exercise. After the mock disaster is completed, representatives from each agency, if not all participants of the exercise, are invited to a debriefing to review the observers' comments. It must be stressed to all participants that many mistakes are always made during exercises, and that traditionally, should the real incident occur, it will run smoother. No one should take the critique personally but should reflect on it as a mechanism for improvement.

Although mass casualty incidents and disasters occur infrequently, their effect on the community can be devastating. With proper planning and practice, the effect of this devastation can be minimized so that the community can gain some sense of normalcy in a short period of time.

SPECIAL EVENTS
Preparing for the Very Important Person (VIP)

Planning for visits from VIPs presents a unique set of circumstances that the EMS system must be prepared to handle. As with any other EMS event or incident, careful community planning and teamwork will create an atmosphere that will facilitate the safe response to any emergency that arises. Usually the dignitary (VIP) provides a group of people who are specially trained to assist in development of a plan before their visit. For example, the Secret Service will coordinate the security and EMS that will be used during a visit from the President or Vice President of the United States. They will meet with community leaders, as well as fire, police, and EMS officials weeks to months before an event and explain exactly what they want and how it is to be carried out. Each official, then, goes back to their respective departments and begins educating staff as to what their role will be on the day of the visit. When the President or Vice President visits the greater Cincinnati area, a paramedic unit from the Cincinnati Fire Division accompanies the motorcade from its origin at the airport to its multiple destinations. Secret Service agents accompany the EMS unit and instruct them as to where to go and what to do should some disaster arise. Because of the high security involved with the protection of the President, most EMS personnel are kept in the dark as to exactly what the nature of their service will be until some injury or illness occurs.

Predetermined treatment centers are designated ahead of time so that specialized physicians and extra security personnel can be commandeered and put on standby at the institution in case their services should be needed. It is important that each person carefully follow instructions, and not deviate unless instructed to do so by a superior. A carefully planned, coordinated effort between fire, police, EMS, community leaders, and the representatives of the VIP will facilitate the creation of a system that is capable and ready to handle any type of problem.

Mass Gatherings

Supplying EMS services to large gatherings of people can be intimidating and frightening. With careful planning and practice it is possible to provide service to hundreds of thousands of people. The main goals of EMS at any mass gathering are to gain rapid access to and triage of casualties, provide resources for stabilization and transfer of seriously ill or injured patients, provide sufficient facilities on site to deal adequately with minor complaints, coordinate patient evacuation, and help relieve the local hospitals of what otherwise could be an intolerable patient load (Farrow, 1972).

Methods described by Hnatow and Gordon (1991) for the planning and implementation of a medical system for a mass gathering include the following:

1. *Organization of medical care,* bringing all the agencies together who will be assuming responsibility for the health of the crowd. This would involve local EMS agencies, hospitals, American Red Cross, fire protection, and law enforcement.
2. *Planning elements.* Estimating the size, type, and condition of the crowd is absolute before plans can be developed. This can be accomplished by studying recent similar gatherings and evaluating their system and what problems transpired. It is estimated that approximately 1% to 2% of people attending large events will need medical care (Hnatow & Gordon, 1991). It is important to keep in mind variables such as why people are attending the event, alcohol use, and the weather.
3. *Personnel.* Variables such as the age of the audience, length of the event, movement

of the crowd, type of event, and the use of alcohol or drugs must be considered when determining the type and number of EMS personnel necessary for proper coverage. A ratio of one physician for every 16,000 attendees, one registered nurse for every 8000 attendees, and one paramedic for every 7000 attendees is suggested (Hnatow & Gordon, 1991).

4. *Medical triage and facilities.* A four-tiered triage response can be used and adapted so that critically ill or injured people may be transferred to an off-site tertiary care center. Tier one uses observers, such as police, ushers, and security personnel who can monitor the crowd and identify potential medical problems. If the patient is stable and ambulatory, they can direct them to local medical stations or call for assistance from tier two. Tier two involves a mobile treatment team that consists of a paramedic and assistants who can conduct triage on patients and transport them to the most appropriate facility. This transportation may be either by ambulance, golf cart, or on foot if the terrain or crowd density will not allow a motorized vehicle. The goal of the mobile treatment team is to transport the patient to the medical facility safely and expeditiously. Tier three involves medical facilities that are stations placed strategically throughout the event area that have the capability to provide first aid and triage to hospitals for those requiring more involved assessment or treatment. These facilities can be basic first-aid stations equipped with bandages and oxygen or more complex centers that can manage cardiac arrest until transportation can be arranged to an outside facility. The more-advanced stations ideally should be staffed with physicians, registered nurses, and EMT-paramedics. The fourth tier involves local hospitals that receive victims who are triaged and transported out of their facilities.

It is essential that transportation needs, communications, and public education are addressed in the preplanning phase. All medical areas and EMS personnel must be easily identified by any person who is seeking their assistance. A common error made in most large crowd events is the lack of record keeping for future data and medicolegal protection. The name, social security number, injury/illness, treatment rendered, and disposition of any person who is triaged or treated must be documented.

HAZARDOUS MATERIALS

It is 4:00 AM. You have just completed an interfacility transport and are returning to your base hospital. While driving on the interstate you notice that a tanker truck approximately 1 mile ahead of you has turned over. Naturally, you are concerned that someone may be injured, but you are also aware that if this tanker contains hazardous material you could jeopardize your own safety as well as that of your crew.

This situation is only one of a host of ways in which prehospital nurses could find themselves face-to-face with a hazardous materials incident. Unless special training is sought by the prehospital nurse, knowledge of hazardous materials is extremely limited.

Concern about the harmful effects of hazardous materials incidents has led to a demand for greater levels of emergency preparedness. Laws, such as Title III of the Superfund Amendments and Reauthorization Act (SARA) of 1986, the Environmental Protection Agency's "Chemical Emergency Preparedness Program," and Occupational Safety and Health Administration (OSHA) regulations, were enacted to enhance the skills and knowledge of emergency response personnel who might be involved in and respond to a hazardous materials incident. SARA Title III requires development of local emergency response plans that include training programs of local emergency response and medical personnel. Other sections of SARA Title III encompass emergency planning, emergency notification, community right-to-know reporting requirements, and toxic chemical release reporting/emissions inventory (Superfund Amendments and Reauthorization Act, 1986). OSHA states that training is required for all personnel who participate or are expected to participate in emergency response to hazardous materials accidents (Federal Register, 1989). OSHA has developed a four-tier training scheme that incorporates four different levels of emergency response skills. They include first responder awareness, first responder operations, hazardous materials technician, and hazardous materials specialist.

The first responder awareness program is aimed at "those persons who are likely to witness or discover a hazardous substance release,

and who have been trained to initiate an emergency response sequence by notifying the proper authorities of the release" (Borak, Callan, G Albott, 1991). Personnel at this level would not be caring for victims but would be restricted to observing and reporting only. This is the minimum level of training.

First responder operations respond to releases or potential releases of hazardous substances as part of the initial response for the purpose of protecting nearby persons, property, or the environment from the effects of the release. This would include EMS functions. EMS personnel at this response level work at a safe distance from the incident.

The next level, hazardous materials technician, involves individuals who are trained to enter the hazardous zone to plug, patch, or otherwise stop the release of the hazardous substance. Although the EMS system's goal would be to go in and safely extricate the victim from the hot zone, the person trained at this level may function far beyond that capacity. How-

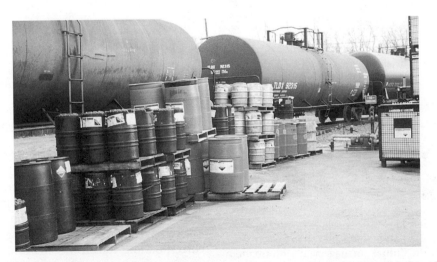

Fig. 3-18 Hazardous materials can be found in containers of any size in solid, liquid, or gaseous form. Here, multiple-size barrels are stacked next to train tankers filled with hazardous materials. If a spill would occur here, the rescuer would be faced with a myriad of different chemicals to which the patient and rescuer could be exposed.

ever, it is necessary for any EMS provider, be it a physician, nurse, paramedic, or EMT, who will be entering the point of release of the hazardous substance to be trained in both theory and practice at the hazardous materials technician level.

Hazardous materials specialists are expected to provide support and advanced knowledge to the hazardous materials technicians. Since their expertise incorporates the training of the hazardous materials technician and the advanced knowledge of hazardous materials incidents, they may be called on to be the authority at a hazardous materials scene (Borak, Callan, & Albott, 1991).

Identifying Potential Hazardous Materials

What exactly is a hazardous material? A hazardous material is any substance that, in its present state or changed state, endangers life,

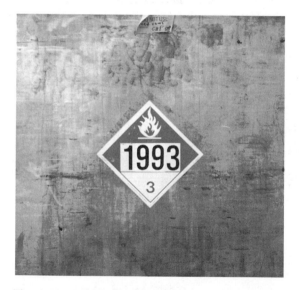

Fig. 3-19 This placard identifies the chemical in the container as a flammable liquid *(#3 in lower corner) (red)* with initial management information found in guide 27 of the DOT *Emergency Response Guide (middle # 1993).* The flame in the top corner identifies it as a flammable, either solid, liquid, or gas.

property, or the environment. Therefore any substance has the potential to be a hazardous material given the right set of circumstances. With this fact in mind, a high degree of suspicion is important, since any run may have the potential to become a hazardous materials incident. This may involve an overturned car with gasoline leaking, or perhaps chemical workers overcome by anhydrous ammonia. Because some hazardous materials may not be immediately identifiable or may have the potential to be misidentified, ways to identify hazardous materials are reviewed in the following sections (Figure 3-18).

Hazardous materials are given an international classification number that may be displayed in the bottom of placards or in the hazardous materials description on shipping papers (Figure 3-19). Each class is broken down into divisions that further delineate the potential properties of the substance, as shown by the following (U.S. DOT, 1990):

Class	Substance
I	Explosives
II	Gases
III	Flammable liquids
IV	Flammable solids, including spontaneously combustible materials, and materials that are dangerous when wet
V	Oxidizers and organic peroxides
VI	Poisonous and etiologic (infectious) materials
VII	Radioactive materials
VIII	Corrosives
IX	Miscellaneous hazardous materials

If the substance cannot be identified by the number in the lower corner of the placard or from the shipping papers, the symbol on the placards and the color code can provide valuable information about the contents. The following list identifies the placard color and the corresponding hazardous material (U.S. Environmental Protection Agency, 1986):

Color	Hazardous material
Orange	Explosives
Red	Flammables

Green	Nonflammable gas
White and red stripes	Flammable solid
Yellow	Oxidizers/peroxides
White	Poisons
Yellow over white	Radioactive materials
White over black	Corrosives
White (blank)	Other regulated material

The following coding system for placards and labels uses symbols to indicate dangers and hazards (U.S. Environmental Protection Agency, 1986):

Symbol	Hazardous material
Bursting ball	Explosives
Flame	Flammables
Cylinder	Nonflammable gas
"O" with flames	Oxidizers
Skull and crossbones	Poisons
Propeller	Radioactive materials
Tipped test tube	Corrosives

All placards and labels must contain a United Nations identification number. This number can be used to identify a chemical or it may indicate groups of chemicals with similar hazards. When this four-digit number is obtained, the first responder can refer to the *Emergency Response Guidebook (ERG),* published by the U.S. Department of Transportation, Research and Special Programs Administration, to obtain information on the type of chemical, potential hazards, and emergency action needed. If the four-digit number is not available and the placard is visible, the *ERG* can give the first responder direction until more information is gained. After a material is identified using the *ERG,* the rescuer may refer to the National Institute for Occupational Safety and Health (NIOSH) *Pocket Guide to Chemical Hazards.* This reference guide provides more information than the *ERG,* allowing the rescuer to obtain exposure limits, chemical and physical properties, personal protection, health hazards, and so forth (U.S. Department of Health and Human Services, 1990) (Figures 3-20 to 3-22).

The National Fire Protection Association (NFPA) has developed a marking system for

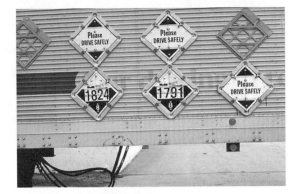

Fig. 3-20 Using the 1990 *Emergency Response Guidebook,* the contents of this trailer can be identified by the placards. The symbol at the top of the triangle identifies the ingredients as a corrosive. The numbers 1824 and 1791 identify the substances as lye, sodium hydrate, or caustic soda solution (#1824) and a hypochlorite solution (#1791).

identifying hazardous materials. Information is provided as to the health, flammability, and reactivity risks of a chemical. The severity of each risk is ranked on a scale from 4 to 0, with 4 representing the greatest risk, and 0 no risk. The information is color coded. Health information is blue, flammability information is red, and reactivity information is yellow. The square diamond with its identifiable points of blue, red, and yellow can be found on most chemical containers. The fourth corner at the bottom is white, containing special information such as "radioactive," or "dangerous when wet" (Borak, Callan, & Albott, 1991) (Figures 3-23 and 3-24). If a Bill of Lading or a placard is not available, the prehospital nurse must consider the materials hazardous and take the proper precautions until proven otherwise.

Hazardous Materials—Plan of Action

The first rule of medicine is "do no harm." This axiom holds particularly true when dealing with hazardous materials. The worse-case

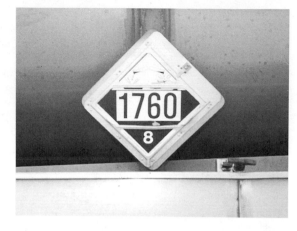

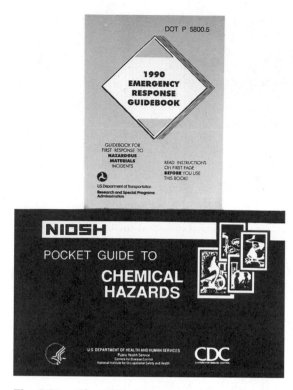

Fig. 3-21 The 1990 *Emergency Response Guidebook* (ERG) and the NIOSH *Pocket Guide to Chemical Hazards* are only two examples of numerous texts available to rescuers that help them make decisions during the advent of a hazardous materials incident. The *ERG* is useful in the immediate identification of a substance, and the NIOSH guide provides more detail about the properties of the chemical and how to protect the rescuer and patient.

Fig. 3-22 Using the *Emergency Response Guidebook*, the rescuer can identify the container contents by the placard. The top of the triangle (test tubes spilling on the hand and piece of solid material) and number 8 in the lower part of the triangle identifies the contents as a corrosive. The UN number (1760) identifies it as one of 31 corrosive materials. It would be necessary to gain more information from the Material Safety Data Sheet or Bill of Lading.

scenario is not one where a victim succumbs to and dies of exposure to a hazardous material, but rather the victim *and* "heroic" rescuers succumb to and die of exposure to a hazardous material. Until the properly trained personnel and equipment become available, distance is the greatest ally. Actions to be taken by first responders, along with identification of the hazardous material, is to set up isolation and protective action distances. Using the *ERG* the first

responder can quickly determine the isolation distance and the protective action distance. According to the *ERG*, 150 feet is the minimum distance required for isolating the unprotected public from any spilled material. The smallest protective action distance is 1000 feet. These distances are approximated from the gases that could be released airborne, traveling in 30 minutes with a 10 mile per hour wind speed (U.S. Department of Transportation, Research and Special Programs Administration, 1990). It is important to note that these are calculated for a no-fire spill incident during transport.

The protective action area is the area where steps need to be taken to preserve the health and safety of emergency responders and the public during an incident involving the release of hazardous materials. People in this area may need to be evacuated, protected in place, inside

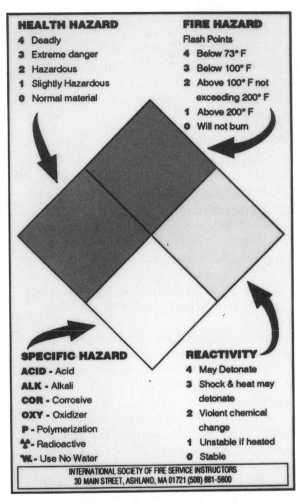

Fig. 3-23 Breakdown of National Fire Protection Association Marking system for hazardous materials (reprinted from *Haz Mat Incident Guide* with permission of ISFSI, 30 Main Street, Ashland, MA 01721. The complete *Haz Mat Incident Guide* may be purchased through ISFSI by calling 800-435-0005.)

buildings, or both. No one should enter the isolation area unless protected by the proper equipment, garb, self-contained breathing apparatus, and the like (Figure 3-25).

During the identification of the hazardous

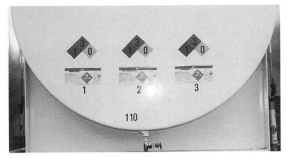

Fig. 3-24 National Fire Protection Association marking system for hazardous materials providing health (blue), flammability (red), reactivity (yellow), and special information (white) information on hazardous chemicals. The number system 0 to 4 rates the risk, with 4 being severe and 0 being no risk.

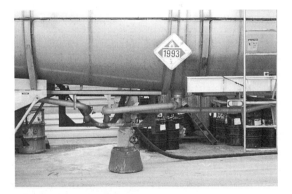

Fig. 3-25 Accidental spills of hazardous materials most commonly occur during the transfer of substances from one container to another.

material and the set up of the isolation and protective action zones, it is necessary to call the Chemical Transportation Emergency Center (CHEMTREC). CHEMTREC is a service of the Chemical Manufacturer's Association and operates around the clock to receive toll-free calls from the United States and Canada, providing immediate advice for the on-scene commander. CHEMTREC can usually provide immediate

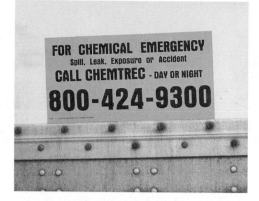

Fig. 3-26 Sometimes the phone number of CHEMTREC may be located on the side of the containers, as seen on this truck. The CHEMTREC phone number must be readily available for the EMS first responder.

hazard information, warnings, and guidance when given the identification number, the name of the product, and the nature of the problem. If this information is not available, the CHEMTREC communicator needs as much information about the incident as possible. The CHEMTREC number can be dialed directly at 1-800-424-9300. If your phone line cannot receive calls, it is important that the line be maintained with the CHEMTREC communicator continuously (Figure 3-26). Information to give CHEMTREC includes the following:

1. Name and callback number
2. Nature and location of the problem
3. Name of carrier, shipper, or facility operator and responsible party
4. Container type, rail car or truck number, vessel name, or other identifying information (U.S. Department of Transportation, Research and Special Programs Administration, 1990).

The National Response Center (NRC), operated by the U.S. Coast Guard, receives reports required from spillers of hazardous substances. The NRC also acts as the notification, commu-

nications, technical assistance, and coordination center for the National Response Team. After receiving a report, the NRC immediately relays the information to the responsible federal on-scene coordinator. The NRC can telephonically connect the caller with the coordinator or other official.

Decontamination

The isolation area commonly referred to as the *hot zone* is set up, and the hazardous material technicians enter the zone to perform rescue, containment of the spill, and cleanup. This team, which has now made contact with the chemical, must not spread it outside of the hot zone, thereby contaminating other people and the environment. A single point of entry is made whereby the people leaving the hot zone are decontaminated before entering unprotected areas.

Decontamination is the process by which personnel, apparatus, equipment, and supplies are made safe by the removal of hazardous substances. The procedure may be as simple as a wash down with water from a small hose to a more complex and time-consuming event. No matter what the scenario, the hazardous materials team must be prepared to carry out the decontamination procedure at any level. There are five general methods of decontamination; they include:

Dilution—A method of reducing the concentration of the contaminant to a level at which it is no longer harmful. Water is used except when the potential exists for a chemical reaction.

Absorption—A process of picking up the hazardous substance with an absorbent material. Kitty litter, clay, soil, and commercially available products may be used. When complete, the absorbent must be disposed of properly.

Degradation—A process of altering the chemical structure of the hazardous material by mixing it with another reactive chemical. The purpose is to render the hazardous material into a less harmful substance. (Degradation is seldom used for decontamination of victims with acid or alkali exposure because of the potential for burns from the chemical reaction.)

Isolation and disposal—Methods used for any equipment that cannot be decontaminated by other methods.

Special equipment may be needed to complete the decontamination process. Showers may need to be constructed, and all run-off must be collected for disposal. The decontamination area must be upwind from the incident and not in the potential path of run-off from the chemical.

When leaving the hot zone, workers enter the decontamination area. Borak and colleagues (1991) have broken down the steps of decontamination into a nine-station decontamination procedure.

- *Station I, entry point from the hot zone.* The team mechanically removes as much of the contaminants as possible from the victims and rescuers. Equipment used in the hot zone is left in a tool drop area located in station I.
- *Station II, gross decontamination.* The rescue personnel and victims are showered or scrubbed by the decontamination personnel. At this point, victims may be transported directly to station VI for full body washing; if not, they proceed to station III with the rescuers.
- *Station III, protective clothing removal.* All protective clothing is removed and placed in a plastic bag, labeled, and then moved to the side for later disposal. If the rescuer has donned multiple layers of protective clothing, the station can be divided into multiple sections to accommodate the removal of each layer of clothing.
- *Station IV, self-contained breathing apparatus (SCBA) removal.* SCBAs are removed and isolated. If reentry is necessary, change

over and replacement of SCBAs may be accomplished in station IV.
- *Station V, personal clothing removal.* All personal clothing and items such as rings and watches are removed and bagged. Victims not undressed at station II should be totally undressed at this station.
- *Station VI, body washing.* Full body washing is performed using soft scrub brushes or sponges and soap or mild detergents. Liberal rinsing with water should be performed.
- *Station VII, dry off.* Disposable towels and sheets are used to dry the entire body. Disposable coveralls or hospital gowns may be used and placed on the rescuer and victim.
- *Station VIII, medical assessment.* At this station the prehospital nurse has the first contact with the patient. A rapid patient assessment should be completed with all wounds being cleansed and bandaged. Stabilization and poison control recommendations should be followed at this time.
- *Station IX, transport to definitive care.* The rescuers or victims are transported to receiving hospitals for further medical attention or to areas for rest and observation. It is important to note that rescuers in fully encapsulated suits run the risk of heat-related emergencies. During the rescue the suit isolates them from the external environment. Normal mechanisms for cooling, such as convection, are inhibited. After decontamination, rest and fluid replacement are usually needed.

The material presented has been a brief overview of the decontamination procedure. It is important to remember that this is not all inclusive, and proper training and practice as recommended by OSHA are necessary before undertaking such a task.

Protection of EMS Personnel

When prehospital nurses are notified that they will be receiving a victim from a hazardous material incident, it is important that they begin to take the steps necessary to prevent contamination of themselves, their equipment, the public, and the receiving hospital. While in the field, it is important that access to the patients and contaminated area be limited to as few personnel as needed. Decontamination of all personnel is mandatory before loading onto the ambulance. Depending on the type of contaminating chemicals, rescuers should use disposable chemical-protective clothing, goggles, shoe covers, masks, and latex or vinyl gloves. The ambulance should be protected by lining the interior with heavy-duty plastic sheets and duct tape. All equipment that is nonessential and portable must be removed from the vehicle.

Since residual contaminants may remain on a victim despite the most aggressive decontamination procedures, ambulance ventilation is vital during transport to prevent contamination and injury of the prehospital worker. If the victim is in dire straits and a full decontamination process could not take place before loading on the ambulance, then the prehospital nurse may need to don a self-containing breathing apparatus for the transport. Early notification of the emergency department at the receiving hospital is necessary so that proper precautions may be implemented.

The charge nurse at the receiving institution must commandeer personnel who will be strictly dedicated to the incoming contaminated victim and will have no other patient care responsibilities. A triage area is set up outside of the hospital to control the flow of contaminated victims inside the hospital proper. A single, separate emergency department entrance is designated leading to an area where further decontamination along with patient assessment and treatment can be started.

Proper garb, such as chemical-resistant suits, goggles, boots, gloves, and masks, should be worn until complete decontamination and removal of the contaminant have been accomplished. All garbage and used items must be bagged and labeled as *contaminated* for proper disposal.

A personal exposure log must be kept on all personnel, both prehospital and emergency, who have had direct contact with hazardous materials victims and their contaminants. All personnel exposed to a documented hazardous material must have a medical examination to detect the possible effects of that exposure. Education of the possible untoward side effects of the contaminant and follow-up are mandatory.

As evidenced by the potential complexity of a hazardous materials incident, education, training, and practice are vital to the proper handling of a hazardous material incident. Professional rescuers must always be concerned with their safety as well as that of fellow rescuers, the public, and the environment, taking precautions to prevent further harm from such materials.

REFERENCES

Academy of Medicine of Cincinnati. (1993). *Protocols and standing orders for paramedic services.* Cincinnati, OH: Academy of Medicine.

American College of Emergency Medical Services Committee. (1984). Control of advanced life support at the scene of medical emergencies. *Annals of Emergency Medicine, 13*(7), 547-548.

Association of Air Medical Services. (1990). Position paper on the appropriate use of emergency air medical services. *The Journal of Air Medical Transport, 9*(9), 29-33.

Bledsoe, B.E., Porter, R.S., & Shade, B.R. (1991). Gynecological emergencies. *Paramedic emergency care* (pp. 921-922). Englewood Cliffs, NJ: Prentice-Hall/Brady.

Borak, J., Callan, M., & Albott, W. (1991). *Hazardous materials exposure: Emergency response and patient care.* Englewood Cliffs, NJ: Prentice-Hall/Brady.

Butman, A.M. (1985). *Responding to the mass casualty incident: A guide for EMS personnel.* Akron, OH: Emergency Training.

Campbell, J.E. (1988a). Field evaluation and management of the trauma patient. *Basic trauma life support advanced prehospital care* (2nd ed.). (pp. 21-41). Englewood Cliffs, NJ: Prentice-Hall/Brady.

Campbell, J.E. (1988b). Mechanism of injuries due to motion. *Basic trauma life support advanced prehospital care* (2nd ed.). (pp. 1-20). Englewood Cliffs, NJ: Prentice-Hall/Brady.

Campbell, J.E. (1988c). Spinal trauma. *Basic trauma life support advanced prehospital care* (2nd ed.). (pp. 120-132). Englewood Cliffs, NJ: Prentice-Hall/Brady.

Childs, B.J., & Ptacnik, D.J. (1986). Emergency driving. *Emergency ambulance driving* (pp. 141-142). Englewood Cliffs, NJ: Prentice-Hall/Brady.

Clawson, J.J. (1991). Running "hot" and the case of Sharon Rose. *Journal of Emergency Medical Services, 16*(7), 11-13.

Clawson, J.J., & Dernocoeur, K.B. (1988). Dispatch priority card concepts. *Principles of emergency medical dispatch.* (pp. 58-61). Englewood Cliffs, NJ: Prentice-Hall/Brady.

DeLorenzo, R.A. (1992). Bright lights, big noise: how effective are vehicle warning systems? *Journal of Emergency Medical Services, 17*(6), 57-62.

Emergency Nurses Association. (1991). *National standard guidelines for prehospital nursing curriculum.* Chicago: The Author.

Farrow, R.J. (1972). Pop music festivals. *Practitioner,* pp. 208, 380-386.

Federal Emergency Management Agency. (1989). *National Fire Academy—Incident command system—student manual.* Washington, DC: U.S. Government Printing Office.

Federal Register, 54 (March 6, 1989), 9294-9330.

Garcia, L.M. (1985). *Disaster nursing planning, assessment, and intervention.* Rockville, MD: Aspen.

General Services Administration. (1990). *KKK-A-1822C federal specification for ambulances.* Washington, DC: U.S. Government Printing Office.

Grant, H.D., Murray, R.H., & Bergeron, J.D. (1994a). Breathing aids and oxygen therapy. *Emergency care* (6th ed.). (pp. 188-191). Englewood Cliffs, NJ: Prentice-Hall/Brady.

Grant, H.D., Murray, R.H., & Bergeron, J.D. (1994b). Vehicle rescue. *Emergency care* (6th ed.). (pp. 706-729). Englewood Cliffs, NJ: Prentice-Hall/Brady.

Hafen, B.Q., & Frandsen, K.J. (1985). Psychological aspects of disaster. *Psychological emergencies and crisis intervention* (pp. 304-305). Englewood, CO: Morton.

Hafen, B.Q., & Karren, K.J. (1989). Stabilization and transportation. *Prehospital emergency care and crisis intervention* (pp. 639-661). Englewood, CO: Morton.

Heckman, J.D. (Ed.). (1992a). Extrication. *Emergency care and transportation of the sick and injured* (5th ed.). (pp. 700-731). Park Ridge, IL: American Academy of Orthopaedic Surgeons.

Heckman, J.D. (Ed.). (1992b). The modern emergency vehicle. *Emergency care and transportation of the sick and injured* (5th ed.). (pp. 735-747). Park Ridge, IL: American Academy of Orthopaedic Surgeons.

Henry, M.C., & Stapleton, E.R. (1992a). Ambulance operations. *EMT prehospital care* (pp. 755-792). Philadelphia: W.B. Saunders.

Henry, M.C., & Stapleton, E.R. (1992b). Extrication. *EMT prehospital care* (pp. 735-753). Philadelphia: W.B. Saunders.

Hnatow, D.A., & Gordon, D.J. (1991). Medical planning for mass gatherings: A retrospective review of the San Antonio papal mass. *Prehospital and Disaster Medicine, 6*(4), 443-450.

Holmquist, P., Lee, G., & Songne, E.A. (1989). Field photography: An aid to trauma patient evaluation. *Journal of Emergency Nursing, 15*(5), 434-435.

Jones, S.A., Weigel, A., White, R.D., McSwain, N.E., & Breiter, M. (1992). The Emergency Medical Services system. *Advanced emergency care for paramedic practice* (pp. 9-18). Philadelphia: J.B. Lippincott.

Lucia, J. (1993). On the ball behind the wheel. *Journal of Emergency Medical Services, 18*(4), 50-59.

Natt, D. (1989). Nonsystem physicians. In A. Kuehle (Ed.), *Emergency medical director's handbook* (pp. 267-270). St. Louis: Mosby.

Noose, G. (1989). A second set of victims: Search and rescue perspectives. *Emergency Medical Services, 18*(8), 81-87.

Superfund Amendments and Reauthorization Act of 1986, Title III, S 303(c) (8), 100 STAT, 1732.

U.S. Department of Health and Human Services. (1990). *National Institute for Occupational Safety and Health pocket guide to chemical hazards.* Washington, DC: U.S. Government Printing Office.

U.S. Department of Transportation, National Highway Traffic Safety Administration. (1978). *Training program for operation of emergency vehicles.* Washington, DC: U.S. Government Printing Office.

U.S. Department of Transportation, Research and Special Programs Administration. (1990). *1990 Emergency response guidebook (DOT p 5800.5).* Washington, DC: U.S. Government Printing Office.

U.S. Environmental Protection Agency. (1986). Identification of hazardous materials. *Emergency response to hazardous materials incidents (165.15). 9,* pp. 5-55.

PART TWO

The Practice of Prehospital Nursing

CHAPTER 4

Patient Transport

OBJECTIVES

1. Identify the history of patient transport
2. Discuss indications for patient transport
3. Describe the impact of transport on the patient

COMPETENCIES

1. Identify indications for patient transport
2. Name the advantages and disadvantages of patient transport
3. Identify equipment that is necessary for safe patient transport

One of the major roles that nurses play in the care of the patient in the prehospital nursing environment is patient transport. Over the past 20 years patient transport has evolved into a well-established specialty involving the use of sophisticated equipment and techniques. There are no longer any patients who are too sick to move.

This chapter discusses the history, indications, related legal implications, methods, and risks of patient transport. A list of equipment for patient transport, whether by air or ground, is provided at the end of the chapter.

HISTORICAL PERSPECTIVE

Early accounts of transport of wounded soldiers cited the need to move victims from the battlefield. As early as 1500 BC records were kept regarding triage systems for injured patients (Cales & Heilig, 1988; Carter, Couch, &

O'Brien, 1988). The Code of Hammurabi regulated fees for the trauma surgeon. Romans and Greeks always had a physician in attendance on the battlefield to identify the severely wounded and direct their evacuation.

The first modern method of patient transport employed a horsedrawn cart. This method was developed and directed by Napoleon's surgeon, Dominique Larrey (Carter et al., 1988). The first air transport of injured patients was believed to have occurred in 1870 in France (McNab, 1992), but actually the first air ambulance transports were conducted by the United States Army in 1918 (Carter et al., 1988).

The United States military recognized early the benefits of rapid transport from the battlefield to more definitive care. Patient mortality and morbidity decreased after each world war because of the use of transport. After World War I there was an 8% decrease in mortality and morbidity, and after World War II there was a 4.5% decrease. A 2.5% decrease occurred after the Korean and Vietnam conflicts, during which time helicopter transport of the wounded from the battlefield and mobile army surgical hospitals (MASH) were begun (Cales & Heilig, 1988; Carter et al., 1988).

In the 1950s research was initiated that looked at the mortality and morbidity of civilian trauma in the United States. Two issues continued to be identified as major factors contributing to an increase in mortality and morbidity: (1) the amount of time it took to transport an injured individual to definitive care and (2) the skills of the individuals who were providing prehospital care.

In 1966 a White Paper entitled "Accidental Death and Disability—the Neglected Disease of Modern Society" was published by the National Academy of Sciences/National Research Council and pointed to the need for a more organized system to provide care for the injured. This landmark paper paved the way for President Johnson's signing of the National Traffic and Motor Vehicle Safety Act and the Highway Safety Act, which tied federal funding in with the development of state Emergency Medical Service (EMS) agencies (Cales & Heilig, 1986). Federal monies continue to be tied to safety issues such as seat belt and helmet usage, as witnessed in the 1992 bill that provides for state highway funding contingent on the passage of state seat belt and helmet laws.

In 1973 the EMS Act was signed into law. This began the organization of emergency medical services by providing guidelines and a curriculum for the education of prehospital care providers (Blackwell, 1993). Even though there is a specific curriculum that outlines the basic education for all emergency medical technician—ambulance (EMTAs) and paramedics, the types of procedures and medications they may administer vary from state to state.

In 1972 the first hospital-based helicopter program was created using a nurse to deliver patient care in Denver, Colorado (Semonin-

Holleran, 1993). In 1975 the Children's Hospital in Columbus, Ohio, reported using a National Guard helicopter to transport critically ill and injured children (Harris, Orr, & Boles, 1975). A specific transport system that used pediatric nurses and physicians was developed in Denver in 1980 (Dobrin, Block, & Gilman, 1980).

Patient transport using both air and ground methods was developed in the 1980s. Today there are multiple public and private services that offer patient transport.

INDICATIONS FOR PATIENT TRANSPORT

Indications for patient transport range from those based on specific research to the need for resources not obtainable at certain health-care facilities. As for a national standard that dictates the need for patient transport, there is currently not one available.

In general, patient transport or transfer is needed in the following situations (Rea, 1991; Hart, Haynes, Schwaitzberg, & Harris, 1987; Haley, 1993):

- Nursing and medical expertise are not available at the referring health-care facility.
- Diagnostic procedures are not available at the referring health-care facility.
- The benefits of transfer outweigh its risks.
- The family requests that their family member be transferred.

In addition to these general guidelines, certain illnesses or injuries necessitate patient transport to another facility or to a definite location. The following is a summary of some of these indications.

The Trauma Patient

The greatest amount of research into the need for transport has focused on the patient who has been traumatically injured. As noted in the section on the history of transport, the first transport of patients involved those who had been injured during battle.

General guidelines that indicate the need for the trauma patient to be transported to a higher level of care such as a level I or II trauma center are presented in an article by Hart et al. (1987). These include:

1. Serious injury to one or more organ systems
2. Hypovolemic shock requiring more than one transfusion
3. Orthopedic injuries involving:
   a. Two or more long bone fractures
   b. Fractures of the thoracic cage
   c. Compromised neurovascular status
   d. Fracture of the axial skeleton
   e. Spinal cord injuries
   f. Blunt abdominal trauma with hemodynamic instability
   g. Patients requiring advanced ventilatory support
   h. Extremity reimplantation
4. Head injuries involving:
   a. Cerebral/spinal leak
   b. Altered mental status
   c. Deteriorating neurological status
   d. Increased intracranial pressure

Specific guidelines for the transport of trauma patients by helicopter include (Baxt, 1986; Boyd, Corse, & Campbell, 1989; Burney et al., 1990; Champion, 1986; Garrison, Benson, & Whitley, 1986):

1. Transport time by ground to a trauma center is greater than 15 minutes
2. Ground transport is impeded either to access or egress from the scene of injury
3. Presence of multiple victims
4. Time to local hospital via ambulance is greater than the time to the trauma center via helicopter
5. Wilderness rescue
6. Ground transport will delay local response capability

Additional methods that have been used to identify indications for transport or transfer of trauma patients include mechanism of injury and scoring systems. Mechanisms of injury that may indicate a severely injured patient and the need for transfer and transport to a higher level of care include (NAEMSP, 1992):

1. Accident at speeds greater than 55 miles per hour
2. Patient entrapment
3. Death of others involved in the same accident
4. Falls from heights greater than 15 feet
5. Penetrating trauma to the abdomen, pelvis, chest, neck, or head
6. Crushing injuries to the abdomen, chest, or head
7. Major burns of the body surface area, burns involving the face, hands, feet, or perineum, or burns with significant respiratory involvement or major electric or chemical burns
8. Patients who have been involved in a serious traumatic event who are younger than 12 or older than 55 years of age
9. Patients with near-drowning injuries, with or without existing hypothermia
10. Adult patients with any of the following vital sign changes: systolic blood pressure <90 mm Hg; respiratory rate <10 or >35 breaths per minute; heart rate <60 or >120 beats per minute; unresponsive to verbal stimuli

Scoring systems that have been used include:
- Trauma/Revised Trauma Score
- CRAMS (see Table 6-7)
- Trauma Triage Rule
- Glasgow Coma Scale

Cardiovascular Emergencies

Some research has identified reasons to transfer and transport the patient with a cardiovascular emergency. These indications include (Gabram, Piancentini, & Jacobs, 1990; Burney et al., 1990):

1. The need for cardiac intensive care that is not available at the referring facility

2. The need for cardiac catheterization and definitive surgery
3. Treatment for cardiogenic shock that may include insertion of a balloon pump, mechanical assist devices, or experimental medications
4. The need for organ transplant

Other Patient Examples

Other patients that are transferred and transported include the pregnant patient and the neonate. Indications for maternal transport include:

- Placenta previa or placenta abruptio
- Fetal distress
- Maternal trauma
- Prenatal complications such as diabetes and eclampsia
- Perimortem delivery

Indications for neonatal transport include:

- Premature and low–birth weight infants
- Neonatal illness
- Neonatal injury

PRINCIPLES OF APPROPRIATE PATIENT TRANSFER
Legal Implications

In 1986 the Consolidated Omnibus Reconciliation Act (COBRA) was implemented. This legislation furnishes guidelines, regulations, and penalties that govern patient transfer and transport. Included in the COBRA are the following provisions that govern the legal implications of patient transport (Southard, 1989):

1. All hospitals must examine all patients who come to the emergency department and must provide the necessary medical care.
2. Patients are not to be transferred until stabilized.
3. Documentation must be provided that the patient will receive better care at the receiving facility.
4. Ambulances, fixed-wing aircraft, and he-

Box 4-1
AMERICAN COLLEGE OF EMERGENCY PHYSICIANS GUIDELINES FOR TRANSFER

1. The health and well-being of the patient must be the overriding concern when any patient transport is considered.
2. The patient should be evaluated before transfer.
3. The patient should be stabilized as much as possible by the referring facility before transport.
4. The patient and patient's family should be informed about the reasons for and the risks of transport.
5. The patient should be transferred to a facility appropriate to the medical needs of the patient, with adequate space and personnel available.
6. The receiving facility must agree to accept the patient.
7. Economic reasons should not be the basis for transferring or refusing a patient at a receiving facility.
8. Communication about the patient's condition and initial care to the receiving facility must occur.
9. The patient should be transferred in a vehicle that is staffed by quality personnel and contains appropriate equipment for the patient who is being transferred.
10. When possible, written protocols and transfer agreements should be in place.

From "Principles of Appropriate Transfer" by American College of Emergency Physicians, 1990, *Annals of Emergency Medicine, 3,* p. 337.

licopters must have appropriate personnel and equipment to make the transfer.

The American College of Surgeons (ACEP) has developed guidelines for the appropriate transfer of the patient. These guidelines are summarized in Box 4-1. Currently, the American Association of Critical Care Nurses and the

---

Box 4-2

SUMMARY OF THE GUIDELINES FOR THE TRANSPORT OF THE CRITICALLY ILL PATIENT

1. The benefits of patient transfer should outweigh the risks.
2. The practitioner needs to be aware of the legal implications of patient transfer and transport.
3. Pretransport coordination and communication should include physician-to-physician contact, decision about the mode of transportation, nurse-to-nurse contact and communication, and securing a copy of all medical records relevant to the patient's care.
4. Accompanying transport personnel should be a minimum of two patient care providers and a vehicle operator. At least one care provider should be a registered nurse.
5. Equipment should be available to manage the patient's airway, breathing, and circulation, including monitors and medications. Communication equipment that is used during transport should be available.
6. Continuous monitoring should occur during transport. Minimal monitoring includes EKG monitoring and vital sign monitoring. Patients with specific problems may require additional monitoring such as capnography and invasive monitoring.

From "Guidelines for the Transport of the Critically Ill Patient" by Guidelines Committee of the American College of Critical Care Medicine and Transfer Guidelines Task Force American Association of Critical Care Nurses, 1993.

American College of Critical Care Medicine have proposed guidelines for the transport of the critically ill patient. Box 4-2 contains a summary of these guidelines that address both the interhospital and intrahospital transport of critically ill patients.

In addition to the legal implications and appropriate transfer guidelines, several other factors need to be considered when a decision has been made to transfer and transport a particular patient. The first factor is identification of a receiving facility. When choosing a receiving facility, nursing and medical personnel need to look at available resources at a potential receiving facility. Such resources as specialized staff, equipment, and expertise need to be considered. The distance of the receiving facility from the referring facility is also an important consideration.

A second factor that should be appraised involves the existence of written policies and agreements between receiving and referring facilities. Identification of centers that are capable of providing certain types of services and generating triage guidelines could save time.

The third factor involves what mode of transportation should be used to get the patient to more definitive care. Both ground and air offer advantages and disadvantages (see Modes of Transport).

In summary, when transporting ill or injured patients, transport services should provide the following (Crippen, 1990):

- The expertise necessary for safe initial assessment and stabilization before and during transport
- A staff capable of using the equipment and technology necessary to deliver care during transport to specific groups of patients such as critically ill or injured patients
- A reason why the transport will make a difference in patient outcome

MODES OF TRANSPORT

Several variables need to be contemplated when selecting a mode of transportation (Boyd & Hungerpiller, 1990; Blunt & Crowther, 1992). These include the following:

- The surrounding geography of both the referring and receiving facilities

- The distance the patient will need to be transported
- The amount of time it will take to get to the receiving facility
- The patient's condition and potential problems that may develop before arriving at the receiving facility
- Traffic and road conditions
- Weather conditions at referring and receiving facilities and en route
- The number of patients a particular transport vehicle can transport
- The crew composition of each mode of transportation

There are advantages and disadvantages to what mode of transportation is selected for a particular type of patient or patient problem.

Ground Transport

As previously discussed, the first method of transport of the ill or injured patient was by ground. Ground transport methods included being carried by another person, on an animal, or in a wagon or cart. Vehicles designated as ambulances were used in the early twentieth century in New York and Cincinnati. Today, ground transport vehicles not only may provide basic transport services but also may be

equipped as intensive care units capable of allowing the delivery of complicated technical care during transport (Figure 4-1).

Advantages of ground transport include the following (Boyd & Hungerpiller, 1990):

- Availability of ground vehicles
- Adequate work space
- Capable of traveling in any kind of weather
- Space may allow the capability to carry more personnel
- Sensitive monitoring equipment may function better

Disadvantages of ground transport include the following (Boyd & Hungerpiller, 1990):

- May take three times longer to transport a person by ground than by air (rotor wing)
- Poor road conditions may make ground transport uncomfortable for the patient, as well as potentially dangerous
- In some communities when the ground service is providing patient transfer and transport, there is not a vehicle available for emergency response

Air Transport

Hospital-based air transport began in 1972. Today, patient transport by air may be accom-

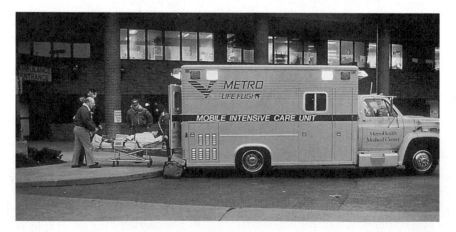

Fig. 4-1   Critical care ground ambulance, Metro Life Flight, Cleveland, Ohio.

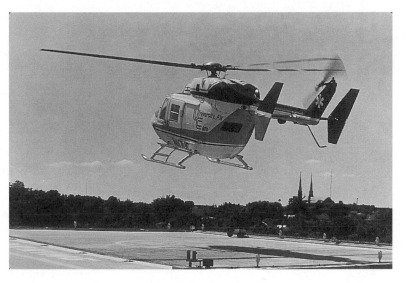

Fig. 4-2   BK 117 helicopter, University Air Care, Cincinnati, Ohio.

plished in either a rotor- or fixed-wing aircraft (Figure 4-2).

Advantages of air transport include the following (Boyd & Hungerpiller, 1990):
- Saves time
- Crew composition generally provides advanced levels of care
- Improved communication capability
- Heightened emergency response at the receiving facility
- Continued availability of ground EMS resources within the referral area

Disadvantages of air transport include the following: (Boyd & Hungerpiller, 1990):
- Weather restrictions may impede the availability of rotor- and fixed-wing transport
- Potentially more costly
- Physiological impact may be detrimental to the patient
- Psychological impact, particularly fear of flying, may be detrimental to the patient

RISKS OF TRANSPORT

No matter what method is chosen for the transport of the ill or injured patient, risks may be involved. Some of these risks include the possibility of an accident during transport, the potential for death or further injury during transport because of inadequate equipment or inexperienced transport crew(s), delay in arriving at the definitive care facility because of vehicle failure or environmental obstacles such as a snow or rain storm, and loss of communication during transport with medical direction (Boyd & Hungerpiller, 1990; Preston, 1992).

IMPACT OF TRANSPORT

Whenever a patient needs to be moved from one location to another, whether it is from the scene of injury or from an intensive care unit to another intensive care unit, the patient is potentially at risk to develop additional problems and complications. Both ground and air transport can potentially have an impact on the patient and the equipment that is used during transport. Sources of additional stress on the patient during transport may come from atmospheric changes and vibration during air transport, noise, and environmental temperature changes, which can occur during both ground

Table 4-1   Physiological Impact of Air Transport

Physiological Change	Effects	Interventions
1. Altitude changes	1. Hypoxia	1. Apply supplemental oxygen Place patient on pulse oximeter Use end tidal CO_2 monitor to monitor tube placement
2. Changes in barometric pressure	2. Expansion of gases as altitude increases; changes in equipment containing air, such as PSAGs, endotracheal tubes, air splints, IV bags, and bottles	2. Monitor air expansion effects on equipment and adjust as needed Place saline in endotracheal tube Vent IV bottles Monitor IV rates on ascent and descent
3. Temperature changes	3. Hypothermia, heat stress	3. Keep patients warm by applying blankets Remove any wet dressings before transport If warm, be sure there is adequate ventilation
4. Dehydration	4. Less moisture at higher altitude	4. Fluid administration as needed
5. Noise	5. Increase in metabolic rate and oxygen consumption	5. Apply hearing protection
6. Vibration	6. Increase in metabolic rate and oxygen consumption	6. Explain events to patient to decrease the impact of vibration

and air transport. Some potential complications or problems that may develop from these additional stresses include hypoxia, loss of temperature control, and nausea and vomiting. Table 4-1 contains a summary of the physiological impact of air transport (Semonin-Holleran, 1993; Blumen & Dunne, 1992).

EQUIPMENT FOR TRANSPORT

A comprehensive list of equipment necessary to stock both ground and air transport services consists of a core set of supplies with more similarities than differences. The following equipment list serves as a guide for any or all of these services, yet must be adapted for special patient considerations, as well as streamlined for cost containment.

1. Airway equipment
   Ambu bags (infant, child, adult)
   All sizes of masks for Ambu bags
   Simple and complex oxygen masks
   Nasal cannula
   Oral and nasopharynx airways
   Nebulizer setup
   Portable suction unit
   Tonsil suction
   Suction catheters (5/6, 8, 10, 14, 18 Fr)
   Magill forceps (pediatric and adult)
   Laryngoscope handles (child and adult)

Laryngoscope blades
  Miller 0, 1, 2, 3
  MAC 2, 3, 4
Spare laryngoscope batteries and bulbs
Endotracheal tubes

Uncuffed		Cuffed		Endotrol
2.5	4.0	5.5	7.0	7.0
3.0	4.5	6.0	7.5	8.0
3.5	5.0	6.5	8.0	

Stylets
Benzoin, adhesive tape, tracheostomy tape
CO_2 detector
PEEP valve
Pulse oximeter
Ventilator and filter and spirometer
Cricothyrotomy tray
Tracheostomy tubes
Needle cricothyrotomy setup
Nasogastric tubes, sizes 5 to 18
Catheter tip syringe
Surgilube

2. Cardiothoracic equipment
  Cardiac monitor and supplies, including extra batteries
  Defibrillator and supplies, including adult and pediatric paddles
  External pacer and supplies (pacer pads)
  Transvenous pulse generator and cable
  Automatic blood pressure machine
  Manual blood pressure equipment (pediatric, adult, and obese)
  Doppler
  Pressure monitor and transducer and tubing kit
  MAST pants (?)
  Thoracotomy tray and drainage system
  Chest tubes, sizes 12 Fr to 36 Fr
  Vaseline gauze
  Needle decompression supplies
  Pericardiocentesis setup
  Multiple adapters (sims, connectors, small and large Y)

3. Intravenous equipment
  Intravenous solution (normal saline, Ringer's lactate, 5% aqueous dextrose solution)
  Blood tubing
  Minidrip tubing
  Extension tubing
  Intravenous needles (24 to 14 gauge)
  Butterfly needles (27 to 19 gauge)
  Intraosseous needles (15 and 18 gauge)
  Syringes of multiple sizes
  IV start packs
  Razors
  Arm boards
  Laboratory blood tubes
  Stopcocks
  Pressure bag
  7 Fr conversion kit
  IV controllers or pumps and setup
  Blood products and blood cooler

4. Medications
  Advanced cardiac life support medications
  Antianginal agents
  Antiarrhythmics
  Anticonvulsants
  Antiemetics
  Antihistamines
  Antihypertensives
  Diuretics
  Local anesthetics
  Narcotics/narcan
  Nasal decongestants
  Paralytic agents
  Steroids
  Tocolytics
  Vasopressor agents

5. Miscellaneous
  Oxygen
  Stethoscope
  Isolation equipment (gloves, masks, goggles)
  Disposable needle boxes
  Instruments (bandage scissors, trauma scissors, hemostats, ring cutter)
  Tape
  Betadine solution

Dressing supplies (4 × 4's, Kling, Ace, cravats)
Eye shields
Burn sheets
Burn cable and electrodes
Cervical collars
Cervical immobilization device
Pediatric transport board
Car seat
Isolette
OB delivery tray
Bubble bag
Stockinette cap
Stuffed toys
Emergidose cards
Soft/leather restraints
Linens, blankets, towels
Flashlight
Cellular phone
Two-way radio
Thermometer
Instant camera and film
Disposable needle boxes
Paperwork
Information and map to receiving facilities

Additional equipment specific to the mode of transport and the type of service may include the following:

Ambulance
Immobilization devices (because space and weight are less of a consideration).
Backboard
Traction splint
Vacuum splints

Helicopter
Ear protection for patient and crew
Survival bag (stocked with equipment in case of an emergency landing).

Fixed-wing aircraft
Certain bulk supplies (because of extended transport times).
IV solutions, medications
Food and drink for the crew
Patient "comfort kit" (e.g., bedpan, urinal, Foley catheter)
More versatile type of ventilator (i.e., allows for patient assist, PEEP)
IV controller capable of infusing IV bag setup (precluding need to change syringes multiple times).

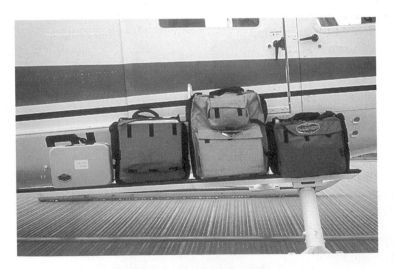

Fig. 4-3 Equipment bags.

It is imperative in any of these systems that the caregiver be familiar with the location and operation of all of their equipment. The prehospital nurse does not have the luxury in this setting to call down to Central Service and order additional equipment if something is missing or nonfunctional. It should be everyone's intent at the onset of their shift to inventory the equipment that they may be responsible to use. A comprehensive yet functional checklist may facilitate this process.

There should be a set of back-up bags, if your budget allows, to aid in safe and efficient restocking practices for quick turnarounds. This will provide for a more controlled inventory and subsequent replacement of used equipment at the nearest convenient time (Figure 4-3). Provisions also need to be made for a periodic overview and exchange of all items showing expiration dates (medications, IV solution, procedure trays, and so forth).

One last bit of advice is to always expect the unexpected! If you prepare yourself for the worst scenario, you will seldom be caught off guard; therefore optimize your patient management abilities.

SUMMARY

The process of patient transport is made up of multiple components. These include the indications, the mode, the risks, and the impact of transport. When preparing for patient transport, the nurse needs to consider all of these factors and their impact on both the patient and the care they may require.

REFERENCES

Baxt, W. (1986). Measuring the impact of rotorcraft aeromedical services. *Emergency Care Quarterly, 11,* 59-65.

Blackwell, T. (1993). Prehospital care. In J. Marx (Ed.). Advances in trauma. *Emergency Medicine Clinics of North America, 11*(1), 1-14.

Blumen, I., Dunne, M. (1992). Altitude and flight physiology. *Emergency, 24,* 36-43.

Blunt, E., & Crowther, E. (1992). Trauma transport. In E. Bayley & S. Turcke (Eds.), *A comprehensive core curriculum for trauma nursing* (pp. 81-97). Boston: Jones & Bartlett.

Boyd, C., Corse, K., & Campbell, R. (1989). Emergency interhospital of the major trauma patient: Air vs. ground. *Journal of Trauma, 29*(6), 789-794.

Boyd, C., & Hungerpiller, J. (1990). Patient risk in prehospital transport: Air versus ground. *Emergency Care Quarterly, 5*(4), 48-55.

Burney, R., Rhee, K., Cornell, R., Bowman, M., Storer, D., & Moylan, J. (1990). Evaluation of hospital-based aeromedical programs using therapeutic intervention scoring. *Aviation, Space, and Environmental Medicine, 6,* 563-566.

Cales, R., & Heilig, R. (1988). *Trauma care systems.* Rockville, MD: Aspen Publications.

Carter, G., Couch, R., & O'Brien, R. (1988). The evolution of air transport systems: A pictorial review. *Journal of Emergency Nursing, 6,* 499-504.

Champion, H. (1986). Helicopter triage. *Emergency Care Quarterly, 11,* 13-21.

Crippen, D. (1990). Critical care transportation medicine: New concepts in pretransport stabilization of the critically ill patient. *American Journal of Emergency Medicine, 11,* 551-554.

Dobrin, R., Block, B., & Gilman, J. (1980). The development of a pediatric transport system. *Pediatric Clinics of North America, 3,* 633.

Gabram, S., Piancentini, L., & Jacobs, L. (1990). The risk of aeromedical transport for the cardiac patient, *Emergency Care Quarterly, 15*(2), 72-81.

Garrison, H., Benson, N., & Whitley, T. (1986). Helicopter use by rural emergency departments to transfer trauma victims: A study of time-to-request intervals. *American Journal of Emergency Medicine, 7,* 384-386.

Haley, K. (1993). Emergency nursing core course. Park Ridge, IL: Emergency Nurses Association.

Harris, B., Orr, R., & Boles, E. (1975). Aeromedical transportation for children. *Journal of Pediatric Surgery, 10,* 719.

Hart, M., Haynes, D., Schwaitzberg, S., & Harris, B. (1987). Air transport of the pediatric trauma patient. *Emergency Care Quarterly, 3,* 21-26.

McNab, A. (1992). Air medical transport: "Hot air" and a French lesson. *Journal of Air Medical Transport, 11*(8), 15-18.

National Association of Emergency Medical Services Physicians. (1992). Air medical dispatch: guidelines for scene response. *Prehospital and Disaster Medicine, 7*(1), 75-78.

Preston, N. (1992). 1991 air medical helicopter accident rates. *Journal of Air Medical Transport, 2,* 14-15.

Rea, R. (1991). *Trauma nursing core course.* Chicago: Emergency Nurses Association.

Semonin-Holleran, R. (1993). Air medical transport of the trauma patient. In J. Neff & P. Kidd (Eds.), *Trauma nursing: Art and science* (pp. 625-642). St. Louis: Mosby–Year Book.

Southard, P. (1989). COBRA legislation: Complying with ED provisins. *Journal of Emergency Nursing, 1,* 23-25.

CHAPTER 5

Prehospital Safety

OBJECTIVES

1. Discuss key components of a safety awareness program and how those components are integrated into the prehospital practice
2. Identify the risks involved in situations with no ongoing safety program
3. Describe the purpose and goals of a safety committee, as well as the responsibilities of its members
4. Describe the internal and external environment and risk of personal injury associated with each
5. List the three areas of protective practices and describe examples specific to each
6. Describe design changes that can improve crashworthiness in the EMS helicopter
7. Describe design features that improve occupant safety in a ground ambulance
8. Describe personal protective equipment in use today
9. List and describe safety practices incorporated into the daily routine of the prehospital nurse
10. Describe the practice of ground flight following and how it relates to the safety of the prehospital nurse
11. Discuss the importance of scene safety and the added measures taken when working near or around a crime scene
12. Describe the preparation and training of the prehospital nurse

COMPETENCIES

1. Identify occupant safety hazards in a ground or air ambulance
2. Properly secure an adult and pediatric patient to a stretcher
3. Evaluate the requirements of specific protective equipment relative to the environment

As a society we have come to expect a safe working environment for all workers regardless of the inherent risk of the work. In working environments where the potential for injury exists, those risks must be identified and steps implemented to reduce the risk to a level that will not interfere with job performance and will protect the health and safety of the worker.

In many working environments the risk to personal safety can never be completely eliminated. In those instances safety measures must be taken to reduce the risk to an acceptable level, and then an ongoing monitoring program that evaluates the effectiveness of safety practices should begin. As time goes on, changes in safety practices may be required to meet new demands brought on by a changing work environment, or new information may dictate new approaches to old problems. Through monitoring and reevaluation the working environment is fine tuned to eliminate or reduce risk to an acceptable level. The challenge for organizations is to define "acceptable risk." Therein also lies the challenge for each member or potential member of the organization.

Individuals with serious doubts regarding their personal safety may find the stress created by those concerns interfering with the performance of their duties.

DEVELOPING A SAFETY AWARENESS PROGRAM

A key to providing a safe environment is development of a safety awareness program. The program should begin with a mission statement, in which the organization states up front its commitment to provide a safe, professional environment. The program must be aggressive and involve all members of the organization. Management personnel must be involved because of the financial commitment involved in purchasing equipment and providing "down" time for training, education, and retraining. Safety costs may seem excessive, but considering the cost of compensation for medical care and wages during recuperation from a job-related injury, they pale in comparison. Consider, for instance, costs associated with lifetime compensation for a permanent disabling injury, rescue units out of service because of injury, the erosive effect of the potential for injury on performance, and the high turnover of personnel. The total safety approach involves developing meaningful measures of safety for vehicle safety, equipment safety, team training, protocols and policies, quality assurance tools, and annual reviews.

The Safety Committee

A component of safety programs being used today, especially in air medical programs, is the safety committee. Many programs have safety committees made up of a cross section of representatives who meet to discuss significant safety issues. The committee can be helpful in keeping dialogue about safety open and nonthreatening. Each member of the safety committee serves as a conduit by which individuals in the program may channel concerns for further discussion and action where indicated, unencumbered by management. Safety information is reviewed frequently, changes made as required, and new information disseminated during regularly scheduled safety meetings where all members of the program are present. Also gaining in popularity are statewide safety councils made up of local programs working together to address common concerns.

A comprehensive safety program critically evaluates training, equipment, and policies and procedures to create a constancy of purpose toward improving safety, with the aim of developing a safe and injury-free environment, potentially reducing system cost and increasing job satisfaction.

THE PREHOSPITAL ENVIRONMENT

The prehospital nurse's role is evolving in many directions: from the nurse who works in emergency, intensive care, and critical care units, and in the nursery unit, who occasionally, out of necessity, is involved in an interfacility transport, to the highly specialized nurse involved in search and rescue operations.

When assessing safety risk in the environment, it is helpful to think of the external environment and the internal environment. The external environment includes the outside physical response area such as terrain and climate. Also included in the external environment is the population density: urban, suburban, or rural. The greater the geographical response area, the more likely variations in terrains and population densities will be encountered. For example, a busy metropolitan Emergency Medical Service (EMS) helicopter program may also cover an area that would require frequent flights over a large body of water requiring training in water-ditching emergencies. A prehospital program has little control over the external environment, and planning and training must be conducted to meet the challenges to personal safety (see Personal Survival).

The internal environment is the transport vehicle (ground or air ambulance) in which the prehospital nurse practices. The internal environment is the environment over which a program has the most control. It is also the environment that presents the most immediate dangers to personal safety. According to the National Safety Council (1992), for the years 1989 and 1990 there were 5900 accidents involving ambulances; 53 of those accidents involved fatalities. From 1978 to 1990 there have been 75 EMS helicopter crashes involving 76 fatalities and 30 serious injuries (Dodd, 1992). It is clear that a substantial number of deaths and serious injuries could be averted by recognizing and addressing internal environmental factors.

MAKING THE WORKING ENVIRONMENT SAFE

In exploring ways of improving the safety environment of the prehospital nurse, there are three primary areas of concern: interior design issues related to occupant protection, personal protective gear, and safety practices. Although it is helpful to look at each area independently, no single area can stand alone in a total safety approach. Each area must be analyzed and combined with the other two to achieve a complete safety program.

Occupant Protection

Of primary concern to all prehospital practitioners is the ability to survive an accident whether it involves a ground or air vehicle. To date, there is no government specification for crashworthiness and occupant protection for EMS helicopter design. The Federal Aviation Administration (FAA) sets minimum crashworthy standards that are strictly adhered to by all helicopter manufacturers, domestic or foreign. All EMS configurations must also meet those minimum standards. The United States General Services Administration (GSA) has produced a document in conjunction with the ambulance manufacturers that establishes criteria for ground ambulance design. The document, KKK-A-1822C, defines an ambulance, outlines the operational requirements, and addresses safety design features of ambulances purchased by the federal government. These specifications data have become the gold standard for ambulance design, performance, equipment, and test parameters and provide a practical degree of standardization. The specification document, KKK-1822C, is available from the GSA for a nominal charge.

Design features that contribute to occupant safety include available seat belts at each position; round, padded corners on built-in cabinets; hand grasp bars positioned throughout the patient compartment; and an adequate electrical system that affords good lighting and meets requirements for operating medical equipment from on-board electrical sources. Fire extinguishers should be present and mounted in easily accessible places within the patient compartment. Reputable manufacturers should be able to produce information on the structural integrity of the vehicle, as well as information regarding rollover protection, safety restraints, stopping distances, and required maintenance and inspection intervals.

For the past 30 years the U.S. Army has been conducting and compiling research on helicopter crashworthiness (Dodd, 1992). Crashworthiness has been defined as "the relative ability of a particular vehicle design to withstand crash impact forces with minimal structural damage.

Progressive structural collapse may be engineered to reduce the loads on the occupant through energy-absorbent techniques. Thus, crashworthiness relates to the protection of the occupants" (Snyder, as quoted by Dodd, 1992). The Army, through its research, has successfully developed designs that reduce injuries and deaths from crashes of relatively moderate impacts deemed "survival impacts." For example, improvements in the designs of fuel systems have significantly decreased deaths and injuries in postcrash fires since their introduction in the 1970s on army helicopters (Springate, McMeekin, & Ruehle, 1989). Additional crashworthy components of the army helicopter include landing gear and cabin floors that are designed to absorb energy as they progressively collapse. Unfortunately, modifications to existing helicopters incorporating such designs are extremely expensive. However, as new helicopter designs are introduced, cost alone should not be the determining factor in designing a helicopter using existing technology that minimizes crash-impact forces and maximizes occupant survival chances.

A 1988 study conducted by the NTSB on EMS helicopter accidents found that poor weather conditions were the "greatest single hazard to EMS helicopter operations." In addition, it found that in numerous EMS helicopters, the interior was not modified to meet applicable FAA standards for crashworthiness or good engineering practices. Some findings cited a lack of shoulder harnesses, seats improperly attached to the floor, seats constructed from nonapproved materials, medical equipment not properly restrained, fixed intravenous hooks projecting from the interiors, and loosely stored or mounted equipment. The study further concluded that the lack of crashworthiness considerations in the majority of EMS helicopter designs may be a factor in the 3.5 increase in fatality rates when compared with helicopters that have been modified (Dodd, 1992).

Army helicopter research has also been conducted on energy-attenuating seats, restraint systems, and reducing interior hazards such as projections in occupant strike zones. EMS helicopters currently flying could easily be retrofitted with these designs to improve their crashworthiness. Perhaps the easiest modification to make is installing a double shoulder harness together with a lap belt, which the army found to be much more effective in protecting occupants than lap belts alone. In addition, energy-attenuating seats, which are available as standard equipment in the pilot's and co-pilot's positions in some aircraft, are seldom incorporated into the EMS completion package. The combination of lap belts with shoulder harnesses and energy-attenuating seats can dramatically improve occupant injury tolerance (Dodd, 1992).

A final area in improving crashworthiness is in the EMS completion of the patient care area. Completion designs have centered on such concerns as increased space, reduced weight, and increased sophistication of on-board medical equipment. Crashworthiness and occupant protection must likewise be of equal concern. Efforts should be made to eliminate fixed objects in the head strike area. Similar to their ground counterparts, the EMS completion should use rounded corners, free of sharp edges. All supports for equipment should be mounted flush or allow for recessing the equipment into the med wall where possible. Oxygen and suction gauges should be recessed. Padding should be placed where possible on any head strike obstruction that cannot be totally eliminated. Light bulbs should be covered by shatterproof globes that prevent the bulb from vibrating loose in flight and scattering slivers of glass. Fluorescent tubes, if used, should be locked into place to prevent loosening caused by vibration. At least one multipurpose halon fire extinguisher mounted in a quick-release bracket should be available. In large aircraft, a fire extinguisher should be located in the pilot compartment and in the patient compartment.

Protective Equipment

The topic of personal protective equipment for prehospital providers is subject to interpretation by individual organizations. To date, no national standards exist. The selection of a uniform varies among organizations according to the program's mission and budget and the climate and terrain. The uniform should be selected with the following factors in mind: safety, efficiency, comfort, and appearance.

Uniforms made of flame-retardant material are currently used by many flight programs. In 1985, Kruppa's survey found that 29% of civilian EMS programs wore flame-retardant uniforms. If a program decides on flame-retardant apparel, the uniform should be long-sleeved and loose fitting and worn only with cotton underwear. Flame-retardant uniforms have been criticized for being uncomfortably hot in warm climates and requiring special laundering to maintain their flame-retardant properties. They are also more expensive. A complete flame-retardant uniform includes gloves, with pant legs tucked into leather boots. A flame-resistant uniform is designed to protect the wearer from a flash fire and provide enough time (<20 seconds) to evacuate a burning aircraft. Recently, Galey and Lord introduced a lower-cost, fire-retardant, cotton-polyester fabric that it markets under the name Flamex. Among the most commonly used fire-resistant fabrics in use today are Nomex III from Du Pont and Monsanto's SEF Modacrylic (Colver & Colver, 1991).

Footwear is an important consideration for the prehospital nurse. For the nurse who responds to scene work, a leather boot that provides ankle protection is important. The sole should be thick and oil resistant. If job performance involves rescue work or extrication, steel toes are advisable. In situations where the prehospital nurse actually is involved in extrication and rescue, full turnout gear including a helmet and leather gloves should be used.

Of particular interest to flight nurses is the use of helmets to protect against head injuries. A study of helmet use by Hoffman and Shinskie (1990) found that 21% of civilian EMS programs used helmets, an increase of 7% over the 1989 study done by Kruppa. Crowley (1992) found that in military occupants of survivable helicopter crashes, those without helmets were almost four times as likely to incur a serious head injury and six times as likely to have fatal head injuries as those with helmets. It is important to remember that Crowley (1992) studied military personnel, but he went on to state that it seems reasonable to assume the findings would be applicable to the EMS population with similar crash profiles as those in the study. Dodd (1992) in his study concluded that the modification of the EMS interior for the transport and care of patients seems to be the factor most strongly associated with an increase in injury risk for EMS occupants.

Perhaps the most important factor in purchasing a helmet is selecting a knowledgeable vendor who is familiar with custom-fitting helmets. The SPH-5 helmet is a civilian version of the army's SPH-4B and is a popular choice of programs that choose to use helmets. Many lightweight helmets designed for fixed-wing use will not provide sufficient protection in a rotary-wing accident and therefore should not be used by helicopter flight teams (Gambin, 1987). The helmet shell should be lightweight, weighing less than 4.4 pounds, and the center of gravity of the helmeted head should match that of the unhelmeted head. A heavy or unbalanced helmet will rapidly cause fatigue or neck pain. The helmet's liner should absorb energy and fit comfortably. Quality helmets have energy-absorbing earcups that also aid in reducing noise. The chin strap should hold the helmet firmly in place. A helmet's characteristics should match or exceed the U.S. military specifications for the SPH-4B. Some manufacturers have created a system that incorporates a personalized insert that snaps into the hard outer shell of the helmet, thus reducing the cost of a complete helmet for each member of the organization.

Safety Practices

Safety practices can range from what appear to be seemingly minor daily tasks to practices that, although not performed as a daily routine, could potentially save a life—that life being your own. A good example of an important daily task familiar to all prehospital nurses is the practice of equipment checks. Reliance on equipment is vitally important to the care of critical patients. Equipment must be present, accessible, and in working order. Training and regular preventive maintenance and calibration must be incorporated into the organization's quality assurance program. The goal of such a practice is to protect the nurse and organization from litigation by detecting and addressing malfunctioning or missing equipment before that situation causes patient harm.

Another safety factor probably given little thought during the course of a shift's activity is securing the patient and equipment in transport. Medical equipment such as monitors, IV controllers, and equipment and medication boxes must be secured en route to decrease the likelihood of these becoming projectiles and inflicting injuries to the patient or crew members. Patients must be securely restrained with stretcher restraint belts at the chest, hips, and knees. It may be difficult to secure infants and small children to a stretcher. Pediatric patients must never be held during transport. An infant carrier that conforms to applicable federal motor vehicle safety standards should be used. The child should be snugly restrained with the belts provided with the carrier, and the carrier should then be secured to the stretcher in a rear-facing position. Pediatric immobilization devices are available for those patients who require spinal immobilization.

Combative patients can present a serious risk to the safety of the prehospital care nurse. The cramped confines of a ground ambulance or helicopter are not an ideal environment for restraining a combative individual. Restraints must be applied before leaving for the intended destination. Protocols regarding chemical restraints and their use must be in place before these issues arise. In areas where paralytic agents are used to control combativeness in patients with head injuries, both patient care and crew safety have benefited.

Ground Flight Following

The practice of flight following is a standard by which most air medical programs operate. A specially trained communication specialist is in constant contact with the pilot during a flight. Where distances between the aircraft and base are too great, the pilot makes contact with other programs along the flight path or airports and has them make phone calls to the communication specialist back at the base hospital. In this manner the communication specialist can keep abreast of the progress of the flight. More important, the communication specialist can recognize early on when an aircraft is overdue and institute efforts to identify potential problems. Policies and procedures must be in place in the event of an overdue or downed aircraft with precise, detailed instructions as to who to call to institute a search, as well as alerting the program's administrative personnel of the situation. In view of the great distances covered by many ground units, the use of a similar program with properly trained personnel and well-designed policies would potentially benefit EMS systems.

Securing the Scene: Violence

Prehospital nurses involved in caring for injured victims at scenes must be aware of the hectic and potentially dangerous situations that can threaten their safety. The first concern of prehospital care providers should be their own safety. A prehospital nurse who becomes injured at a scene becomes another victim that further stresses the available resources and may render the unit out of service, further complicating patient rescue and treatment efforts. Unless specifically trained, the prehospital nurse should not engage in the extrication or rescue effort. These efforts generally require the understanding of rescue principles and equipment, as well as protective equipment to ensure the safety of the rescuer. A good practice is not to interfere with an extrication. Attempting assessment or IVs on an entrapped patient, even if the situation is judged to pose no safety risk to the nurse, usually results in a longer extrication time. Instead, as extrication continues, measures to ensure a rapid as possible departure should be taken. The only possible exception is a delayed extrication with a patient who needs an airway established. Again, this situation should pose no safety risk to the nurse.

Particular caution needs to be exercised when responding to the scene of a violent crime. Crime has become commonplace in our society, not only in large cities but also in small towns and rural areas. In some cities, bulletproof vests are being worn by EMS providers because of concerns for their personal safety (Garza, 1993). Prehospital nurses must receive assurances from law enforcement personnel present that the scene is safe. They should never enter a crime scene before the arrival of the police. Since a crime scene may contain evidence, it should not be disturbed more than is absolutely necessary to perform patient care. The local coroner can help a prehospital program develop specific guidelines for preserving the crime scene.

Preparation and Training

Most organizations provide an orientation program to new employees in which the new employee is introduced to the program's mission statement, administrative structure, and specific policies and procedures. It is also dur-ing this period that the new employee should receive a safety orientation, which should include an introduction to all policies and practices related to maintaining a safe environment for the nurse and patient. Responsibilities and obligations must be stated clearly, and the new employee's understanding should be evaluated.

For the ground prehospital nurse, orientation topics should include emergency vehicle driver education classes; scene safety; the use of driver, passenger, and patient safety restraints; and the location and use of on-board fire extinguishers. Some organizations also provide a back injury prevention program for their employees (Terribilini & Dernocoeur, 1989). Baseline audiometric examinations can also be conducted at this time. Johnson, Hammond, and Sherman (1980) found that ambulance cab noise during siren use could exceed 105 dBa. OSHA currently requires employers to provide hearing conservation programs for employees exposed to a time-weighted average sound level of 85 dBa or greater.

A similar program specific to flight nursing would include a helicopter safety orientation that addresses issues of working around a running aircraft, emergency landing procedures, emergency fuel shutoff procedures, and emergency power shutdown procedures. The location and activation procedures of the emergency locator transmitter should also be included. These are specific tasks that the flight nurse needs to be able to perform in case the pilot is incapacitated. The location and use of fire extinguishers should also be a part of the orientation. A baseline audiometric examination should be performed with yearly follow-ups. The availability and use of hearing protectors must be stressed. Many programs carry a survival packet or bag on the aircraft that contains signaling devices, matches, space blankets, a compass, and additional survival equipment. Opportunities should be made available to practice survival techniques (see Personal Survival).

It is important that the orientation process include and stress safety practices in both ground and air organizations. However, a single orientation program, not matter how thorough, is not enough. A continuing education and evaluation program should be established. The program should include a mandatory annual review and an ongoing quarterly review of selected topics.

QUALITY MANAGEMENT

Quality management (QM) programs or quality improvement programs are an essential element of EMS organization today. Regardless of the model or process, their goal is to document effectiveness and to examine and improve in problem areas.

Safety is an area that can and should be examined using the existing QM model chosen by the organization. The key to evaluating safety using a QM program is documentation. If documentation does not exist to support the claim of effectiveness, then the organization cannot prove effectiveness. Many times documentation can come directly from the run summary or patient records. Such information would be related to steps taken to ensure patient safety, such as documenting measures used to secure the patient en route. The documentation may come from other available sources as well. In the example given earlier in the chapter regarding daily equipment checks, the expectation is that a daily or start-of-shift check will be performed to detect and correct malfunctioning or missing equipment to prevent patient harm. The documentation that the check took place might include a log with all equipment within the ambulance listed and a space available for date and signature of the person performing the check. These logs could then be used later in a formal audit and review. A way of proving that training and yearly safety updates occur would be to record the content of the program together with names and signatures of those who attended.

A final evaluation tool is direct observation. An example might have to do with the expectation that hearing protectors be used when working around a helicopter while the engines are running. Because it is impractical to document every time hearing protectors are worn in this situation, a violation of this standard would have to be observed by a manager or QM officer. In this case, the process of individual counseling and reevaluation would meet ongoing quality assurance goals.

Safety is a topic that easily lends itself to QM studies. The parameter can be related to patient or employee safety. The difficulty in evaluating safety topics is in developing useful tools to document practice.

Personal Survival

Survival in the prehospital environment is essential for the delivery of good care. Most medical transfers and scene runs are routine, and survival consists solely of operating a vehicle, whether a ground ambulance or air ambulance, safely. However, there are more and more situations where medical teams are going into wilderness areas and disaster areas. Because of weather or terrain, it is necessary for medical teams to have at least a basic understanding of survival principles.

Survival training has been an integral part of military training since World War II. Pilots and aircrews, ships' personnel, soldiers, marines, airmen, and sailors who must go into jungles, deserts, and mountains all must know survival skills to carry out their mission. All search and rescue teams must be familiar with survival techniques to keep themselves and their patients alive until transport to a hospital setting. Most people view wilderness settings from their automobile or fly over in aircraft. If their automobile should become disabled or their aircraft make an emergency landing, then they are in a survival situation. Vehicles can end up in lakes or rivers, on fire, or with injuries to the crew.

They may be in mountainous terrain, desert with temperatures of 120°, or rain forests with a 300 foot tree canopy. Obviously it is better to avoid being in such situations if possible.

Preventive measures should always be used with the safety of the crew and the patients in mind. All vehicle and equipment inspections should be done before their use. Safety equipment such as seatbelts, helmets, communication devices, and life jackets should be used at all times, used correctly, and not modified. All personnel who may be expected to use any equipment should be familiar with that equipment and have used it. Someone unfamiliar with a defibrillator is not expected to be able to use it in a situation that calls for one. They may be able to figure it out, but in a survival situation they may not have that time. All skills, medical or survival, must be practiced to maintain a high level of expertise. Many people take a basic survival training course but never practice their skills. When the time comes for them to use their survival training, their skills have degenerated, so they are unable to use what they have learned. Survival can be divided into two main areas. The first is preparation, or what a person does before they are in a survival situation. The second is prioritization, or determining the most important things to do once a person is in a survival situation.

PREPARATION
Physical and Mental

Preparation for survival has several stages. Physical preparation involves maintaining a high level of physical fitness, both aerobic and upper body strength. Most survival situations will stress the individual physically, and better conditioning increases the chance for survival. It is said that in long-term survival situations the fat people get skinny and skinny people die. In the short term, however, the person who can avoid injury, swim or hike long distances, climb into a life raft, or build a shelter in a snowstorm will survive. Many people have died in survival situations for one reason—they could not swim. This is a basic skill that everyone involved in search and rescue or transport must have, especially over large bodies of water. Mental preparation involves being familiar with various types of terrain, climate, and environment and knowing the variations in temperature and the potential for flooding, dust storms, sandstorms, hurricanes, and tornadoes. The principles of weather prediction should be understood, and the latest forecast and severe weather warnings should be monitored. A midwestern ambulance service may use a road for transport that in heavy rains may be under water. A mountain rescue service may be trapped by a summer snowstorm in the Rockies. A Gulf Coast ambulance may be isolated because of hurricane winds knocking down trees and washing out bridges. Running out of gas in the Southwest desert can be fatal. It is necessary to avoid things that cannot be controlled and control those things that can be. Mental preparation also involves reading survival texts and personal experiences of people in survival situations who have survived. We can learn from the experience of others and gain some insight into what they had to contend with and how we might perform in the same situation.

The most important mental conditioning—the will to live—cannot be learned, but fortunately this potential is in all of us. In almost every single survival story the most important factor in whether the people involved lived or died was their attitude. Those who refused to give up, who kept trying in the face of adversity, even when they made stupid errors and didn't do things by the book, survived. Those who gave up, died. Many people interviewed after being rescued mentioned two things that seemed to make a difference: their determination not to give up and maintaining a sense of humor.

Clothing

Choice of clothing is important especially in cold weather, since a person's clothing may be the only shelter from the environment and protection against hypothermia. Clothing should be of an appropriate material and design. It should protect the wearer against the environment yet be comfortable and practical. The layering principle should be followed when selecting clothing for cold weather. This allows maximum trapping of warm air near the body and permits the person to remove a layer to prevent overheating and sweating during exertion. The first layer should be long underwear of a polypropylene material. Modern polypropylene is very soft, similar to cotton, and comes in three basic weights. It maintains approximately 80% of its insulating ability even when wet and is also used for gloves, socks, and head coverings. The lightweight should be worn as the first layer in fall or spring and the middleweight or expedition weight in the winter or in the mountains. The next layer should be either wool or synthetic fleece. Wool has been the standard material for the outdoors against which all other materials are judged, but modern synthetics have superior insulating properties when wet. The third layer should be Goretex, which is a waterproof material that allows water vapor to escape from the body but does not allow water droplets through. Two pairs of socks should be worn; this not only prevents friction and blisters, but also gives the individual the option to use one pair as mittens if necessary. The socks should be either polypropylene or wool/polypropylene blend. If wet weather is a certainty, then Goretex socks are quite beneficial and may help to prevent trench foot and frostbite. Shoes should be ankle high to prevent them being pulled off in mud or water. This also prevents rocks, sand, and snow from entering the top of the shoe and gives more support to the ankle during stress. Shoes should be made of a waterproof material such as Goretex, which allows the feet to breathe, or should be treated with a waterproof coating.

Hand protection is essential in a survival situation. If a person is unable to build a fire because of frostbitten hands, then they might quickly succumb to hypothermia. Gloves do not protect the hands adequately from cold; only mittens can insulate the fingers and allow each finger to help keep the adjacent fingers warm. Goretex mittens with pile linings that come up to the mid forearm are ideal. The problem with mittens is that they make it impossible to do any type of fine work such as starting an intravenous line or taking a pulse. A solution to this problem is to wear a polypropylene glove inside the mitten and to remove the mitten to do work, replacing it when it becomes cold. Mittens should be fastened to the person by a string or other connector so that they are not easily misplaced. If the mittens or gloves are lost, the hands must be protected. Socks make reasonable mittens, and if one portion of the anatomy must be exposed to cold, it is better to have frostbitten feet than hands. Most heat is lost through the head and neck, and therefore protecting these areas is essential. A balaclava made of expedition weight polypropylene takes up little room yet is very efficient at retaining warmth. A hood attached to the Goretex parka completes the head covering in cold, wet, windy weather.

Hot environments create different demands. Here the person must be protected from heat gain and water loss, and the head must be protected from sun, wind, and insects. Ripstop cotton is good material for desert environments. Long-sleeve shirts and long trousers should always be worn. Leather gloves will protect the hands from thorns, spines, and hot objects. Eye protection is necessary in almost every situation, since snow blindness or blowing sand can cause corneal injury. The rule of thumb is to minimize the amount of skin exposed to the environment.

Survival Kits

The individual survival kit must meet the following criteriae: (1) It must be compact enough so that it can be carried at all times; (2) it must include essential items and yet be flexible enough to be used in various environments; and

---

Box 5-1
BASIC SURVIVAL KIT

Pocketknife, Swiss army type	Penlight
Signal mirror	Cravat
Waterproof matchbox	Bandaids
Space blanket	Parachute cord
Compass/map	Needle/thread
Insect repellant	Sunglasses
Metal match	Iodine crystals
Candle	Aluminum foil
Mosquito headnet	Whistle
Canteen	

---

(3) it must contain high-quality items that must be protected from the elements. Many of the items will be carried in the individual's pockets; the remainder can be carried on a belt pack or similar container. A heavy-duty plastic bag can be used to store the items, and this bag can also be used as a water container, solar still, or rain hat. See Box 5-1 for the contents of a basic survival kit.

A vehicle survival kit should include spare clothing and food and water, as well as signaling equipment, a tool kit for self-rescue (shovel, rope, axe, and jack), and communication equipment such as a radio or cellular telephone. Aircraft flying in remote areas or over large bodies of water should have adequate survival and rescue equipment including flotation devices, life rafts, shelters, sleeping bags, and signaling devices.

PRIORITIES
The Rule of Threes

An average person can survive 3 minutes without oxygen, 3 hours without warmth, 3 days without water, and 3 weeks without food. This rule gives us our priorities in a survival situation. Obviously, medical concerns and safety are more important in an accident, but once

these are addressed then the rules of threes is invoked. A person trapped in a vehicle underwater must know how to escape within a relatively short time. A person who has clothing, water, and shelter can spend several days trying to obtain food with minimal adverse consequences. The basic skills that we need are based on our priorities and include shelter building, fire building, signaling, obtaining water, and direction finding.

Basic Survival Skills

Survival kits are not designed to replace survival skills but to augment them. Survival skills must be practiced periodically to maintain a minimum level of expertise. For example, building a fire in the backyard in the snow or rain, erecting an emergency shelter during a picnic, or identifying edible or poisonous plants on a day hike in the park familiarizes the individual with some of the problems associated with these activities in a nonsurvival situation. If it becomes necessary to perform these tasks in a survival situation, the performance, it is hoped, will be easier.

Obtaining oxygen is clearly an important skill but difficult to teach and more difficult to practice. Sometimes just envisioning a situation and determining what to do in that situation is the first step. For example, your vehicle is caught in an avalanche that comes across a road in the mountains; you are in a building that is on fire and filled with smoke; your ambulance is upside down in a lake after skidding off of the road. Perhaps you could escape from these situations without difficulty, but how about your injured partner or a patient? Deciding what to do or at least thinking about it beforehand is helpful. Knowing that air is usually trapped in a vehicle underwater, that smoke may rise and provide a clear crawl route at floor level, and that providing an air space with the hands and arms when buried in snow may allow you to dig yourself out may give you an advantage in these situations.

The prevention of hypothermia, the number one killer of people in survival situations, begins with the proper selection of clothing, as previously discussed. Obviously, dry clothing is a better insulator than wet clothing. A person in water should always try to get as much of their body out of the water as possible. Using personal flotation devices, floating debris, or preferably a life raft for support is a good idea. Even in a strong wind, the wind chill will not be as deleterious as the water. Field expedients can be used to decrease heat loss. Seat covers can be used as ponchos or blankets, seat cushions for insulation, and plastic bags for vapor barriers. Grass and leaves inside clothing can also provide insulation. The head, neck, and hands should have priority for preventing heat loss. The head and neck because this is where most heat escapes, and the hands because simple lifesaving tasks are impossible to perform once the hands are frozen.

Shelter construction should be based on three main principles. First, the structure should provide shelter on all sides. Building a roof is not enough. If not enough material is available to build a complete shelter and it is not possible to build a snow shelter, then the sequence of priorities is a roof, floor, windward side, and leeward side. The roof is obviously essential to protect from rain and snow, which increase the chance of hypothermia through radiation heat loss. The floor, insulated if possible, prevents heat loss through conduction. The sides protect against wind and blowing precipitation and heat loss through evaporation and convection. The second principle is to make a fire if possible to keep the shelter warm. With lean-to shelters a fire can be built outside the shelter with a reflector (either a rock, piece of metal, or wood) set up about 2 feet from the fire to reflect the heat into the shelter. A candle or stove can be used inside a snow shelter and can supply an amazing amount of heat. Precautions should be taken to allow carbon monoxide to escape from any shelter so that the occupants are not poisoned. A shelter designed to fit the number of individuals present is easier to heat and more efficiently contains the heat produced by the people in it. The third principle is to design the shelter to match the environment. Desert shelters must protect from heat gain, water loss, and blowing sand. Sometimes, digging a hole in the ground works better than building a lean-to above ground. Take advantage of caves, rock overhangs, trees, and other natural shelters. Be aware of potential dangers when selecting a shelter site, for example, dead trees or tree limbs that may fall in a strong wind, rockslides, caves with other inhabitants such as bears, skunks, or cougars, and trees or rocks that may conduct lightning. Vehicles make good shelters in many cases and are more easily spotted by rescuers. Wrecked vehicles still may have many parts that can be used to construct a shelter. Airplanes have little insulation, and automobiles can become ovens in the desert, so common sense should prevail in all decisions concerning shelter. Perhaps using the automobile during a sandstorm or at night and a shade trench during the day would be the optimum shelter if stranded in the desert (Figs. 5-1 to 5-3).

Fire building is a skill that has gone out of vogue in Western civilization. Camping stoves

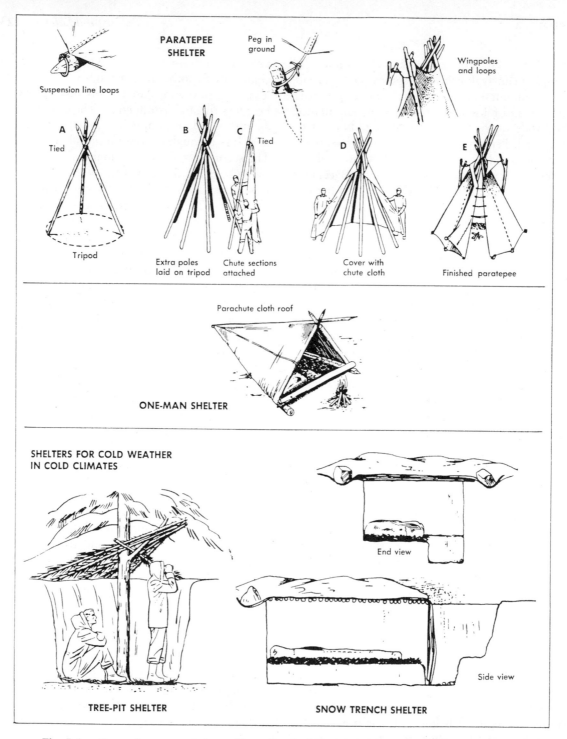

Fig. 5-1 General purpose shelters. (From *Survival-Training Edition AFM 64-3,* by Department of the Air Force, 1969, Washington, DC: US Government Printing Office.)

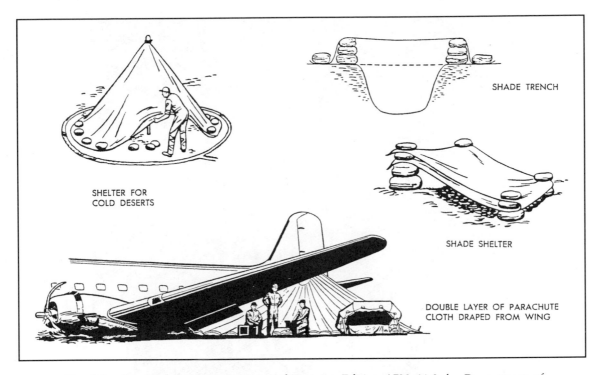

SHELTER FOR
COLD DESERTS

SHADE TRENCH

SHADE SHELTER

DOUBLE LAYER OF PARACHUTE
CLOTH DRAPED FROM WING

Fig. 5-2   Desert shelters. (From *Survival-Training Edition AFM 64-3,* by Department of the Air Force, 1969, Washington, DC: US Government Printing Office.)

have replaced campfires, gas starters or treated logs are used in fireplaces, and gas or electric ovens are used in nearly every home. Everyone could build a fire 100 years ago, and this skill was taken for granted. A fire meant warmth, light, a hot meal, pure water, and a way to keep wild animals away. In a survival situation, a fire can be all this and more. It can be used as a signal to rescuers. A fire needs three elements, fuel, heat source, and oxygen. If any element is missing the fire will be extinguished. Many types of fuel can be used. Wood is the most obvious, but oil or fuel from a vehicle, animal fat, cardboard, and paper may all be available in a survival situation. Wood that is dead and dry makes the best firewood, and a good source is dead limbs still attached to trees. Dead limbs on the ground are often wet but are a second choice. To ignite the wood some form of tinder

is needed. Tinder may be thin sticks about the size of a match, dry leaves, birch bark, dry grass, or an old bird's nest. The tinder should be about the size of a softball and placed against a base log 6 to 10 inches in diameter. Next, small sticks, the diameter of a pencil or smaller, should be layered over the tinder, then sticks about finger size. More sticks, gradually increasing in size up to 4 to 5 inches in diameter, should be readily available to place on the fire once the initial sticks are burning. This principle must be used throughout; it is impossible to light a 2-inch-diameter stick with a match, but if you gradually increase the size of the stick from match size, you can ignite an 18-inch-diameter log. There are many types of heat sources also. Wooden, strike-anywhere matches in a waterproof container are the best. Metal matches, flint sticks, butane lighters, paper

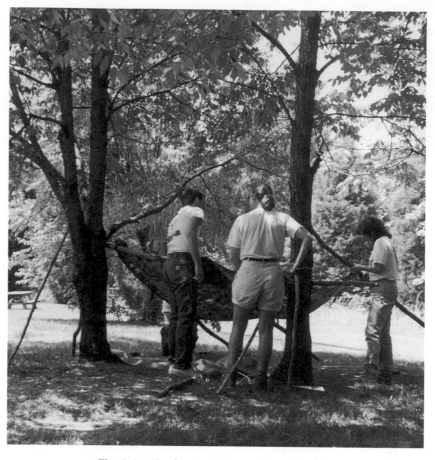

Fig. 5-3   Students erecting a lean-to shelter.

matches, and magnifying lenses will work but are not as reliable. Wooden matches should be replaced yearly, and a piece of sandpaper can be glued inside the lid of the matchbox to provide a strike surface. Candles, paraffin-soaked tinder, steel wool, magnesium ribbons, and other adjuncts to fire starting are helpful but not essential. Expedient methods include using a battery from a vehicle or two D-cell flashlight batteries, soaking a can full of sand with oil or kerosene (gasoline is explosive and extremely dangerous to use for this purpose), and using alcohol wipes, insect repellent, or other flam-

mable substances that can be found in an ambulance or aircraft (Figs. 5-4 and 5-5).

Water is found nearly everywhere on the earth, but unfortunately most of it is either contaminated or cannot be used by the human body. All ground water should be considered contaminated and must be purified before use. The easiest way to purify water is to bring it to a boil. This kills all pathogens but of course does not remove chemical contaminants or solutes. Iodine, sodium hypochlorite (bleach), and other commercial water purification tablets kill most organisms, and filters remove most but

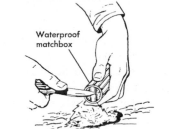

FLINT AND STEEL

This is the easiest and most reliable way of making a fire without matches. Use the flint fastened to the bottom of your waterproof match case. If you have no flint, look for a piece of hard rock from which you can strike sparks. If no sparks fly when it is struck with steel, find another. Hold your hands close over the dry tinder; strike flat with a knife blade or other small piece of steel with a sharp, scraping, downward motion so that the sparks fall in the center of the tinder. The addition of a few drops of gasoline before striking the flint will make the tinder flame up — FOR SAFETY, KEEP YOUR HEAD TO ONE SIDE. When tinder begins to smolder, fan or blow it gently into a flame. Then transfer blazing tinder to your kindling pile or add kindling gradually to the tinder.

One way to start a fire is with flint and lint ball.
1. Imbed a ¼-inch piece of lighter flint (pyrophoric alloy-large size) in a ½" X ¼" X 2" piece of soft wood or plastic. Flint should be imbedded close to one end and centered.
2. Wind 2- to 3-feet of 8-strand flax (linen) harness maker's thread at the end opposite the flint.
3. To use, unwind about 1 inch of linen, and on a smooth dry surface, scrape the strands of linen into a ball of lint using the sharp edge of a knife.
4. Place lint ball in contact with flint. With the sharp edge of the knife, use pressure and strike a spark directly into the lint ball. Lint will quickly blaze.

One of the distinct advantages of this piece of equipment is its usefulness, even after complete immersion in water. The linen dries very quickly and 5 minutes of air drying after a thorough wetting is sufficient to make it usable.

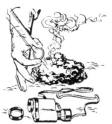

BURNING GLASS

A convex lens can be used in bright sunlight to concentrate the sun's rays on the tinder. A 2-inch lens will start a fire most any time the sun is shining. Smaller lenses will work if the sun is high and the air is clear.

ELECTRIC SPARK

If you have a live storage battery, direct a spark onto the tinder by scatching the ends of wires together, to produce an arc.

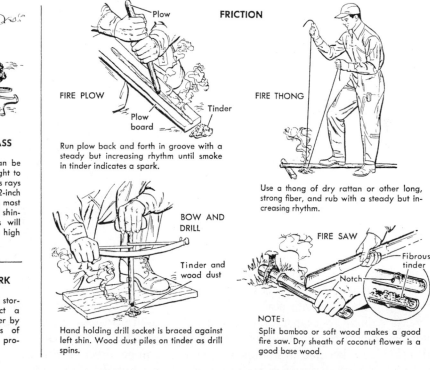

FRICTION

FIRE PLOW

Run plow back and forth in groove with a steady but increasing rhythm until smoke in tinder indicates a spark.

BOW AND DRILL

Hand holding drill socket is braced against left shin. Wood dust piles on tinder as drill spins.

FIRE THONG

Use a thong of dry rattan or other long, strong fiber, and rub with a steady but increasing rhythm.

FIRE SAW

NOTE:
Split bamboo or soft wood makes a good fire saw. Dry sheath of coconut flower is a good base wood.

Fig. 5-4 Fire making without matches. (From *Survival-Training Edition AFM 64-3*, by Department of the Air Force, 1969, Washington, DC: US Government Printing Office.)

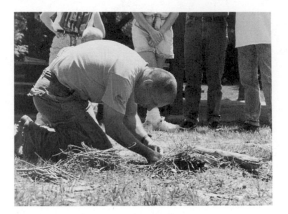

Fig. 5-5   Instructor lighting a fire.

not all pathogens. Some combination filters use iodine plus a ceramic filter, and this removes all pathogens. Solar stills and vegetable stills can be used to produce distilled water by using the energy of the sun to evaporate and condense water from plants, sea water, and ground water (Fig. 5-6). Snow and old (gray) sea ice can be melted and used for drinking water. Snow or ice should not be eaten directly but should be melted or heated first to avoid lowering body temperature. Rainwater and dew can be collected in tarps, on vehicles, or wiped from plants. Sea water, brackish water, and urine should never be drunk, but can be used in solar stills. Animals and plants can be a source of water, but a general rule is not to eat if water is scarce because water is used in metabolizing most proteins and fats. Conserve your sweat, not your water. Prevent water loss in hot climates by keeping as much skin covered as possible, wetting clothing with nonpotable water to increase cooling by evaporation, and drinking whenever possible. In a survival situation dehydration can become a serious problem. Thirst is not a good indicator of hydration status. Urine concentration and flow is better, and a small amount of dark urine is a sign of dehydration.

Food can become a problem in prolonged survival situations. Hard candy, pemmican, and peanut butter can be included in the survival kit in cold climates where calories become more important for maintaining heat production. Many common plants such as blueberries, prickly pears, coconuts, blackberries, and acorns can be used for food relatively safely. It is best to avoid eating unknown plants and mushrooms; a case of gastroenteritis may be fatal in a survival situation, especially in hot climates. Plants with milky saps or that cause burning when rubbed on the skin or inside the lip should not be eaten. Plants eaten by animals may not be safe for humans. Most animals and fish can be eaten, but all should be cooked if possible to destroy parasites.

The best way out of a survival situation is to be rescued. All aircraft and most ships are required to carry emergency locator transmitters (ELT) or emergency position indicating radio beacons (EPIRB). These transmitters are designed to emit a radio signal when activated that will be received by satellites and relayed to rescue personnel. This gives the rescuers a general area in which to search but will not pinpoint the victims. The ability to signal rescuers is relatively simple if the victim(s) has a radio and can guide the rescuer to his or her position. Flares, smoke grenades, flashlights, signal fires, gun shots, and whistles are all good signaling devices when used appropriately. These methods should be employed when rescuers are seen or heard, but using them to attract attention when no one is around is wasteful because they will not be available when needed. A mirror, however, can be used to flash a signal into the sky or toward the horizon at sea. It cannot be used up (until the sun burns out) and can be seen by aircraft flying at 30,000 feet. The flash can be directed with a little practice, and once an aircraft is attracted the flash should not be held on the aircraft, since this makes it difficult for the crew to see. If possible, geometric patterns can be placed on the ground near where

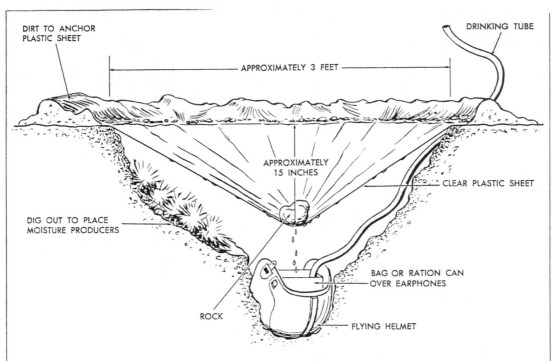

Dig a bowl-shaped hole in the soil about 40 inches in diameter and 20 inches deep. Add a smaller, deeper sump in the center bottom of the hole to accommodate the container. If polluted waters, such as body waste, are to be purified, a small trough can be dug around the side of the hole about half way down from the top. The trough insures that the soil wetted by the polluted water will be exposed to the sunlight and at the same time that the polluted water is prevented from running down around or into the container. If plant material is to be used, line the sides of the hole with pieces of the plant or its fleshy stems and leaves. Place the plastic film over the hole and put a little soil on its edges to hold it in place. Place a rock no larger than your fist in the center of the plastic and lower the plastic until it is about 15 inches below ground level. The plastic will now have the shape of a cone.

CAUTION
Make sure the plastic cone does not touch the earth anywhere causing loss of water.

Put more soil on the plastic around the rim of the hole to hold the cone securely in place and to prevent water vapor losses. Straighten the plastic to form a neat cone with an angle of about 30 degrees so that the water drops will run down and fall into the container in the bottom of the hole. It takes about one hour for the air to become saturated and start condensing on the underside of the plastic cone.

Fig. 5-6 Solar still. (From *Survival-Training Edition AFM 64-3,* by Department of the Air Force, 1969, Washington, DC: US Government Printing Office.)

the victims are to attract attention. Either a large **X** or SOS is standard. The patterns can be made from brush or vehicle parts or stamped out in the snow. Trenches can be dug in the sand and filled with oil and ignited. Smudge fires can be made by throwing wet leaves or grass onto a fire.

Direction finding is relatively simple. What is more important is knowing which way to travel and how to travel. A compass points to magnetic north, but true north may be east or west of that position depending where on earth you are located. At night the North Star (Polaris) can be easily found in the Northern Hemisphere

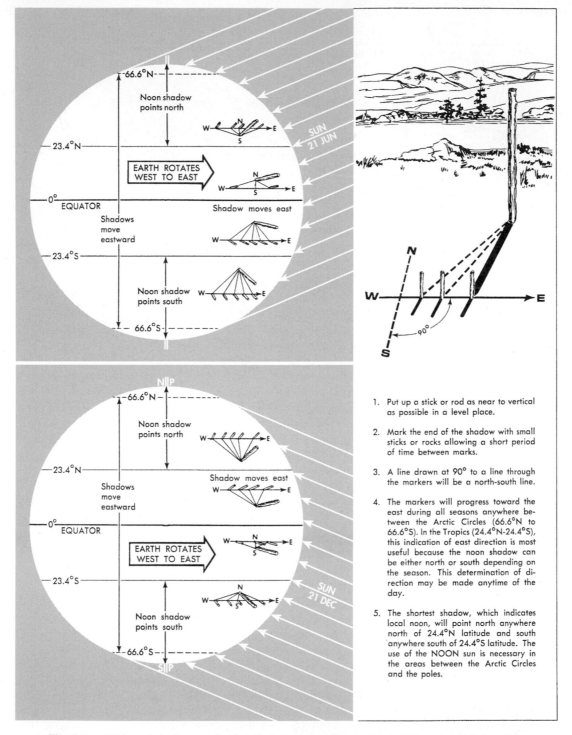

1. Put up a stick or rod as near to vertical as possible in a level place.

2. Mark the end of the shadow with small sticks or rocks allowing a short period of time between marks.

3. A line drawn at 90° to a line through the markers will be a north-south line.

4. The markers will progress toward the east during all seasons anywhere between the Arctic Circles (66.6°N to 66.6°S). In the Tropics (24.4°N-24.4°S), this indication of east direction is most useful because the noon shadow can be either north or south depending on the season. This determination of direction may be made anytime of the day.

5. The shortest shadow, which indicates local noon, will point north anywhere north of 24.4°N latitude and south anywhere south of 24.4°S latitude. The use of the NOON sun is necessary in the areas between the Arctic Circles and the poles.

Fig. 5-7 Stick and shadow method to find direction. (From *Survival-Training Edition AFM 64-3*, by Department of the Air Force, 1969, Washington, DC: US Government Printing Office.)

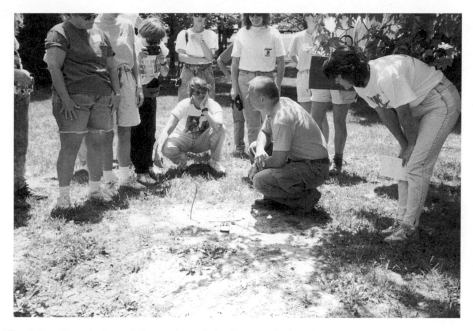

Fig. 5-8   Correlation of the stick and shadow method with a compass to find direction.

halfway between the Big Dipper (Ursa Major) and the Big "W" or "M" (Cassiopeia). A non-digital watch or the stick and shadow method can be used to find direction during the day using the sun (Figures 5-7 and 5-8). Once direction has been determined, then which direction to travel must be decided. If you have previously identified key terrain features on a map in the area that you are operating in, then you will know which direction to travel. For example, if you know that an interstate highway runs north and southwest of your operating area, then by traveling west you will cross the highway and reach help. Knowing the position of rivers, mountain ranges, electric wires, and roads will help you decide which direction to travel. If you have shelter, water, food, and signaling devices and do not know which way to travel it is better to stay where you are and signal. Rescuers will start their search in the general area where you were thought to have been

or along your planned route. Not only the direction of travel but how and when to travel are also important. Deserts are best crossed at night to conserve water, mountains are difficult to cross at any time, mangrove swamps, marshes, and snow crevices are impassable. Sometimes river travel is the best method if a raft can be constructed. Most large rivers have towns or villages along them, but currents, rapids, and waterfalls can be dangerous. If you decide to travel, leave a note outlining your plans and direction of travel so that rescuers will know where to look.

Bibliography

Auerbach, P.S., & Geehr, E.C. (1989). *Management of Wilderness and environmental emergencies* (2nd ed.). St. Louis: Mosby.

Boy Scouts of America. (1984). *Fieldbook* (3rd ed.). Irving, TX: Author.

Craighead, F.C., & Craighead, J.J. (1984). *How to survive on land and sea* (4th ed.). Annapolis: Naval Institute Press.

Department of the Air Force. (1969). *Survival training edition AFM 64-3*. Washington, DC: US Government Printing Office.

Wiseman, J. (1986). *Survive safely anywhere: The SAS survival manual*. New York: Crown Publishing.

REFERENCES

Colver, C.P., & Colver, J.C. (1991). Managers, workers must realize the need for flame-retardant clothing. *Journal of Occupational Health and Safety, 60*(1), 20-23.

Crowley, J.S. (1992). Flight helmets: How they work and why you should wear one. *Journal of Air Medical Transport, 4*(10), 10-21.

Dodd, R.S. (1992). *Factors related to occupant crash survival in emergency medical service helicopters*. Unpublished doctoral dissertation, Johns Hopkins University, Maryland.

Gambin, R.W. (1987). Flight helmet user requirements and how they are achieved. In *Proceedings of the Twenty-Fifth Annual SAFE Symposium*. Newhall: Safe Association.

Garza, M.A. (1989). Bulletproof vests. The latest fashion in EMS. *Journal of Emergency Medical Services, 14*(6), 20-21.

Hoffman, D.J., & Shinskie, D.W. (1990). Evaluation of helmet wearing by medical helicopter services. (Abstract) *Journal of Air Medical Transport, 9*(9), 79.

Johnson, D.W., Hammond, R.J., & Sherman, R.E. (1980). Hearing in an ambulance paramedic population, *Annals of Emergency Medicine, 9*, 557-561.

Kruppa, R.M. (1989). Air medical safety—A follow-up survey. *Journal of Air Medical Transport, 4*(10), 10-21.

National Safety Council. (1992). *Accident Facts*. Chicago.

Snyder, R.G. (1978). *General aviation crash survivability*. Paper 780017, p. 4. Warrendale: Society of Automotive Engineers.

Springate, C.S., McMeekin, R.R., & Ruehle, C.J. (1989). Fire deaths in aircraft without the crashworthy fuel system. *Aviation, Space Environmental Medicine, 10*(2), B35-38.

Terribilini D.C., & Dernocoeur, K. (1989). Save your back: Injury prevention for EMS providers. *Journal of Emergency Medical Services, 14*(10), 34-47.

National Organizations and Associations

American Ambulance Association
3814 Auburn Blvd Ste 70
Sacramento CA 95821-2123
916-483-3827

American Association of Critical-Care Nurses
101 Columbia
Aliso Viejo CA 92656-1491
800-899-2226

American Association of Women Emergency Physicians
21 West Colony Place Ste 150
Durham NC 27705
919-490-5891

American Board of Emergency Medicine
200 Woodland Pass Ste D
East Lansing MI 48823
517-332-4800

American Burn Association
Baltimore Regional Burn Center
Baltimore MD 21224
800-548-2876

American College of Emergency Physicians
1125 Executive Circle
Irving TX 75038
214-550-0911

American College of Surgeons, Committee on Trauma
55 E Erie St
Chicago IL 60611
312-664-4050

American Critical Incident Stress Foundation
5018 Corsey Hall Dr Ste 104
Ellicott City MD 21042
410-730-4311

American Red Cross
430 17th St NW
Washington DC 20006
202-737-8300

American Trauma Society
8903 Presidential Pkwy Ste 512
Upper Marlboro MD 20772
800-556-7890

Association of Air Medical Services
35 S Raymond Ave Ste 205
Pasadena CA 91105
818-793-1232

Associated Public-Safety Communications Officers
2040 S Ridgewood Ave
Daytona Beach FL 32119
904-322-2500

Center for International Emergency Medical Services
Humboldtstr 12A
Germany
49-611-307891

Commission on Accreditation of Air Medical Services
PO Box 1305
Anderson SC 29622
803-287-4177

Commission of Accreditation of Ambulance Services
PO Box 619911
Dallas TX 75261
214-580-2829

Disaster Research Center
University of Delaware
Newark DE 19716
302-831-6618

Doctors for Disaster Preparedness
   2509 N Campbell Box 272
   Tucson AZ 85716
   602-325-2680
Emergency Care Research Institute
   5200 Butler Pike
   Plymouth Meeting PA 91462
   215-825-6000
Emergency Management Institute
   16825 S Seton Ave
   Emmitsburg MD 21727
   301-447-1286
Emergency Medical Service Institute
   4240 Greensburg Pike
   Pittsburgh PA 15221
   412-351-6604
Emergency Medicine Foundation
   PO Box 619911
   Dallas TX 75261-9911
   214-550-0911
Emergency Nurses Association
   216 Higgins Rd
   Park Ridge IL 60068
   312-649-0297
Farmedic Training Inc
   Alfred State College
   Alfred NY 14802
   607-587-4734
Federal Emergency Management Agency
   500 C St SW
   Federal Center Plaza Rm 801
   Washington DC 20472
   202-646-2442
International Association of Dive Rescue Specialists Inc
   201 N Link Ln
   Fort Collins CO 80524-2712
   303-224-9101
International Association of Fire Chiefs
   4025 Fair Ridge Dr Ste 300
   Fairfax VA 22033-2868
   703-273-0911
International Critical Incident Stress Foundation Inc
   5018 Dorsey Hall Dr Ste 104
   Ellicott City MD 21042
   410-730-4311
Mountain Rescue Association
   2144 S 1100 E Ste 150-375
   Salt Lake City UT 84106
   801-328-0523
National Association for Search & Rescue
   PO Box 3709
   1120 Waples Mill Rd Ste 300
   Fairfax VA 22030
   703-352-1349

National Association of Air-Medical Communication Specialists
   PO Box 34531
   Phoenix AZ 85067-4531
   602-230-9117
National Association of Emergency Medical Technicians
   9410 Ward Parkway
   Kansas City MO 64114
   816-444-3500
National Association of Emergency Vehicle Technicians
   PO Box 790
   Hauppauge NY 11788
   800-638-8265 ext 232
National Association of EMS Physicians
   230 McKee Place Ste 500
   Pittsburgh PA 15213
   412-578-3222
National Association of First Responders
   5334 Armadillo Ave
   Orange Beach AL 36561
   205-981-3383
National Disaster Medical System
   5600 Fishers Ln Parklawn Bldg Rm 4-81
   Rockville MD 20857
   800-USA-NDMS
National Emergency Management Association
   PO Box 11910 Iron Works Pike
   Lexington KY 40578-1910
   606-231-1876
National EMS Pilots Association
   35 South Raymond Ave Ste 205
   Pasadena CA 91105-1931
   605-341-0273
National Fire Academy
   16825 S Seton Ave
   Emmitsburg MD 21727
   301-447-1117
National Flight Nurses Association
   6900 Grove Rd
   Thorofare NJ 08096
   609-384-6725
National Flight Paramedics Association
   35 S Raymond Ave Ste 205
   Pasadena CA 91105
   818-405-9851
National Head Injury Foundation
   1776 Massachusetts Ave NW Ste 100
   Washington DC 20036
   202-296-6443
National Institute for Burn Medicine
   909 E Ann St
   Ann Arbor MI 48104
   313-769-9000

National Institution of Emergency Vehicle Safety
17155 Robey Mail Code B
Castro Valley CA 94546-3852
510-276-4300
National Study Center for Trauma & EMS
22 S Green St
Baltimore MD 21201
410-328-5085
Professional Aeromedical Transport Association
PO Box 7519
Alexandria VA 22307
800-541-7517

React International Inc
242 Cleveland St
Wichita KS 67214
316-262-2100
Society for Pediatric Emergency Medicine
4567 E Ninth
Rose Medical Center
Denver CO 80220
303-320-2492
World Association for Emergency & Disaster Medicine
230 McKee Place Ste 500
Pittsburgh PA 15213
412-578-3222

CHAPTER 6

Patient Assessment and Preparation for Transport

OBJECTIVES

1. Identify the components of a primary and secondary assessment
2. Discuss patient preparation for transport
3. Identify potential problems that may develop during transport
4. Discuss the role of the family in the transport process
5. List some of the equipment needed for transport

COMPETENCIES

1. Perform a primary and secondary assessment before transport
2. Evaluate and perform primary airway interventions
3. Provide information for the family of a patient to be transported
4. Identify the equipment that is needed for transport
5. Employ techniques to manage the patient's pain during transport

Patient assessment is the first step in patient preparation for transport. It provides the nurse with an opportunity to identify patient problems and to assess the patient's condition before transport. The initial assessment contributes to patient preparation for transport and identifies the potential effects of transport.

Once the initial assessment and stabilization of the patient have been completed, the nurse prepares the patient for transport. The data collected during the initial assessment provide the framework for the plan of care the nurse uses during transport. Preparation is made not only for the specific problems that have been identified, but also for the potential problems that may arise during transport. Plans also are for-

mulated for the effects that transport may have on the patient.

The assessment of the patient in the prehospital care environment can be an intense challenge. Patient location (e.g., entrapped in a vehicle) (Figure 6-1), limited personnel and equipment, and the specific illness or injury present potential barriers to successful prehospital patient assessment.

The environment poses additional barriers to assessment. Lack of light, noise, space, vehicle movement, speed, and weather can make normal assessment maneuvers such as auscultation difficult to perform (Lazear, 1992).

The type of transport vehicle may also make it difficult to assess the patient. The location of

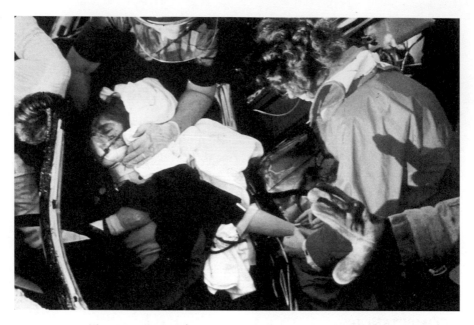

Fig. 6-1   Patient location can make assessment difficult.

the patient in the ground ambulance, helicopter, or fixed-wing aircraft poses potential problems in assessment. Although more portable equipment has become available, some pieces are still susceptible to movement and vibrations that may affect their reliability.

Patient assessment provides the framework for patient preparation for transport. The assessment needs to be organized, rapid, and complete. Patient problems must be identified, interventions performed, and their effectiveness evaluated. Patient assessment is a continuous process that occurs before, during, and after transport.

PATIENT ASSESSMENT

Patient assessment in the prehospital care environment begins with scene assessment whether the nurse responds directly to the patient or to another facility (Emergency Nurses Association, 1991). The nurse should assess the

surrounding environment for hazards. Box 6-1 summarizes some of the potential hazards that may be found at the scene.

Upon arrival at a referring facility, the prehospital nurse should survey available resources for patient preparation. Equipment and supplies necessary for patient stabilization may be limited, so the prehospital nurse must be prepared.

The principles of prehospital nursing assessment are no different from those governing assessment within the hospital. However, the prehospital environment dictates that the assessment be organized, direct, and rapid. Adaptation and flexibility are key concepts when performing patient assessment in the prehospital care environment. Tight spaces, darkness, noise, and equipment that may or may not be functioning can and do present challenges in the prehospital care environment.

Patient assessment begins with the primary survey and obtaining information about the pa-

---

Box 6-1
POTENTIAL HAZARDS

Scene Hazards

Wires
Uneven ground
Vehicles
Accident itself
People
Signs
Light poles
Water
Loose debris

Referring Facility Hazards

Buildings
Wires
People

---

tient's illness or injury. Depending on the patient's illness or injury and the time constraints of transport, a secondary survey may be performed. The following information provides a summary of how to obtain a patient history and perform a primary survey, initial patient care, and secondary survey before transport.

History

As previously stated, the principles of patient assessment in the prehospital care environment are essentially the same as those within the hospital. The history of the illness or injury provides a guide for initial stabilization, preparation for transport, and ongoing assessment.

Generally, the nurse is given some information en route to the patient. However, what the nurse finds on arrival may be quite different from the information received.

General Principles of History Gathering

According to Henry and Stapleton (1992, p. 56), "history is the patient's story of significant events related to and surrounding the present problem." When gathering historical information related to the patient's illness or injury, some general principles should be followed including identifying the patient's chief complaint or problem. If the patient is unable to provide that information, then the nurse needs to obtain it from others at the scene (prehospital care providers, police, bystanders), referring personnel (nurses, physicians), or from individuals who may be with the patient. Scene survey may also provide information. If the patient is unconscious, the nurse should look for medic alert jewelry or information in the patient's wallet.

A common mnemonic used to collect general history information is AMPLE:

A	Allergies and alcohol or substance abuse
M	Medications/immunizations for the child
P	Past medical history
L	Last meal
E	Events leading to the emergency
	Everything that has been done up until the transport team's arrival

If the patient's chief complaint or problem is related to pain, the *PQRST* method is useful when collecting historical information. *PQRST* (Lee, 1992; Kidd, 1993) represents the following:

P	Provoking Factors: What caused or causes the pain? Does anything relieve the pain or make it worse? What was the patient doing when the pain began?
Q	Quality of the Pain: Many words may be used to describe the pain, which may also provide the nurse with clues to what may be the origin of the pain. For example, words such as *burning* or *crushing* are used by patients to describe chest pain.
R	Region and Radiation: Ask the patient to point to the area where the pain is felt. Elicit if there is a pattern to the pain.
S	Severity: Numbering, for example from 1 to 10, can be used to describe the severity of the pain.
T	Time: Words that describe the temporal nature of the pain, such as how long, when, what time of day.

Specific factors may prevent the nurse from obtaining a history in the prehospital care environment. These include the patient's inability to provide information because of illness or injury, the lack of witnesses to a particular event, and the absence of family or significant others before transport.

When the patient is being transported from a referring facility, as much information as possible should be collected and communicated with the receiving facility (see Patient Preparation). Sometimes this may be nearly impossible, particularly when patients are transported directly from the scene. The prehospital nurse needs to keep in mind that a history may provide as much information about the patient's condition as the primary survey. A history also alerts the nurse to problems that may develop during transport.

Trauma History

History gathering is different for the trauma patient than for the patient with a medical illness (Hart, 1988). Exploring the mechanism of injury is the first step in obtaining a trauma history. When, where, how, and by what was the patient injured? Many times a complete de-

scription of the event is limited. The prehospital nurse should not devote a great deal of time and energy to securing a complete description. However, a general idea of the mechanism of injury provides clues to potential injuries and complications that may occur during transport. Box 6-2 contains a description of predictable injuries that may occur with motor vehicle crashes (Kidd, 1993).

In recent years instant photographs have been used to enhance information related to the mechanism of injury. Dickinson, Krett, and O'Connor (1992) reported that when prehospital photography was used to enhance the details related to a motor vehicle crash, the receiving physicians altered their perceptions about the patient's injuries 46% of the time. In 22 of 26 cases (85%) the receiving physician upgraded the severity of the motor vehicle crash based on the photographs.

When obtaining a trauma history, the nurse should also gather information that describes the scene of the accident. Are there multiple victims? Are all victims accounted for? If the victims are unable to provide information about additional victims, schoolbooks, clothing, or toys may suggest the presence of additional vic-

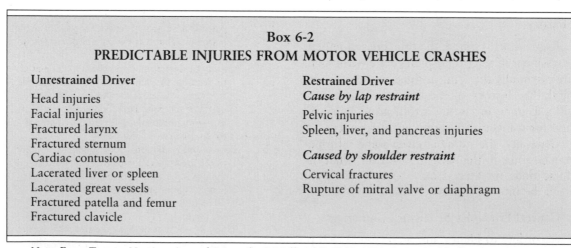

Box 6-2

PREDICTABLE INJURIES FROM MOTOR VEHICLE CRASHES

Unrestrained Driver

Head injuries
Facial injuries
Fractured larynx
Fractured sternum
Cardiac contusion
Lacerated liver or spleen
Lacerated great vessels
Fractured patella and femur
Fractured clavicle

Restrained Driver
Cause by lap restraint

Pelvic injuries
Spleen, liver, and pancreas injuries

Caused by shoulder restraint

Cervical fractures
Rupture of mitral valve or diaphragm

Note. From *Trauma Nursing: Art and Science* by J. Neff and P. Kidd, 1993, St. Louis: Mosby.

tims (Campbell, 1988). A more in-depth discussion about obtaining a trauma history is contained in Chapter 7.

Medical Illness History

The medical history begins with the chief complaint or current patient problem. The mnemonic *PQRST* previously described can be of great assistance when obtaining a medical history. History related to the present illness including related signs and symptoms should be collected. Significant past medical history and risk factors for a particular disease process (smoking and chronic obstructive pulmonary disease) can provide additional pieces of meaningful information.

Care initiated before the arrival of the prehospital nurse needs to be gathered. These data (Hart, 1988) should include the following:

- Initial physical findings
- Initial treatments and results
- Vital sign trends
- Medications given
- Laboratory results
- X rays
- EKGs
- Intravenous infusions
- Intake and output
- Family notification

Primary Survey and Initial Patient Care

The primary survey is based on the assessment of the patient's airway, breathing, circulation, and neurological disability and exposure. Whether the nurse performs the primary survey and provides initial patient care at the scene of the injury or illness or within the walls of a referring facility, the basic steps remain the same.

Airway

The patient's airway is assessed to determine if it is patent, maintainable, or not maintainable. For any patient who has a suspected traumatic injury, the airway is evaluated while using cervical spine precautions. An assessment of

---

Box 6-3
AIRWAY INTERVENTIONS

Basic Life Support

Positioning the airway (cervical spine precautions in suspected trauma)
    Head tilt–chin lift
    Jaw thrust
    Modified jaw thrust
Ventilation
    Bag-valve-mask ventilation
Airway adjuncts
    Nasopharyngeal airways
    Oropharyngeal airways
Suctioning
Foreign body upper airway obstruction

Oxygen Delivery Systems

Nasal cannula
Simple masks
Partial rebreathing masks
Nonrebreathing masks

Esophageal Airways

Esophageal obturator airway
Esophageal gastric tube airway
Pharyngeotracheal lumen airway
Esophageal tracheal combitube
Tracheoesophageal airway

Advanced Life Support

Endotracheal intubation
Nasotracheal intubation
Digital manual intubation
Retrograde intubation
Cricothyrotomy
Transtracheal ventilation

Advanced Airway Adjuncts

CO_2 detectors
BAM devices
Lighted stylets

Note. From *The Airway: Emergency Management* by R. Dailey, B. Simon, G. Young, and R. Stewart, 1992, St. Louis: Mosby.

the patient's level of consciousness in concert with the airway status provides the nurse with an impression of the effectiveness of the patient's current airway.

Summary of Primary Airway Assessment
- Patent, maintainable, nonmaintainable
- Level of consciousness
- Skin: ashen, pale, gray, cyanotic, mottled
- Preferred posture to maintain airway (e.g., child with epiglottitis, patient in pulmonary edema)   ient in pulmonary
- Airway clearance
- Sounds of obstruction

If an airway problem is identified, the appro-priate intervention should be used. The decision to use a particular intervention depends on the patient's problem and the potential for complications during transport. Box 6-3 contains a summary of airway interventions.

Supplemental oxygen should be given to all patients before transport. Specific equipment such as a pulse oximeter or CO_2 detector provides continuous airway evaluation during transport (see Patient Preparation).

Pharmacological Adjuncts for Airway Management
Specific pharmacological agents are useful in prehospital airway management. These include

Table 6-1   Pharmacological Adjuncts for Intubation

Drug	Dosage	Indications	Potential Problems
Sedation			
Diazepam	2-10 mg bolus Repeat 1.0-2.5 mg IV every 10 min.	Amnesia, muscle relaxation	May potentiate action of other drugs
Midazolam	1-5 mg titrate in 0.5 increments	Amnesia, sedation	Response to drug is related to how fast the drug is given
Thiopental	3-5 mg/kg bolus	Sedation	May cause hypotension and apnea
Etomidate	0.2-0.4 mg/kg	Sedation	Myoclonic muscle spasms; may produce pain with injection and cause nausea and vomiting
Fentanyl	2-3 mcg/kg 1 mcg/kg every 5 min.	Sedation, analgesia	May cause respiratory depression, excessive sedation, and nausea; also may cause chest rigidity and nasal itching
Neuromuscular Blocking Agents			
Succinylcholine	1.0-1.5 mg/kg (adult)	Rapid sequence intubation	Inability to intubate patient, hyperkalemia, malignant hyperthermia
Pancuronium	0.1 mg/kg	Prolonged muscle relaxation	Tachycardia, prolonged muscle relaxation
Vecuronium	0.1 mg/kg	Intermediate-duration muscle relaxation	Prolonged relaxation
Atracurium	0.5 mg/kg	Intermediate-duration muscle relaxation	Histamine release, prolonged relaxation

Note. From *Emergency Drug Therapy* by W. Barsan, M. Jastremski, and S. Syverud, 1991, Philadelphia: W.B. Saunders; and *The Airway: Emergency Management* by R. Daily, G. Young, and R. Stewart, 1992, St. Louis: Mosby.

drugs that provide sedation and amnesia, as well as neuromuscular blocking agents that facilitate intubation. Table 6-1 contains a list of drugs that may be used to facilitate airway management. Box 6-4 contains an example of a protocol for the use of neuromuscular blocking agents.

Breathing

Assessment of ventilation begins with observing whether the patient is breathing. If the patient is apneic or in severe respiratory distress, immediate interventions are indicated. If the patient is having any difficulty with ventilation, the nurse needs to identify the problem and proceed with the appropriate interventions.

Box 6-4
PROTOCOL FOR THE USE OF NEUROMUSCULAR BLOCKING AGENTS
UNIVERSITY AIR CARE

Neuromuscular blocking agents facilitate endotracheal intubation of patients with conditions such as head injury, drug overdose, and status epilepticus. They can also be used for agitation control, CT scanning, and to prevent sudden rises in intracranial pressure associated with head trauma. This protocol outlines one approach to the proper use of these agents. Final decision-making responsibility for how these agents are used remains in the hands of the flight physician. Specific protocols for intubation and postintubation paralysis follow this overview and introduction.

Once a neuromuscular blocker has been administered, paralysis of the muscles of respiration rapidly follows. Administration of these agents commits the flight crew to manually ventilating the patient once paralysis has occurred. Endotracheal intubation should follow shortly thereafter. In the unlikely event that endotracheal intubation is not possible and bag mask ventilations do not adequately ventilate the patient after paralysis, the airway must be secured by cricothyrotomy. This procedure is rarely necessary, but the required equipment for cricothyrotomy should always be at hand whenever neuromuscular blockers are used. These agents should not be used for endotracheal intubation in cases where a cricothyrotomy would be difficult or impossible (e.g., children < 2 years of age, massive neck swelling) or in cases where ventilation and intubation will be difficult after

paralysis (e.g., epiglottitis, upper airway obstruction).

Succinylcholine is the drug of choice for endotracheal intubation in the patient requiring paralysis. Its use should be preceded by atropine in children and by lidocaine in patients with head trauma or cardiac irritability. Patient who are awake and oriented at the time of paralysis should be sedated with an agent such as diazepam before and during paralysis, unless their condition contraindicates sedation. Pancuronium, administered after endotracheal intubation, is useful for continued paralysis lasting 30 minutes or longer in the agitated patient (i.e., head-injured patient). Vecuronium, like pancuronium, can be used after intubation. Vecuronium is particularly useful when short-term paralysis is required for procedures or transfers lasting 40 minutes or less.

For review purposes, descriptions of these neuromuscular blocking agents (succinylcholine, pancuronium, vecuronium), precede the protocol that follows.

Neuromuscular Blockade with Succinylcholine for Endotracheal Intubation
Succinylcholine (Anectine)

Type: Depolarizing (fasciculations occur initially, not reversible)
Primary indication
    Endotracheal intubation in the patient requiring paralysis

Continued.

Box 6-4, cont'd
PROTOCOL FOR THE USE OF NEUROMUSCULAR BLOCKING AGENTS
UNIVERSITY AIR CARE

Absolute contraindications
1. Patients in whom a cricothyrotomy would be difficult/impossible
   - Children less than 2 years old
   - Massive neck swelling
2. Patients who would be difficult/impossible to intubate/ventilates40after paralysis
   - Acute epiglottitis
   - Upper airway obstruction

Relative contraindications
   NOTE: The benefit of obtaining airway control must be weighed against the risk of complications in these patients.
   - Hyperkalemia (K+ rises after succinylcholine administration)
   - Penetrating eye injuries (increased intraocular pressure with IV use)
   - Known hypersensitivity to the drug
   - Unstable fractures that may be displaced by fasciculations
   - History of malignant hyperthermia
   - Known pseudocholinesterase deficiency

Dosage/route
   1.5 mg/kg IV push
   (In normal-sized adults, an initial dose of 100 mg is usually adequate.)
   A less desirable alternative is the IM route (2.0 mg/kg IM)

Pediatric dosage
   1.5 mg/kg IV push
   Children should be premedicated with atropine (0.01 mg/kg IV push) before succinylcholine

Repeat dosage
   If inadequate relaxation occurs after the first IV dose, a second dose of 1.0 to 1.5 times the first dose may be administered. An increased incidence of complications (hyperkalemia, bradycardia) is associated with more than two doses.

Onset of paralysis
   IV: 20-50 sec; IM: 2-5 min
Duration of paralysis
   IV: complete—2-5 min
     partial—10-20 min
   IM: complete—4-6 min
     partial—10-40 min
Metabolized by plasma pseudocholinesterases
Complications
   Inability to intubate/ventilate
   Hyperkalemia in susceptible patients:
     Extensive burns (more than 3 days after injury)
     Trauma (more than 3 days after injury)
     Neuromuscular disease (CVA, tetanus, MS, MD)
   Hypotension
   Bradycardia/asystole
     Vagally or hypoxia mediated, particularly frequent after multiple doses or in children not pretreated with atropine
   Aspiration
   Increased intraocular pressure
   Prolonged paralysis in pseudocholinesterase-deficient patients
   Malignant hyperthermia

Procedure for endotracheal intubation using succinylcholine

Use of succinylcholine requires the presence of a physician and flight nurse who have competence in endotracheal intubation and cricothyrotomy, as well as familiarity with the contraindications and pharmacological effects of the drug.

Any patient requiring emergent endotracheal intubation is assumed to have a full stomach. To prevent aspiration of gastric contents, all intubations should be done in a "crash sequence" with continuous cricoid pressure until ET tube position is confirmed

Box 6-4, cont'd
PROTOCOL FOR THE USE OF NEUROMUSCULAR BLOCKING AGENTS
UNIVERSITY AIR CARE

and the cuff inflated. Sedation, using an agent such as diazepam or lorazepam, should be administered before paralyzing any alert/oriented patient. A brief neurological examination including best motor response and pupilary examination should be performed before paralysis.

Intubation sequence

1. Assemble required equipment
   - Bag-valve-mask connected to functioning oxygen delivery system
   - Working suction with Yonker suction tip attached
   - Endotracheal tube(s) with stylet and intact cuff
   - Laryngoscope with blades and bright light
   - Cricothyrotomy tray
   - Atropine 1.0 mg, succinylcholine (enough for two doses) drawn up in labeled syringes
2. Check to be sure that a good, functioning, secure IV line is in place and running.
3. Connect patient to a cardiac monitor. If a third medical team member is available, assign him the sole responsibility of watching the monitor for dysrhythmias during subsequent steps. This person should immediately alert the flight physician and flight nurse if bradycardia or other dysrhythmia occurs.
4. Allow the patient to breath 100% O_2 via the mask (gently assist ventilations if necessary).
5. Premedicate as appropriate.
   - Valium 3-5 mg IV push for sedation of awake patients
   - Atropine 0.01 mg/kg IV push for children/adolescents

   - Lidocaine 1 mg/kg IV push for intracranial pressure control in head-injured patients, patients with CNS injury (hypertensive crisis, bleed), or for dysrhythmia control in patients at risk for ventricular arrhythmias
6. Give succinylcholine 1.5 mg/kg IV push.
7. Apply cricoid pressure to occlude the esophagus until intubation is successfully completed and the ET tube cuff is inflated (usually done by flight nurse).
8. After fasciculations stop (if they occur), demonstrate adequate relaxation by ventilating the patient four to five times with the bag-mask. Jaw relaxation and decreased resistance to bag-mask ventilations indicate that the cords are paralyzed and that it is time to proceed with intubation.
9. Perform endotracheal intubation. If unable to intubate during first 20-second attempt, stop and ventilate the patient with the bag-mask for 30-60 seconds. If inadequate relaxation is present, give a second dose of succinylcholine (1.0 to 1.5 times the initial dose). If repeated intubation attempts fail, ventilate the patient with the bag-mask until spontaneous ventilations return (usually 6-10 minutes after succinylcholine administration). If endotracheal intubation fails and you are unable to adequately ventilate patient with the bag-mask, perform cricothyrotomy.
10. Treat bradycardia occurring during intubation with atropine 0.5 mg IV push and by temporarily halting intubation attempts and hyperventilating the patient with the bag-mask and 100% O_2.
11. Once intubation is completed, inflate the cuff and confirm ET tube placement by auscultating for bilateral breath sounds

Continued.

Box 6-4, cont'd
PROTOCOL FOR THE USE OF NEUROMUSCULAR BLOCKING AGENTS UNIVERSITY AIR CARE

(and by subsequently obtaining a chest radiograph).

12. Release cricoid pressure, secure ET tube.

Neuromuscular Blocking Agents for Use after Endotracheal Intubation
Pancuronium bromide (Pavulon), vecuronium bromide (Norcuron)

Type: Nondepolarizing (no fasciculations, partially reversible)

Primary indication
  Induction and maintenance of skeletal muscle relaxation after endotracheal intubation has been completed

Absolute contraindications
  Known hypersensitivity
  Inexperience in airway management

Relative contraindications
  Myasthenia gravis (a small dose can last for *days*)
  Use caution in any patient in whom release of histamine could be detrimental, e.g., severe asthma or cardiac disease.
  Vecuronium causes less histamine release and tachycardia than pacuronium.

Complications
  Bronchospasm
  Hypotension
  Prolonged block, especially in myasthenics, also may occur with use of pancuronium in patients with renal failure.
  Bradyarrhythmias
  Tachyarrhythmias

	Pancuronium (Pavulon)	Vecuronium (Norcuron)
Dosage/route	0.06 to 0.1 mg/kg IV push	0.05 to 0.10 mg/kg IV push

Do not administer these agents IM.

Pediatric dosage	0.06 to 0.1 mg/kg IV push	0.04 to 0.06 mg/kg IV push
	Neonates (<4 weeks): start with 0.02 mg/kg	
Onset of paralysis	2-3 minutes	3-5 minutes
Duration of paralysis	35-60 minutes	25-45 minutes
Repeat dosage	0.01 mg/kg	0.01 mg/kg

Note: Repeat dosing significantly lengthens duration of paralysis.

Reversible?	Yes (usually >30 minutes after last dose)	Yes (usually >20 minutes after last dose)

Both agents are reversible only after spontaneous recovery begins.

Metabolized by	Excreted unchanged by kidneys	Hepatic, excreted in bile

Protocol for the Use of Neuromuscular Blockers in Air Care Patients after Endotracheal Intubation

Before these agents (Pavulon, Norcuron) can be used, the patient's airway should be controlled with an endotracheal tube. Sedation, using an agent such as diazepam or midazolam, should be administered before paralyzing any awake/oriented patient. A neurological examination including best motor response and pupillary examination should be performed before paralysis.

Use of these drugs requires the presence of a physician and flight nurse who are familiar

---

Box 6-4, cont'd
PROTOCOL FOR THE USE OF NEUROMUSCULAR BLOCKING AGENTS
UNIVERSITY AIR CARE

with their pharmacological actions and contraindications. A description of the pertinent
characteristics of these drugs follows the
procedure description. For some pediatric
patients, sedation with small doses of intravenous fentanyl may be preferable to prolonged neuromuscular blockade with these
agents.

Paralysis Procedure

1. Ensure that the endotracheal tube is in
   working order and is in proper position
   above the carina. Be sure the patient is receiving supplemental O_2.
2. Assemble required equipment:
   - Bag-valve-mask connected to functioning
     oxygen delivery system (or a working
     ventilator)
   - Working suction with tonsil sucker at-
     tached
   - Labeled syringe drawn up with Pavulon
     or Norcuron
3. The following equipment should be readily
   available for possible use in the event of
   inadvertent extubation after paralysis:
   - Endotracheal tube(s) with stylet and in-
     tact cuff

- Laryngoscope with blades and bright
  light
- Cricothyrotomy tray
4. Check to be sure that a good, functioning,
   secure IV line is in place and running.
5. Connect patient to a cardiac monitor to
   detect dysrhythmias occurring during subsequent steps.
6. In awake/oriented patients, sedate with diazepam 3-5 mg IV push or lorazepam 1-3
   mg IV push.
7. Give Pavulon 0.1 mg/kg or Norcuron 0.1
   mg/kg by slow IV push. If assisted ventilation is not already in progress, begin ventilating the patient as paralysis takes effect
   (usually 1-2 minutes after administration).
8. If inadequate relaxation is present 5 minutes after administration or if paralysis
   wears off earlier than required, additional
   incremental doses (usually 25% of the initial dose) may be administered. Before giving additional doses, ensure that the IV line
   is functioning and is not infiltrated.
9. Repeat sedation (diazepam 3-5 mg) should
   be administered every 30-60 minutes in
   awake patients who require continued
   paralysis.

Summary of Primary Breathing Assessment
- Rate and depth of respirations
- Cyanosis
- Position of the trachea
- Presence of obvious injury or deformity
- Work of breathing
  - Use of accessory muscles
  - Nasal flaring
  - Presence of breath sounds bilaterally

- Presence of adventitious breath sounds
- Asymmetrical chest movements
- Palpation of crepitus

Circulation

Palpation of both peripheral and central
pulses provides information about the patient's
circulatory status. The quality, location, and
rate of the patient's pulses should be noted. The

temperature of the patient's skin can be assessed along with the pulses.

Summary of Primary Circulation Assessment

- Tachycardia, bradycardia
- Skin appearance: cyanotic, dusky, mottled, pale
- Capillary refill greater than 2 seconds
- Diminished peripheral pulses
- Skin temperature
- Level of consciousness
- Decreased urinary output (assessment of patients at a referring facility)
- Hypotension
- Dysrhythmia

Any active bleeding needs to be quickly identified and proper interventions, such as direct pressure, initiated to control bleeding. The nurse should observe the patient for indications of circulatory compromise. Skin color, diaphoresis, and capillary refill are appraised during circulatory assessment.

Intravenous access is obtained for fluid, blood, and drug administration. Depending on patient location and venous accessibility, peripheral, central, or intraosseous access may be used.

Disability: Neurological Assessment

The neurological assessment comprises assessment of level of consciousness, motor sensory function, and pupil size, shape, and response. A simple method to evaluate the patient's level of consciousness is the AVPU method:

A	Alert
V	Responds to verbal stimuli
P	Responds to painful stimuli
U	Unresponsive

Both the Glasgow and pediatric Glasgow coma scales provide an assessment of the patient's level of consciousness and motor function (Tables 6-2 and 6-3).

Table 6-2   The Glasgow Coma Scale (GCS)

Subscale	Description	Score
Eye opening	Spontaneously	4
	To speech	3
	To pain	2
	Do not open	1
Best verbal response	Oriented	5
	Confused	4
	Inappropriate speech	3
	Unintelligible speech	2
	No verbalization	1
Best motor response	Obeys command	6
	Localizes pain	5
	Withdraws from pain	4
	Abnormal flexion	3
	Abnormal extension	2
	No motor response	1

Note. Best total score = 15; E4, V5, M6. Worst score = 3. From *Trauma Nursing* by J. Neff and P. Kidd, 1993, St. Louis: Mosby.

The prehospital nurse needs to discover whether the patient has ingested any toxic substance such as alcohol or other drugs. Patients whose mental status has been altered by drugs or alcohol may pose a potential safety problem during transport and may require chemical paralysis, sedation, or physical restraints.

Exposure

The patient should be exposed as much as possible, keeping in mind the effects of the environment. Discovering hidden problems before the patient is loaded for transport affords the nurse the ability to intervene and prevent disastrous complications. Even though exposure has been emphasized most frequently for the care of the trauma patient, it is just as important in the primary assessment of the patient with a medical illness.

The nurse should always look under dressings or clothing that may conceal important

Table 6-3　Pediatric-Modified Glasgow Coma Scale

Eyes Opening

Score	>1 Year	<1 Year
4	Spontaneously	Spontaneously
3	To verbal command	To shout
2	To pain	To pain
1	No response	No response

Best Motor Response

Score		
6	Obeys	Spontaneous
5	Localizes pain	Localizes pain
4	Flexion-withdrawal	Flexion-withdrawal
3	Flexion-abnormal (decorticate)	Flexion-abnormal (decorticate)
2	Extension (decerebrate)	Extension (decerebrate)
1	No response	No response

Best Verbal Response

Score	>5 Years	2-5 Years	Birth-23 Months
5	Oriented and converses	Appropriate words and phrases	Smiles, coos, appropriately
4	Disoriented and converses	Inappropriate words	Cries; consolable
3	Inappropriate words	Persistent cries or screams	Persistent, inappropriate crying and/or screaming
2	Incomprehensible sounds	Grunts	Grunts; agitated/restless
1	No response	No response	No response

Note. From *Severe Head Trauma* (p. 5) by J. Simon, 1988. Presented at Pediatric Emergencies, Williamsburg: Resource Applications.

pieces of information. Intravenous access can be wrongly assumed when hidden underneath a bulky cover. Clothing can also hide bleeding from thrombolytic therapy.

Another important component of assessment is the nurse's evaluation of all the interventions that have been performed before the prehospital nurse's arrival. This assessment includes evaluating airway, breathing, and circulation interventions.

Summary of Exposure Assessment
- Appropriate tube placement: endotracheal, nasotracheal tubes, chest tubes, nasogastric or orogastric tubes, urinary tract catheters
- Intravenous access: peripheral, central, intraosseous

Equipment Assessment

Even though equipment assessment is not routinely included in descriptions of a patient primary survey, it is an important process that needs to be performed. Whether the appropriate size cervical collar is on the patient, the chest tube drainage system is functioning, or the patient is correctly restrained makes a difference during transport.

Secondary Survey

Depending on the patient's condition and the amount of time needed for transport, a comprehensive secondary survey may not be completed. The secondary survey involves evaluating the patient from head to toe. The skills of inspection, palpation, and auscultation are applied to collect patient information during the secondary assessment. Whether the patient is injured or ill, the nurse should observe, touch, and listen to the patient.

The secondary assessment begins with an evaluation of the patient's general appearance. The nurse should observe the surrounding environment and evaluate its effects on the patient. Is the patient aware of the environment? Is the patient appropriately interacting?

Additional systems and features that should be surveyed include the integumentary (color, presence of wounds, temperature), head and neck (deformities, crepitus, pain), eyes, ears, and nose (drainage), thorax and lungs (chest movement, heart and breath sounds), abdomen, genitourinary, and extremities and back.

Summary of Secondary Survey

Skin
- Presence of petechia, purpura, abrasions, bruises, scars, birthmarks
- Rashes
- Abnormal skin turgor
- Signs of abuse and neglect

Head and Neck
- Presence of lacerations, contusions, raccoon eyes, Battle's sign, drainage from nose, mouth, ears
- In the infant, the anterior fontanelle

- Gross visual examination
- Abnormal extraocular movements
- Position of the trachea
- Neck veins
- Swallowing difficulties
- Nuchal rigidity
- Presence of lymphadenopathy or neck masses

Eyes, Ears, and Nose
- Lack of tearing
- Sunken eyes
- Color of the sclera
- Drainage
- Gross assessment of hearing

Mouth and Throat
- Mucous membranes
- Breath odor
- Injuries to teeth
- Drooling
- Drainage

Thorax, Lungs, and Cardiovascular System
- Breath sounds
- Heart sounds

Abdomen
- Shape and size
- Bowel sounds
- Tenderness
- Firmness
- Masses, suprapubic mass
- Femoral pulses
- Pelvic tenderness
- Color of drainage from nasogastric/orogastric tube

Genitourinary
- Blood at meatus
- Rectal bleeding
- Color of urine in catheter

Extremities and Back
- Gross motor and sensory function
- Peripheral pulses

- Lack of use of an extremity
- Deformity, angulation
- Wounds, abrasions
- Equipment appropriately applied, e.g., traction splints
- Vertebral column, flank, buttocks

Pain Assessment

Assessing the amount of pain the patient has related to the illness or injury is an important component of patient assessment. Physiological indications of pain include the following:

- Tachypnea
- Controlled respirations
- Tachycardia
- Hypotension
- Hypertension

- Nausea and vomiting
- Diaphoresis

Behavioral indications of pain include the following:

- Crying
- Protective behavior
- Guarding
- Moaning
- Self-focusing

Baseline data are collected about the patient's pain experience so that the prehospital nurse will be able to evaluate interventions during transport.

Scoring Systems

Scoring systems were initially developed to identify patients who need care that is unavailable at certain facilities (Emerman, Shade, & Kubincanek, 1992). Scoring systems can be used in the field and for evaluation of patients for interfacility support. The most common scoring systems have been used for the trauma patient. These include the Prehospital Index Score, CRAMS Scale Score, Triage-Revised Trauma Score, and the Pediatric Trauma Score (Cox, 1993). These scoring systems are listed in Tables 6-4 to 6-7.

Little research has been done that provides scoring for conditions other than trauma. However, general guidelines are available to indicate the need for transfer (see Chapter 4).

Table 6-4   Prehospital Index

Components	Value	Score
Blood pressure	>100	0
	86 to 100	1
	75 to 85	2
	0 to 74	5
Pulse	≥120	3
	51 to 119	0
	<50	5
Respirations	Normal	0
	Labored/shallow	3
	<10/min/needs intubation	5
Consciousness	Normal	0
	Confused/combative	3
	No intelligible words	5
Total		0-20

0 to 3—minor trauma
4 to 20—major trauma
(Penetrating abdominal or chest injuries given
   four points in addition to the calculated PHI)

Note. From "Prehospital Index: A Scoring System for Field Triage of Trauma Victims" by J. Koehler et al., 1986, *Annals of Emergency Medicine, 15,* p. 51.

Table 6-5   Revised Trauma Score

Glasgow Coma Scale	Systolic Blood Pressure	Respiratory Rate	Coded Value
13 to 15	>89	10 to 29	4
9 to 12	76 to 89	>29	3
6 to 8	50 to 75	5 to 9	2
4 to 5	1 to 49	1 to 5	1
3	0	0	0
Range 12 to 0			

Note. From "A Revision of the Trauma Score" by H. Champion et al., 1989, *Journal of Trauma, 29,* p. 624.

Table 6-6   Pediatric Trauma Score

Component	Severity Category		
	+2	+1	−1
Size	>20 kg	10 kg to 20 kg	<10 kg
Airway	Normal	Maintainable	Unmaintainable
CNS	Awake	Obtunded	Comatose
Systolic BP	>90 mm Hg	90 mm Hg to 50 mm Hg	<50 mm Hg
Open wounds	None	Closed fracture	Open/multiple fracture
Cutaneous	None	Minor	Major/penetrating

Note. From "The Pediatric Trauma Score as a Predictor of Injury Severity in the Injured Child" by J. Tepas et al., 1987, *Journal of Trauma, 27,* p. 14.

Table 6-7   CRAMS Score

Component	Score		
	2	1	0
Circulation	Normal capillary refill and blood pressure >100 mm Hg systolic	Delayed capillary refill or blood pressure 85 to 95 mm Hg systolic	No capillary refill or blood pressure <85 mm Hg systolic
Respiration	Normal	Abnormal (labored, shallow, or rate >35)	Absent
Abdomen	Abdomen and thorax not tender	Abdomen or thorax tender	Abdomen rigid, thorax flail, or deep penetrating injury to either chest or abdomen
Motor	Normal (obeys commands)	Responds only to pain—no posturing	Postures or no response
Speech	Normal (oriented)	Confused or inappropriate	No or unintelligible sounds

9 or 10—minor trauma
<8—major trauma

Note. From "CRAMS Scale: Field Triage of Trauma Victims" by S. Gormican, 1982, *Annals of Emergency Medicine, 11,* p. 133.

PATIENT PREPARATION

Preparation of the patient for transport is based on the information obtained from the primary and secondary surveys, the type of vehicle the patient will travel in, the amount of time the transport will take, and the potential problems that may develop related to the patient's illness or injury. Patient preparation includes anticipatory planning. Preparing for potential patient problems will make patient care safer and easier.

Over the past 10 years equipment has evolved that has made it easier to monitor and provide care for the patient during transport. Continenza and Hill (1990) recommend that the equipment used for transport meet the following criteria:

1. Should be useful for the transport setting
2. Should be lightweight, portable, and perhaps fulfill several functions such as a monitor with a built-in defibrillator and external pacemaker
3. Should be easily cleaned and maintained
4. Should have the ability to be used both inside and outside the transport vehicle
5. Should be able to withstand the stress of transport such as movement, altitude changes, dropping, water/fluid contamination, weather changes, use by multiple individuals

Tables 6-8 to 6-15 contain descriptions of some of the equipment available for transport. This is not a comprehensive list, but it does offer guidelines. Box 6-5 contains a generic list of equipment that may be used for patient transport. The amount and type of equipment carried by each service are dictated by the kinds of patients cared for. Figure 6-2 shows an example of equipment used by a service that cares for both pediatric and adult patients.

This section discusses general preparation of the patient; the following chapters then address the specific needs based on the patients' problems.

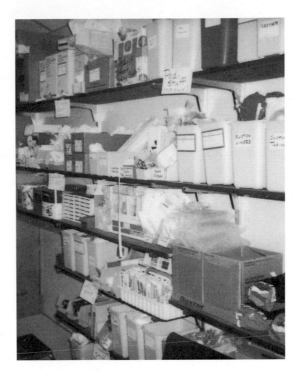

Fig. 6-2   Equipment room.

General Preparation
Airway Management

Patient preparation begins with assessment and management of the patient's airway. The location of the patient influences the type of airway management the nurse will be able to provide. For example, a patient trapped in a vehicle may have limited airway access.

Depending on the type of vehicle and the duration of transport, the nurse may elect to perform more definitive airway management. It is easier to intubate a patient before transport than at 1500 feet or 75 miles per hour. Space limitations and poor lighting may also make definitive airway control more of a challenge during transport.

If the patient is already intubated, tube place-

Text continued on p. 158.

Table 6-8   Pulse Oximeters

Monitor Name	Vendor	H × W × D (in); Weight	Display	Computer Interface	Battery Life (hr)
AD-900	Armstrong Medical	2.8 × 5.8 × 7.5 2.25 lb	LCD pulse strength activity	No	16
Oximeter 100	Life Care	2.5 × 5.8 × 7.5 2.25 lb	LCD pulse strength bar graph	Yes	16
Mini-Ox	MSA Catalyst Research	6 × 3.5 × 1.4 14 oz	LCD	No	200 (9 volt)
N-10	Nellcor	11.13 × 4.25 × 1.87 2.6 lb	LCD pulse display printer	No	*
N-100	Nellcor	4.2 × 12 × 12 16 lb	LED pulse display	No	1
N-200 Cardiosync Oximeter	Nellcor	2.5 × 10 × 10 5 lb	LED pulse display	Yes	2
8500	Nonin	6 × 3 × 1 10 oz	LED printer, color-coded perfusion—green, yellow, red	Yes	80
8604	Nonin Parr Emergency Products	2.5 × 5.5 × 7.5 2.1 lb	LED color coded†	Yes	20
8700 Cardiosync Oximeter	Nonin	8.5 × 3 × 9 3.9 lb	LED	Yes	15
8800 Cardiorespiratory oximeter	Nonin	8.5 × 3 × 3.9 3.7 lb	LED, also contains an apnea monitor	Yes	15
Criticare 503	Criticare	5.5 × 1.5 × 7 1.5 lb	LCD	Yes	6
Biox 3740	Ohmeda	2.8 × 8 × 8.8 5.5 lb	LCD waveform	Yes	3.5
Vitalmax 500	Pace Tech	3.25 × 8.25 × 10.5 11.5 lb	LED pulse strength bar, respiratory rate temperature	Yes	16

*100 cycles.
†Three-color perfusion.

Table 6-9 CO_2 Monitors

Monitor Name	Vendor	H × W × D (in); Weight	Display	Warm-up Time	Battery Life (hr)
FEF	Fenem	Disposable, less than an ounce	Color changes: purple, tan, yellow	Six breaths	2*
MiniCAP 100	MSA Catalyst Research	4 × 10.25 × 15.5 17.5 lb	LED digital display interfaces with a MiniCAP graphic display or an Epson printer	30 sec	1
MiniCAP III	MSA Catalyst Research	5.75 × 2.75 × 1.36 14.3 oz	LED	< 200 ms	8
N-1000/ADAP-C	Nellcor	5.25 × 12.5 × 12.5 25 lb	CRT does display SaO_2, pulse rate, and breathing rate	< 85 ms	15 min
4700 Oxi cap	Ohmeda	5.75 × 10 × 11.75 15 lb	LCD waveforms, 24-hour data trend, apnea alarm	65 sec	45 min
90513 Capnograph	Space Labs	5.4 × 10.25 × 10.25 17 lb	EL,† interfaces with PC Express Monitor	Not listed	2.5
AD-600	Armstrong Medical	5.75 × 7.5 2 lb 8 oz	LED	No warm-up needed	5
Vitalmax 3000	Pace Tech	5.36 × 11.5 × 12 22 lb	LED	Seconds	16

*The FEF can be used up to 2 hours.
†ElectroLuminescent.

Table 6-10 Multiple-Function Monitors

Monitor Name	Vendor	H × W × D (in); Weight	Display	Patient Parameters	Battery Life (hr)
Omega 1445	Invivo Research	4.25 × 9.45 × 10 10.8 lb	LED; does have computer interface	Noninvasive blood pressure (NIBP), SaO_2	45 min
PROPAQ106	Protocol	6.6 × 8.3 × 4.4 5.7 lb, 8.3 lb with SpO_2	LCD	ECG, NIBP, invasive blood pressure (IBP), SpO_2 temperature	6.5
90308 PC Express Monitor	Space Labs	10.3 × 10.1 × 10.3 13.5 lb to 16.3 lb	ElectroLuminescent	ECG, IBP, NIBP, SaO_2, respiratory rate, cardiac output, SvO_2	2.5
Vitalmax 2200	Pace Tech	10 × 9 × 12 28 lb	CRT LED	ECG, NIBP, SaO_2, temperature, respiratory rate	4
Sirecust 630	Siemens	5.1 × 8.3 × 4.2 5.7 lb	LCD	ECG, two invasive pressure channels, NIBP, temperature	30
Escort 100	Medical Data Electronic	6.9 × 7.9 × 10 16.5 lb plus weight for options	CRT	ECG, respiratory rate, NIBP, SaO_2, temperature, IBP, pressure channels	2 to 2.5
Escort 300	Medical Data Electronic	7 × 7 × 8.5	LCD	ECG, respiratory rate, NIBP, SaO_2, temperature, IBP, pressure channels	2.5 to 3

Table 6-11   Cardiac Monitors

Monitor Name	Vendor	H × W × D (in); Weight	Display	Equipment Functions	Battery Life (hr)
TRIAD EP TRIAD EP-II	Cardiotronics	6 × 3.15 × 2 16 oz	Color coded: green, yellow, red	External pacing, hands-off defibrillator, ECG monitoring through a single electrode system	1-2*
LifeDefense Plus	Matrix	4.80 × 13.98 × 15.55 18.7 lb	CRT screen	ECG recorder, hands-off defibrillator, external pacer	†
LIFEPAK 5	Physio Control	Monitor 3.8 × 7.5 × 13.3; defibrillator 3.8 × 7.5 × 13.3; monitor weight 8.25 lb; defibrillator weight 10.5 lb	Cardio Scope	ECG, hands-off defibrillator with FAST Patch attachment	‡
R2 System	Darox	Not listed	Depends on the monitor being used	ECG, external pacing, hands-off defibrillator, and cardioversion	*
90600A Adult/ Neonatal Monitor	Space Labs	6.5 × 11 × 16.75 28 lb	ElectroLuminescent	ECG, Sao_2, noninvasive blood pressure	1
LIFEPAK 10	Physio Control	4 × 16 × 14.6 20 lb	Cardio Scope display	ECG, pacer, defibrillator	‡

*This is an integrated system that operates with an existing monitor such as a LIFEPAK 5.
†Monitor only: 2 hours; monitor and 10 minutes of recorder: 1.5 hours; monitor and pacer (rate 70, 150 Ma): 1.5 hours; 360 joules discharges: 10 minimum.
‡45 minutes of monitoring or 30 minutes of pacing or 25 discharges at 360 joules per battery pack.

Table 6-12   Blood Pressure Monitors

Monitor Name	Vendor	H × W × D (in); Weight	Display	Battery Life (hr)
Digital Electronic	Buffalo Medical Specialties	Not listed	LCD	*
OscilloMate 920/EMS	CAS Medical Systems; Parr Emergency Products	2.75 × 6 × 7.5 3 lb	LCD	†
System 837	Lab Safety Supply	3 × 4.75 × 2 1 lb	LCD	9 volt
Vitalmax 800	Pace Tech	4 × 10 × 10 14 lb	LED	10-15
N-CAT	Nellcor	5 × 11 × 11 15.4 lb	Electro Luminescent	No battery
Lifestat 100	Physio Control	3.5 × 7.9 × 11.7 8 lb	LED	2

*Uses AA batteries; hours of use not listed.
†75 blood pressure measurements when the unit has been fully charged.

Table 6-13   Intravenous Monitors and Pumps

Monitor Name	Vendor	Weight	Accuracy	Battery Life (hr)
MTP/MVP Rotary Peristaltic (requires special tubing)	Armstrong Medical	4 lb	MVP ± 2% MTP ± 5%	8
Auto Syringe Model AS5D	Baxter	7.5 lb	± 3%	4
Auto Syringe Model AS2F	Baxter	19.3 oz		
Auto Syringe Model AS205	Baxter	24 oz	± 3%	24
Auto Syringe AS206GH-2	Baxter	27 oz	± 3%	*
IV-Push Pressure Infuser	MTM Health Products Ltd.	1.9 lb	Flow rate <10 ml/hr; 120 ml/min	†
Rateminder V	Critikon	7 lb	± 3%	‡
MiniMed III	Siemens	3.6 lb	Not listed	6-8§

*24 hours at 2 ml/hr, 5 hours at 100 ml/hr.
†Spring driven; the spring tension simulates the pressure of gravity created if the bag were 36 inches above the patient.
‡Minimum 60 days of continuous operation at 125 ml/hr.
§With all three channels operating at 125 ml/hr each.

Box 6-5
EQUIPMENT FOR TRANSPORT

Airway Equipment

Ambu bags for infant, child, and adult
Anesthesia bag
Oxygen masks in various sizes
Nasal cannula
Intubation equipment for infant, child, and
   adult
Miller blades 0,1,3
MAC blades 2,3,4
Masks for the resuscitation bags
Endotracheal tubes

Uncuffed		Cuffed	
2.5	4.5	4.0	6.5
3.0	5.0	4.5	7.0
3.5	5.5	5.0	7.5
4.0	6.0	5.5	8.0

Magill forceps (pediatric and adult)
Stylets
Tonsil suction
Suction catheters sizes 5/6, 8, 10, 14
Oral airways
Cricothyrotomy tray
Tracheostomy tubes
Portable suction unit
Pulse oximeter
CO_2 detector
Benzoin, adhesive tape, trach tape
Drugs for intubation (succinylcholine, vecuro-
   nium, valium, fentanyl)

Cardiothoracic Equipment

Cardiac monitor
Defibrillator
External pacer
Thoracotomy tray
Needle decompression supplies
Heimlich valves
Chest tubes, 10 Fr to 40 Fr
Automatic blood pressure machine
Manual blood pressure equipment (pediatric
   and adult)
Umbilical catheter trays (3.5 Fr and 5.0 Fr
   catheters)
MAST pants (?)

Nasogastric Tubes

Feeding tubes 5, 8
Salem sumps 10-18
Syringes

Intravenous Equipment/Medications

Intravenous needles (24-14)
7-Fr conversion kits
Blood tubing
Stopcocks
Minidrippers
Syringes
Butterflies
Intraosseous needles
Extension tubing
Intravenous pumps
Pressure bags
Blood and blood cooler
Blood tubes
Cut down tray
Razors
IV start packs
ACLS drugs
Vasopressor agents (dopamine, dobutamine,
   phenylephrine [Neo-Synepherine])
Mannitol
Furosemide (Lasix)
Antihypertensive agents
Others

Additional Equipment

Gloves and masks
Goggles
Surgilube
Sterile water
Flashlight
Disposable needle boxes
Paperwork
Stethoscope
Oxygen
Instant camera and film
Measuring tapes
Emergidose cards
Linen and towels
Dressings
Car seats
Isolette
Cervical collars
Backboards
Pedi transport board
Soft restraints
Bubble bag
Stockinette caps
Maps to receiving facility

Table 6-14   Portable Ventilators

Ventilator Name and Vendor	Powered by	Battery Life (hr)	Weight	Tidal Volume (ml)	Rates (BPM)	PEEP
Auto Vent 2000/3000, Life Support Products Armstrong Medical	Gas	N/A	16 oz	2000: 400-1200; 3000: 200-1200	2000: 8-20; 3000: 16-48	Yes
Uni-Vent 700, Impact	Battery	10	3.2 lb	0-1250	12-16	No
Uni-Vent 750, Impact	Battery	10	<10 lb	Not listed	1-150	Yes
PLV 102 Life Care	Battery	1	28.9 lb	50-2000	2-35	Yes

Table 6-15   CPR Machines

Machine Name	Vendor	H × W × D (in); Weight	Power Source
Heart-Lung Resuscitator	Armstrong Medical Brunswick Biomedical Technologies	17 × 22 × 7 27.1 lb	Oxygen
CARDIOPRESS	Resuscitation Laboratories	* 15 lb	Personnel

*The device consists of two parts. A board made of birch wood and formica is placed under the patient. The dimensions of the board are 34 × 10. The press is 18 × 22. It can be folded and easily stored.

ment should be evaluated and tube security assessed. Securing the endotracheal or nasotracheal tube for transport is important, since movement can potentially cause extubation, endobronchial intubation, mucosal damage, induction of a gag or cough, and increases in the patient's intracranial and intrathoracic pressure (Zecca, Carlascio, Marshall, & Dries, 1991).

Blood, vomit, and other secretions can contribute to tube movement and potential dislodgement. Several devices are available to secure the tube including umbilical tape, adhesive tape and tincture of benzoin, intravenous tubing, and commercial devices such as the Secure-Easy Quickstrap.

Oxygen should be placed on the patient. When available, additional monitoring equipment such as pulse oximeter, CO_2 monitor, or apnea monitor should be used for continuous airway evaluation.

Ventilation Management

A rapid, focused assessment of the patient's ventilatory status needs to be performed during patient preparation. If a chest X-ray film has been obtained before arrival, it needs to be evaluated to anticipate any complications that may occur during the transport process. Breath sounds should be auscultated before placement in the transport vehicle because of noise interference.

If a pneumothorax is suspected or present on the film, appropriate interventions should be taken. If a chest tube or tubes are already in place, the nurse should make sure they are functioning. The drainage system may need to be changed so that it will continue to function during transport.

If the patient is going to be placed on a portable ventilator, the patient's tidal volume, respiratory rate, and forced inspiratory oxygen (FIO_2) need to be calculated before the patient is connected to the ventilator. Some ventilators also provide additional modes including intermittent mandatory ventilation, continuous positive airway pressure, and positive end-expiratory pressure that are useful for critically ill or injured patients (see Box 6-5).

Circulation Management

Initial care is directed at controlling any active bleeding. Bleeding can be controlled with direct pressure by applying gauzepads and elastic tape or bandages (Campbell, 1988). Air splints and pneumatic antishock garments have also been used to help control bleeding. However, the source and the cause of the bleeding should be closely evaluated before transport. Once the patient is packaged, the source of the bleeding can easily be hidden by sheets and blankets.

Intravenous access needs to be ensured. Whether one or two lines are inserted depends on individual protocols. However, secure venous access is critical for fluid resuscitation and blood administration. Additional methods for access include the insertion of central lines and, in the pediatric patient, intraosseous lines.

When medications are infusing, intravenous monitors or pumps must be used to ensure that the medication is being appropriately delivered. Many devices are available (see Table 6-13). Medication concentrations and dosages should always be checked before changing equipment. Some prehospital nurses have found it easier to prepare medications with their own equipment and discard previous concentrations. For more expensive drugs, such as tissue plasminogen activator, that is not an option.

Foley catheters need to be affixed and placed so that they are not pulled during patient movement. It is a good idea to empty the catheter bag before leaving the referring facility. The presence and amount of blood and the color of the urine should be recorded.

If the patient has invasive lines in place such as pulmonary or arterial catheters, the nurse needs to check patency and functioning. In some cases transport monitors that offer specific readings during transport may not be available. The lines need to be secured so that future function is not impaired. If a monitor is available, readings before, during, and after transport should be taken and recorded.

Additional Procedures
Gastric Decompression

To prevent the potential for aspiration and to provide gastric decompression during transport, a nasogastric or orogastric tube should be inserted (Aoki & McCloskey, 1992; Civetta, Taylor, & Kirby, 1992). This procedure is not generally conducted before transport directly from a scene, but it may need to be considered strongly, particularly in the patient who has been given bag-valve-mask ventilation.

As with the Foley catheter, the gastric decompression tube needs to be appropriately placed and secured to prevent dislodgement. If the tube is not going to be placed on suction during transport, it should be capped to prevent it from spilling. When possible, the patient's stomach should be drained before plugging the tube. The presence and amount of blood, as well as the color of the drainage, should be documented.

Patients who are being treated for extensive gastrointestinal bleeding, such as that seen in the patient with liver disease, may have a specific type of gastric tube (e.g., the Blakemore tube) in place. Traction needs to be maintained so that the tube continues to function properly. This tube can place the patient at risk for aspiration, asphyxia, gastric rupture, and erosion of the esophageal wall (Kitt & Kaiser, 1990). When transporting this patient, the airway should be secured by intubation, and the nurse needs to be prepared to intervene if any complications occur. Needless to say, the transport of these patients offers a unique nursing challenge.

Wound Care and Splinting

Wounds and splinting devices require a quick evaluation before the patient is moved. Hidden wounds not only may cause the patient discomfort, but also can place the patient at risk of bleeding and long-term complications. Improperly placed splints or no splinting may also cause problems (Campbell, 1988).

Several types of splints and splint devices are available for transport. The nurse needs to be familiar with the type of equipment being used. How should the splint be placed? What are the potential complications of the device? When should it be removed? These questions are examples of some of the information needed. The neurovascular status of the extremities is to be assessed and documented wherever the splint is applied. Marking where the pulse has been palpated before transport will make it easier to locate and assess during transport.

Courses such as basic trauma life support, advanced trauma life support, trauma nursing core course, and the flight nurse advanced trauma course provide instruction on the use of splints (see Resource List in Chapter 7).

Wound care is provided for patient comfort and protection. Dressing the wound helps control bleeding and keeps it free of debris. If there is concern about additional bleeding or neurovascular compromise, the wound should be dressed so that continuous assessment is possible during transport. Any wet dressings are replaced with dry sterile dressings to prevent heat loss during transport.

An important concept to keep in mind when preparing the patient's wounds for transport is infection control. Many patients who are transported may have infected wounds that leave not only the transport team at risk but anyone else who may need to be transported in the vehicle. Infection control issues are addressed in Chapter 11.

Safety

When preparing the patient for transport, the nurse must consider what safety measures need to be taken. If the patient is combative, chemical paralysis and sedation may be indicated for the safety of both the patient and the transport team (see Table 6-1).

If restraints are needed, a policy should be in place that addresses the use of restraints based on guidelines issued by the Food and Drug Administration (Benson, 1992). These guidelines include the need to:

1. Clearly document the need for the use of restraints during transport
2. Follow the local and state laws regarding the use of patient restraints
3. Closely monitor the patient in restraints
4. Carefully apply the restraining device(s) and adjust them properly so that they maintain body alignment and are not uncomfortable
5. Consider restraints a temporary solution

Appropriate restraint systems must be used for the child. Devices that may be used include care beds, car seats, and pediatric transport boards. Equipment that is used during transport needs to meet federal and state standards.

Pain Management

Pain management in the prehospital setting frequently is not given priority consideration (Stewart, 1989). Several reasons influence the use or lack of use of pain medications in the field. These include the location of the patient, the patient's illness or injury, the possible masking of symptoms, and the effect of pain medications on the patient's vital signs. Movement, noise, changes in temperature, and fear may contribute to causing or increasing the patient's pain during preparation and transport.

In 1992 the United States Department of Health and Human Services published "Clinical Practice Guidelines for Acute Pain Management: Operative or Medical Procedures and Trauma." In these guidelines the need for appropriate pain management is emphasized. Although the prehospital management of pain is not directly addressed, these issues apply to the transport process.

It is pointed out that "the presence of a condition that could eventually result in cardiovascular, hemodynamic, neurologic, or pulmonary instability (e.g., femur fracture, pneumothorax, skull fracture) is not an absolute contraindication to systemic analgesia, although careful titration and monitoring must be provided" (US-DHH, 1992, p. 67).

The prehospital nurse must perform a brief assessment related to the patient's pain. The PQRST mnemonic previously described provides the nurse with a baseline description. If the patient had been medicated before the nurse's arrival, determining which medication was used and how it affected the patient adds important pieces of information to include in the pain assessment.

Pain medications used in the prehospital care environment need to be rapid in onset, short in duration, easy to administer, and easy to store (Stewart, 1989). The intravenous route is the most rapid method of administration. However, intravenous access may not always be available. Alternative methods currently being studied include the use of nasal sprays (Stewart, 1989). Table 6-16 provides a list of drugs that may be used for pain management in the prehospital care environment.

One additional point: it is important to keep in mind the issues related to pain management during transport. Many patients are given paralytic drugs for safe transport or for management of specific problems. The nurse should pay particular attention to the need for sedation and pain management in these patients, since they are unable to communicate. Close monitoring for changes in blood pressure and pulse while under paralysis offers clues to the prehospital nurse of the need for additional sedation or pain medication.

Additional methods that may be used by the nurse to help the patient manage pain during transport include the following:

1. Distraction (e.g., if the patient is alert enough to look out the window, allow them to do so; a child may find a security object such as a stuffed toy of help)
2. Touching and talking to the patient
3. Keeping the patient warm
4. Placing the patient in a position of comfort when possible
5. Explaining events the patient will experience
6. Allowing a family member to accompany the patient

These methods can also be effective in decreasing the patient's pain in conjunction with medication.

Communication

Communication is one of the most important components in the preparation of the patient for transport. It begins before the nurse arrives. Written policies, procedures, and triage guidelines need to be in place at referring facilities

Table 6-16   Drugs for Pain Management

Drug	Dosage	Potential Problems
Morphine sulfate	3-5 mg IV 3-5 mg every 10 minutes	Hypotension Respiratory depression
Fentanyl	2-3 mcg/kg IV 1 mcg/kg every 5 minutes IV	Excessive sedation, chest rigidity, nasal itching, nausea
Meperidine	50-70 mg IV 25-50 mg IV every 15 minutes	Respiratory depression

Note. From *Emergency Drug Therapy* by W. Barsan, M. Jastremski, and S. Syverud, 1991, Philadelphia: W.B. Saunders.

or agencies that identify the type of patient that needs prehospital nursing care, what initial stabilization is required before transport, what modes of transportation are available in the geographical area, and who may accompany the patient.

When the initial contact is made by the referring hospital or agency, information that should be gathered includes the patient's chief complaint or problem (chest pain, multiple trauma, respiratory distress), indications for transport, vital signs, and any interventions that have been performed. The problem, age, and location of the patient are important so that the most suitable nurse(s) can be dispatched. For example, in some areas of the country there are maternal, pediatric, and critical care transport nurses. The equipment required by the patient during transport also influences the nursing skills needed during transport (e.g., intraaortic balloon pump).

Once the team has been assembled and the mode of transport decided, the referring facility or agency needs to be provided with an estimated time of arrival. Before arrival, the nurse prepares for the patient based on the information furnished by the referring facility or agency.

Once the nurse arrives, any information about the patient(s) can be given directly to the nurse and other team members. When arriving at a scene response, the nurse needs to identify the individual in charge and ask what kind of help is needed. During the initial assessment and preparation for transport, the nurse communicates with the other team members and referring individuals. The communication process is composed of both verbal and nonverbal behaviors. Attitudes and actions are important nursing interventions. Always involve those who have been caring for the patient.

If the patient has not received all of the required care, this may afford the prehospital nurse the opportunity to teach, not to preach. The transport team needs to offer explanations about care and interventions, especially when asked. Many times it is useful to establish protocols for transport with referring institutions and agencies. This not only decreases patient preparation time, but also offers an additional method of providing information related to specific patient problems.

Any laboratory results, X-ray studies, or scans need to be copied and sent with the patient. Any valuable items belonging to the patient must be accounted for. Sometimes it is easier to leave them with family members, but it may not be possible. A good way to prevent potential problems is to record a list of what was brought with the patient and to whom it was given upon arrival at the receiving facility. At times, clothing or other valuables may be considered evidence and should be attended to based on an evidence protocol.

The communication process continues during transport. Information that should be conveyed includes a brief description of the patient's chief complaint, problems identified by the nurse's assessment, interventions performed, estimated time of arrival, and the need for any special services or equipment on arrival.

Follow-up communication should occur as soon as possible after the transport has been completed and should include the patient's diagnosis or a summary of injuries, care given at the receiving hospital, and the disposition of the patient. Follow-up communication provides a method of evaluating the care rendered by the prehospital nurse and offers the opportunity for referring agencies and institutions to ask any questions. It is important to keep in mind that patient care is a process and many are a part of it.

The Family

Whenever a family member is ill or injured a crisis is created. Transferring the patient to another facility far away usually increases stress.

Sometimes the nurse does not have the opportunity to interact with the patient's family. When the nurse responds directly to the scene of the illness or injury, the family may not be present or may be injured. When family members are present, the nurse may use them to obtain pertinent patient history.

The nurse needs to be sure that information is provided to the family before, during, and after transport. Policies and procedures should be in place that address when a family member may accompany an injured or ill member. Several reasons have been proposed regarding why family members should not accompany the patient during transport whether by ground or air (Edgington, 1992, p. 13). These include the following:

1. Untrained passengers can be unpredictable and a potential safety problem.
2. Space is limited in the transport vehicle.
3. Risk of legal liability increases if an accident or incident should occur during transport.
4. Family members may not understand patient care interventions.

The following guidelines can be useful when discussing the transport process with a family:

1. Explain to the family why the patient needs to be transported.
2. Obtain consent, when required, before the transport.
3. Encourage the family not to leave until the transport vehicle has left. The patient may not leave the referring facility.
4. If the family is not allowed to accompany the patient, explain why.
5. Advise the family to drive carefully to the receiving facility.
6. Provide maps, directions, and a contact person for the family at the receiving facility.
7. If the family member is alone, encourage them to take someone on the trip.
8. Always allow the family member to see the patient before leaving (Rea, 1991).

Documentation

Copies of any relevant documentation should accompany the patient from the referring facility or agency. If pictures of the scene of the ac-

cident or crash are available, they should be brought along.

Copies of any laboratory results, X-ray studies, scans, and documentation by the referring facility or agency should accompany the patient. If written permission is required for transport, a copy of this document should be included.

The nurse's documentation of the initial assessment, preparation, and interventions can be completed during or after transport. Nursing documentation is based on the specific standards of care for the type of patient being transported. Components of these documents vary based on the information required in each transport service. Some programs use computer documentation and equipment that can download information from the monitor that was used during transport (Hassig, 1992). Figure 6-3 provides an example of a transport document.

PATIENT ASSESSMENT DURING TRANSPORT

The patient's illness or injuries and the initial interventions performed influence the assessment and management needed during transport. Each of the patient care chapters in this text addresses the specific care required during transport related to the patient's illness or injury. Some general care principles of assessment and management during transport include the following:

1. Nurses should position themselves in the transport vehicle so that they can effectively manage the patient's vital functions and reach equipment.
2. Airway equipment, including suction equipment, should be easily accessible.
3. All intravenous, central, or intraosseous lines need to be accessible and functioning.
4. All tubes and drainage systems need to be functioning and secured.
5. If there is any question about cervical

DATE _____ TIME _____

NAME:

FLIGHT

UNIVERSITY OF CINCINNATI HOSPITAL

**UNIVERSITY AIR CARE
FLIGHT RECORD**

REFERRING AGENCY/MD _____

RECEIVING AGENCY/MD _____

INITIAL ASSESSMENT: _____

UAC-4, Rev. 10/91

RESP _____

CIRC _____

NEURO _____

GI/GU _____

EXTREMITIES _____

C COLLAR [ ]   HEAD IMMOBILIZER [ ]   BACKBOARD [ ]   MAST _____

HISTORY, CONTINUED ASSESSMENT & ACTIONS:

TIME	BP	P	R	

I&O Total
Prior to Arrival

I _____ O _____

Flight Totals

I _____ O _____

Lab Values _____

_____

_____

_____

GCS _____

IV FLUIDS/BLOOD PRODUCTS/MEDS
TIME

PAST MEDICAL HISTORY

ALLERGIES _____

DIAGNOSIS _____

RN Signature _____

MD Signature _____

TRAUMA SCORE _____   PARALYTIC AGENTS Yes [ ] No [ ]

WHITE–MEDICAL RECORDS   YELLOW–BILLING   PINK–AIR CARE   GOLDENROD–AIR CARE

Fig. 6-3 University of Cincinnati Hospital Flight Record.

ADULT TRAUMA SCORE

Trauma Score

The Trauma Score is a numerical grading system for estimating the severity of injury. The score is composed of the Glasgow Coma Scale (reduced to approximately one third total value) and measurements of cardiopulmonary function. Each parameter is given a number (high for normal and low for impaired function). Severity of injury is estimated by summing the numbers. The lowest score is 1, and the highest score is 16.

			Before Flight	During Flight	in ER
Respiratory	10-24/min	4			
Rate	24-35/min	3			
	36/min or greater	2			
	1-9/min	1			
	None	0			
Respiratory	Normal	1			
Expansion	Retractive	0			
Systolic	90 mm Hg or greater	4			
Blood Pressure	70-89 mm Hg	3			
	50-69 mm Hg	2			
	0-49 mm Hg	1			
	No Pulse	0			
Capillary	Normal				
Refill	Delayed	1			
	None	0			

Glasgow Coma Scale

Eye Opening	Spontaneous	4	Total	
	To Voice	3	Glasgow	
	To Pain	2	Coma	
	None	1	14 - 15 = 5	
			11 - 13 = 4	
Verbal Response	Oriented	5	8 - 10 = 3	
	Confused	4	5 - 7 = 2	
	Inappropriate		3 - 4 = 1	
	Words	3		
	Incomprehensibled			
	Words	2		
	None	1		
Motor Response	Obeys Command	6		
	Localizes Pain	5		
	Withdraw (pain)	4		
	Flexion (pain)	3		
	Extension (pain)	2		
	None	1		

Total Trauma Score   1 - 16

PEDIATRIC TRAUMA SCORE

Component	Category		
	+2	+1	−1
Size	>20 Kg (40#)	10-20 kg	<10 kg
Airway	Normal	Maintainable	Unmaintainable
Systolic BP	>90 MM Hg	50-90 mm Hg	<50 mm Hg
CNS	Awake LOC	Obtunded/	Coma/decerebrate
Skeletal	None	Closed fracture	Open/multiple fractures
Cutaneous	None	Minor	Najor/penetrating Sum _____ (PTS)

If proper sized BP cuff not available, BP can be assessed by assigning

+2   Pulse palpable at wrist
+1   Pulse palpable at groin
−1   No pulse palpable

Fig. 6-3, cont'd   University of Cincinnati Hospital Flight Record.

Table 6-17 Nursing Diagnoses, Interventions, and Evaluative Criteria in Patient Assessment and Preparation for Transport

Diagnosis	Interventions	Evaluative Criteria
Ineffective airway clearance related to obstruction from blood, foreign bodies, edema, altered mental status as evidenced by the patient's inability to maintain a patent airway	Secure a patent airway by basic and advanced life support maneuvers (Box 6-3) Evaluate effectiveness of present airway by pulse oximeter Check CO_2 monitor regularly Use high flow O_2	*The patient will have the following:* Patent airway Maintainable airway Breath sounds present and equal bilaterally CO_2 readings indicating patent airway Pulse oximeter reading 93% to 100%
Ineffective breathing patterns related to altered mental status, chest injury (pneumothorax), illness (COPD) evidenced by abnormal chest movement, increased work of breathing, presence of adventitious breath sounds (crackles, wheezes)	Establishment of a patent or maintainable airway with BLS and/or ALS maneuvers When indicated: needle decompression, chest tube insertion Evaluation of chest X-ray study when available at the referring facility Place patient on high flow O_2 and on transport ventilator using appropriate settings Use CO_2 and pulse oximeter monitors	*The patient will have the following:* Patent or maintainable airway Breath sounds present and equal bilaterally If chest tube or needle in place, drainage system will be attached and functioning Ventilator will be functioning with appropriate settings CO_2 monitor will indicate a patent airway Pulse oximeter readings will be 93% to 100%
High risk for decreased cardiac output	Control active bleeding with pressure dressings Obtain intravenous, central, or intraosseous access If access is already present, access patency Check the quality and rate of central and peripheral pulses Place patient on a cardiac monitor If invasive lines are present, check placement and functioning	*The patient will have the following:* Active bleeding controlled Patent access either intravenous, central, or intraosseous Cardiac monitor in place Invasive lines functioning

Table 6-17   Nursing Diagnoses, Interventions, and Evaluative Criteria in Patient Assessment and Preparation for Transport—cont'd

Diagnosis	Interventions	Evaluative Criteria
Fear related to the patient's illness or injury and the need to be transferred to another facility	Explain to the patient and family the need to transport patient When possible, consider allowing family to accompany the patient When possible, allow family to see transport vehicle Allow family member to see patient before transport	*The patient will have the following:* The ability to voice their fears Family will be able to see transport vehicle Family will see the patient before transfer

spine injury, immobilize the cervical spine for transport.

6. A combative patient needs to be properly restrained, both chemically and physically.
7. Place all monitors within the nurse's visual field.
8. When indicated, leave wounds and injured limbs exposed for inspection.

SUMMARY

Patient assessment and preparation are the foundations for the care of the patient in the prehospital care area and during transport of the patient to definitive care. The primary and secondary surveys provide the initial information about the patient's current and potential problems.

Patient preparation includes not only care of the obvious, but also anticipation of what may occur. Resources are limited in the prehospital care environment. Anticipatory planning, safety, and prevention are key nursing interventions.

Examples of potential nursing diagnoses that may be used during preparation of the patient for transport are given in Table 6-17. These

nursing diagnoses include ineffective airway clearance, ineffective breathing patterns, high risk for decreased cardiac output, and fear.

REFERENCES

Aoki, B., & McCloskey, K. (1992). *Evaluation, stabilization, and transport of the critically ill child.* St. Louis: Mosby.

Barsan, W., Jastremski, M., & Syverud, S. (1991). *Emergency drug therapy,* Philadelphia: W.B. Saunders.

Benson, J. (1992). *FDA safety alert: Potential hazards with restraint devices.* Rockville, MD: Food and Drug Administration.

Campbell, J. (1988). *Basic trauma life support.* Englewood Cliffs, NJ: Brady Book.

Civetta, J., Taylor, R., & Kirby, R. (1992). *Critical care.* Philadelphia: J.B. Lippincott.

Continenza, K., & Hill, J. (1990). Transport of the critical child. J. Blumer (Ed.). *Pediatric intensive care* (pp. 17-27). St. Louis: Mosby.

Cox, D. (1993). Keeping score. *Emergency, 25*(5), 42-48.

Dailey, R., Simon, B., & Stewart, R. (1992). *The airway: Emergency management.* St. Louis: Mosby.

Dickinson, E., Krett, R., & O'Connor, R. (1992). The impact of prehospital instant photography of motor crashes on physician perception and patient management in the emergency department. *Prehospital and Disaster Medicine, 7,* (Suppl. 1), p. 209.

Edgington, B. (1992). Transporting the family and other concerned parties aboard air medical aircraft. *Journal of Air Medical Transport, 2,* 11-14.

Emergency Nurses Association (1991). *National standard guidelines for prehospital nursing curriculum.* Chicago: The Author.

Emerman, C., Shade, B., & Kubincanek, J. (1992). Comparative performance of the Baxt trauma triage rule. *American Journal of Emergency Medicine 10*(4), 294-297.

Hart, M. (1988). Patient assessment, preparation, and care. In U.S. Department of Transportation. *Air medical crew national standard curriculum.* Pasadena, CA: Association of Air Medical Services.

Hassig, J. (1992). At-the-scene data capture. *Healthcare Informatics, 3,* 18-24.

Henry, M., & Stapleton, E. (1992). *EMT prehospital care.* Philadelphia: W.B. Saunders.

Lazear, S. (1992). Aeromedical transport. In S. Sheehey. *Emergency nursing: Principles and practice.* St. Louis: Mosby.

Kidd, P. (1993). Assessment of the trauma patient. In J. Neff & P. Kidd. *Trauma nursing: Art and science* (pp. 115-142). St. Louis: Mosby.

Kitt, S., & Kaiser, J. (1990). *Emergency nursing.* Philadelphia: WB Saunders.

Lee, G. (1992). *Quick emergency care reference.* St. Louis: Mosby.

Rea, R. (1991). *Trauma nursing core curriculum.* Chicago: Emergency Nurses Association.

Stewart, R. (1989). Analgesia in the field, *Prehospital and Disaster Medicine, 4*(1), 31-34.

U.S. Department of Health and Human Services. (1992). Acute pain management: Operative or medical procedures and trauma. Washington, DC: The Author.

Zecca, A., Carlascio, D., Marshall, W., & Dries, D. (1991). Endotracheal tube stabilization in the air medical setting. *Journal of Air Medical Transport, 3,* 7-10.

CHAPTER 7

Transport Considerations for the Trauma Patient

OBJECTIVES

1. Describe the initial assessment and stabilization of the multiply injured patient
2. Discuss the care of the injured patient during transport
3. Discuss critical trauma triage criteria

COMPETENCIES

1. Demonstrate proficiency in the following assessment skills:
   Scene assessment
   Primary assessment
   Secondary assessment
2. Anticipate and perform needed interventions to transport the trauma patient safely, including:
   Airway control and ventilation
   Chest decompression
   Spinal immobilization
   Fluid resuscitation
3. Demonstrate knowledge of critical trauma triage criteria

Trauma remains the number one killer in the first four decades of life. It does not distinguish between age, race, or gender and usually presents without warning. When working in the prehospital setting, the most important point to remember is that a traumatic injury is a surgical disease, and the ability of the nurse to perform a rapid primary assessment, intervene in life-threatening situations, and facilitate rapid transport to an appropriate facility influence the patient's final outcome. The National Research Council reported in 1985 that each year more than 140,000 Americans die as a result of trauma and approximately 80,000 are permanently disabled from traumatic injury (Snyder, 1993).

Deaths from traumatic injury occur in a trimodal distribution, that is, in three separate peaks. Patients who die within the first seconds to minutes of injury are within the first peak of death. These deaths are usually caused by lacerations to the brain, high spinal cord, heart, aorta, or other large vessels. Deaths occurring within a few minutes to a few hours after injury constitute the second death peak and are usually caused by subdural and epidural hematomas, hemopneumothorax, ruptured spleen, liver lacerations, pelvic fractures, or multisystem trauma associated with severe blood loss (American College of Surgeons Committee on Trauma [ACS], 1989). If patients remain in shock for an extended period of time they may subsequently die of the complications of shock. Hypoperfusion and hypoxia result in anaerobic metabolism and metabolic acidosis. The patient can also develop respiratory acidosis when gas exchange is decreased at the alveolocapillary cellular membrane level. Acidosis results in increased coagulation that blocks the small vessels; platelets aggregate and disseminate, and intravascular coagulation results. As perfusion decreases, myocardial infarction, renal failure, and cerebral edema occur. If shock persists, intestinal mucosa and endothelial cells are damaged and sepsis may result. Decreased intravascular volume, with resulting decreases in blood pressure and colloidal osmotic pressure, may result in adult respiratory distress syndrome (Sheehy, 1992). It is during this period that the nurse in the prehospital setting can make a significant difference. Reducing the time between the initial injury and definitive care can significantly reduce the complications of shock. Rapid assessment, recognition and intervention of life-threatening conditions, and rapid transport can reduce deaths during the second peak of trauma. The third peak occurs several days or weeks after the injury. These deaths are usually the result of sepsis and organ failure (ACS, 1989).

ASSESSMENT

The ability to perform a thorough, rapid assessment is vital in determining life-threatening conditions and anticipating future patient needs. An important aspect of assessment in the prehospital setting includes the scene itself. The nurse can gather many important clues from the scene that influence the entire assessment. The following factors need to be considered during scene evaluation:

1. *Safety.* Every team member is responsible for recognizing all possible dangers and ensuring that none still exist. No one should become a victim. Fire or police should secure the area if the scene is unsafe.
2. *Scene.* What was the mechanism of injury? What is the extent and type of damage?
3. *Situation.* What really happened? Why? Could there be extenuating circumstances (e.g., the driver lost control of the car as a result of a heart attack). Determine the number of patients and their ages (National Association of Emergency Medical Technicians [NAEMT], 1990).

The first priority in the prehospital setting must be the protection of the emergency responders and the patient from further injury. The nurse should evaluate the scene and, if necessary, move the patient to a safe area before initiating treatment. Hazards that may endanger the patient include temperature, rain and snow, water, fire, and proximity of the incident to the highway or other cars (NAEMT, 1990).

During the scene survey the nurse gathers information concerning possible injury patterns by studying the kinematics of the accident. Kinematic energy is energy that changes form because of the incident and is absorbed by the patient's body. By looking at the mechanism, the path of energy can be followed and possible injuries anticipated. Energy is neither created nor destroyed—it is transferred. During an accident, energy is transferred from the vehicle to the body. Two factors affect the amount of energy absorbed by the body: (1) the energy that has already been absorbed by objects from the initial impact and (2) the energy absorbed by protective devices, e.g., airbags, padded dashes and dashboards, and seat belts (Lee, 1991). The slower an object is moving, the less energy is transferred, so the amount of destruction is decreased. This is why it is important to try to de-

Box 7-1
TRAUMA INJURY PATTERNS

Frontal Impact

Trunk	*Head*	*Extremities*
Rib fractures	Scalp lacerations	Knee dislocation
Flail chest	Skull fractures	Femur fracture
Pneumothorax/hemothorax	Cerebral contusion	Hip dislocation
Pulmonary contusion	Cerebral hemorrhage	Acetabular fracture
Cardiac contusion		
Aortic tear		
Lacerated spleen/liver		

Side Impact

Trunk	*Head*	*Extremities*
Clavicle fracture	Cervical spine fracture	Femur fracture
Rib fractures	Cervical ligament sprain	Pelvic fracture
Flail chest	Cervical ligament tear	
Pulmonary contusion	Facial/scalp lacerations	
Lacerated liver/spleen	Skull fractures	
	Cerebral contusion/ hemorrhage	

termine the estimated speed of the vehicle at the time of the accident.

During a lifetime a person is likely to be involved in an automobile accident once every 10 years and has a 33% chance of suffering a disabling injury (Lee, 1991). Autopsy findings, observations by trauma surgeons, and data collected through crash tests with anthropomorphic dummies have provided a correlation between mechanisms of injury with groups of common injuries (Neff & Kidd, 1993). Box 7-1 lists the injuries common to frontal- and side-impact vehicle accidents.

When assessing the patient after a side-impact collision it is important to note the amount of intrusion into the passenger compartment and if the door or post impacted the patient's upper or lower body (Figure 7-1). Vehicles made after 1968 have energy-absorbing

steering columns that have helped to decrease the severity of the injuries in frontal impacts (Figure 7-2) (Neff & Kidd, 1993).

In rear-impact collisions, the trends of injuries depend on whether the vehicle glided to a stop or hit another vehicle or object causing a secondary frontal impact. If it is solely a rear-impact accident and the car seat did not have a headrest or the headrest was malpositioned, hyperextension of the neck with a possible cervical spine injury may result.

When seat belts are worn properly during vehicle accidents, energy should be absorbed by the bony pelvis and chest. If seat belts are not properly positioned, the impact energy is absorbed by soft tissues and may result in injury. Compression injury to intraabdominal organs can occur when seat belts are worn too high, and the increased intraabdominal pressure can

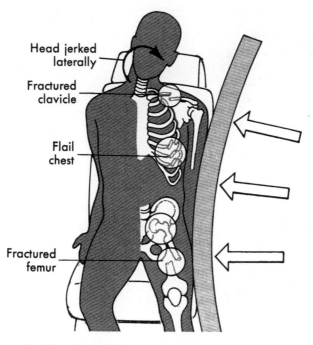

Head jerked
laterally

Fractured
clavicle

Flail
chest

Fractured
femur

Fig. 7-1   Potential injury sites in a side-impact collision. Note that injury is still possible in a side-impact crash, even with airbag inflation, because airbags were designed specifically for frontal crashes. However, injuries are usually fewer in side-impact crashes with airbag inflation than without. (From *Trauma Nursing: The Art and Science* by J.A. Neff and P.S. Kidd, 1992, St. Louis: Mosby.)

cause diaphragmatic rupture. Compression fractures of T12, L1 and L2 may also occur (NFNA, 1990).

Motorcycle accidents also show characteristic injury patterns. The center of gravity is forward on a motorcycle. On frontal impact the body continues forward with the back of the motorcycle raising and the first impact of the body being the thighs onto the handlebars causing bilateral femur fractures. If the initial impact is from the side, the injury patterns usually involve the lower extremity on that side and include open tibia-fibula fractures and dislocation of the ankle. Regardless of the type of impact, the victim is almost always ejected from

the motorcycle. Ejection from either a motor vehicle or motorcycle greatly increases the chances of sustaining a severe injury. The major injury occurs at the point of impact and continues as energy is transferred to the rest of the body (NFNA, 1990).

When struck by a vehicle, it has been shown that adult pedestrians turn to the side to protect themselves (Figure 7-3). Injury patterns include tibia-fibula fractures, femur/pelvis fracture, and cervical spine fracture. Pediatric pedestrians have a tendency to face forward and freeze (Figure 7-4). Depending on the height of the child and the vehicle the injury patterns are femur/pelvis fracture, chest injury, and head injury during second impact (NAEMT, 1990).

Penetrating Trauma

In the assessment of penetrating trauma it is valuable to know what type of weapon was used to determine the velocity and amount of energy transference. Three energy levels that affect injury patterns in penetrating trauma are as follows:

1. *Low energy.* Stab wounds cause a low energy level of injury. It is important to assess for multiple wounds, since nearly one in four patients with abdominal injuries also have an associated thoracic injury. A male attacker tends to stab upward, whereas a female attacker tends to stab downward.
2. *Medium energy.* Handguns and some low-velocity rifles produce a medium energy level. The energy wave that follows the bullet causes pressure waves, called cavitation, around the pathway of the bullet. Small caliber bullets may ricochet off of bone and travel within the body.
3. *High energy.* High-powered rifles produce a much greater energy. Because of this a permanent tract may occur with cavitation and a greater incidence of compression and stretch injuries. With any type of gunshot wound, if the bullet hits bone, the

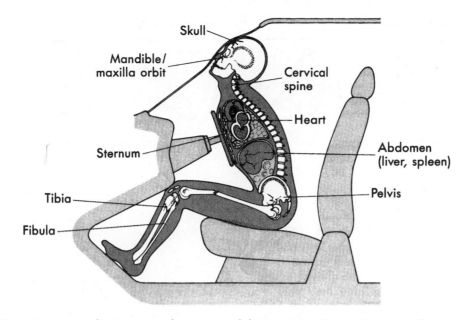

Fig. 7-2   Potential injury sites of unrestrained driver. (From *Trauma Nursing: The Art and Science* by J.A. Neff and P.S. Kidd, 1992, St. Louis: Mosby.)

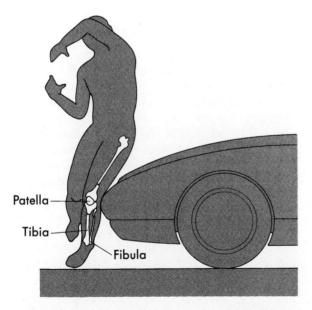

Fig. 7-3   Potential primary injury sites of adult pedestrian. (From *Trauma Nursing: The Art and Science* by J.A. Neff and P.S. Kidd, 1992, St. Louis: Mosby.)

fragments from the bone become secondary missiles and may cause further damage (NFNA, 1990). Because the energy dissipation to the tissues is the change in kinetic energy from entrance to exit, if no exit occurs, then all energy at entrance is absorbed by the surrounding tissues (Boyd, Odom, Campbell, & Martin, 1991).

PRIMARY SURVEY

During the primary survey, any life-threatening conditions that are identified should be managed simultaneously. The primary survey should be performed quickly and with the following priority:

A—airway with cervical spine stabilization
B—breathing and ventilation
C—circulation with hemorrhage control
D—disability: neurological status
E—exposure: undress the patient

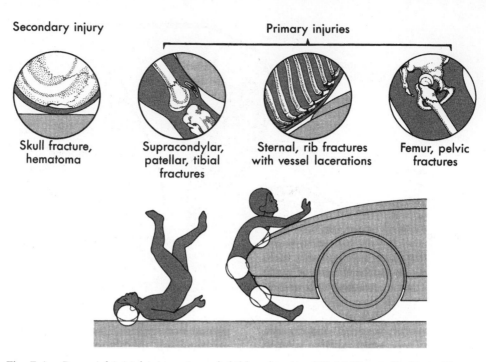

Secondary injury   Primary injuries

Skull fracture,   Supracondylar,   Sternal, rib fractures   Femur, pelvic
hematoma   patellar, tibial   with vessel lacerations   fractures
                       fractures

Fig. 7-4   Potential initial injury sites of child pedestrian (Waddell's triad). (From *Trauma Nursing: The Art and Science* by J.A. Neff and P.S. Kidd, 1992, St. Louis: Mosby.)

Airway

The patient's airway should be assessed for patency. Basic maneuvers should be instituted including suctioning and opening the airway without moving the cervical spine by using a chin-lift or jaw-thrust technique. All multi-trauma patients should be treated as if they have a cervical spine fracture until proven otherwise by x-ray studies. If the patient has a decreased level of consciousness or is unable to protect the airway from aspiration, then intubation should be performed at this time. The nurse in the prehospital setting must be able to recognize the indications for intubation and apply the form of airway management that is optimal for the situation and clinical condition.

Breathing

The patient's chest should be exposed and visually inspected to assess ventilatory exchange.

The chest should be palpated for crepitus and symmetry and auscultated for bilateral breath sounds. Airway patency does not ensure adequate ventilation. All trauma patients should be placed on oxygen, with forced inspiratory oxygen (FIO_2) of 100%. A nonrebreather face mask should be used, since this form of oxygen delivery cannot be accomplished by nasal prongs or a simple face mask. Three conditions that most often affect ventilation are tension pneumothorax, open pneumothorax, and a large flail segment with pulmonary contusion (ACS, 1991). The nurse should suspect respiratory compromise if the patient's respiratory rate is greater than 28 to 30/minute.

Circulation

Three initial observations can give the nurse information regarding the patient's hemodynamic status:

1. *Level of consciousness.* As a person's blood volume decreases, cerebral perfusion is impaired, affecting level of consciousness.
2. *Skin color.* In persons of fair skin color, an ashen gray face and pale, white extremities are ominous signs of hypovolemia. In persons of color, paleness of the mucous membranes is a sign of shock.
3. *Pulse.* A strong, regular peripheral pulse is a good sign. As the shock state progresses the peripheral pulse becomes weak and thready. Absent femoral pulses signify severe blood depletion and the need for immediate resuscitation and transport.

During the primary survey any obvious hemorrhage should be identified and controlled with direct pressure. Tourniquets should not be used because they can produce anaerobic metabolism due to the decreased circulation distal to the tourniquet and actually increase the bleeding if improperly applied (ACS, 1991).

Disability

During the primary survey a rapid neurologic assessment is conducted and pupillary size and function checked. The following mnemonic can be helpful:

A—Alert
V—Responds to *v*erbal stimuli
P—Responds to *p*ainful stimuli
U—Unresponsive

A witnessed decrease in the patient's level of consciousness may indicate intracranial pathology or a decrease in cerebral oxygenation or perfusion. Any change merits immediate reevaluation of the patient's airway, breathing, and circulation status.

Exposure

During the primary survey the patient's clothing should be cut away to facilitate a thorough examination. Although visual assessment is important, care must be taken to protect patients from the elements and to respect their modesty. The primary survey needs to be carried out quickly and efficiently. Much of the primary survey can be completed simultaneously. It is at this time that the nurse decides if the patient has sustained critical trauma requiring immediate transport or noncritical trauma requiring expedient transport. The patient may receive care such as splinting of extremity injuries before transport. Some patients may appear relatively stable during initial assessment but should still be considered critical trauma patients. A triage decision scheme was developed by Dr. Champion to be used as a guideline (Figure 7-5). Once a patient is determined to have suffered critical trauma, only lifesaving measures such as airway establishment and hemorrhage control should be initiated before transport. Initiation of fluid replacement and the secondary survey should be performed en route to the trauma center.

SECONDARY SURVEY

The secondary survey consists of a thorough evaluation beginning at the head and proceeding to the face, neck, chest, abdomen, and extremities. A more detailed neurological examination is performed at this time.

Head

Patients wearing a helmet should have the helmet removed while the head and neck are manually maintained in a neutral position. The head should be palpated for scalp lacerations and possible open skull fractures. The pupils are reassessed and position checked for disconjugate gaze. Contact lenses should be removed if present. The facial bones should be palpated for stabilization. If patients are responsive, they should be asked if they are experiencing malocclusion (imperfect occlusion of the teeth). The ears and nose should be checked for drainage of blood or possible cerebral spinal fluid (CSF) leak. Patients with midface fractures may

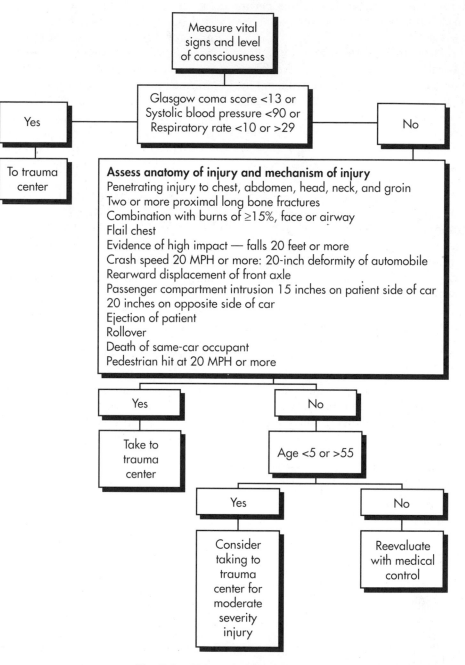

Fig. 7-5   Triage decision scheme.

have a fracture of the cribriform plate. ACS (1989) recommends gastric tubes be placed through the mouth or through a soft nasopharyngeal airway rather than nasally.

Neck

The neck should be visually inspected for contusions, lacerations, or presence of jugular vein distension. Palpation may reveal crepitus or deviation of the trachea.

Chest

Visualization and palpation of the chest wall should be completed to identify sucking chest injuries, flail segments, bruising, or pain on palpation. Pressure exerted on the sternum may elicit pain if any attached ribs are fractured. Auscultation should be carried out high on the anterior chest for pneumothorax and at the posterior bases for hemothorax. Heart tones should also be auscultated at this time, paying particular attention for distant heart sounds that may indicate cardiac tamponade. If not already accomplished, the cardiac monitor and pulse oximeter should be applied and evaluated.

Abdomen

ACS (1989) states that any abdominal injury is potentially dangerous and must be recognized and treated aggressively. The specific diagnosis is not as important as the fact that the injury exists. The abdomen should be palpated for tenderness and observed for any abrasions or contusions. Abdominal injury is not always immediately apparent. Frequent reevaluation is important. The pelvis should be evaluated for instability by slightly rocking and exerting pressure over the iliac crests.

Extremities

The extremities should be visually examined for deformity, contusion, abrasion, and palpated for crepitus, pain, tenderness, or unusual movement. An examination for sensory capa-

---

Box 7-2
GLASGOW COMA SCALE

Eye Opening

Spontaneous eye opening	4 points
Eye opening to verbal stimulus	3 points
Eye opening to painful stimulus	2 points
No eye opening	1 point

Best Verbal Response

Oriented and converses	5 points
Disoriented and converses	4 points
Inappropriate words	3 points
Incomprehensible sounds	2 points
No response	1 point

Best Motor Response

Follows commands	6 points
Localizes to painful stimulus	5 points
Withdraws from painful stimulus	4 points
Flexion—abnormal to painful stimulus	3 points
Extension to painful stimulus	2 points
No response	1 point
Total	**3-15 points**

---

bility and response may be completed simultaneously.

Neurological

Pupillary response and motor and sensory examination should have been completed. At this time a more thorough evaluation of the patient's level of consciousness should be conducted using the Glasgow coma scale (GCS) shown in Box 7-2. Using this scale, with frequent reevaluation, facilitates detection of early changes. Patients with a GCS score less than 8 are considered to be in a coma (ACS, 1989).

INTERVENTION

Airway management is an essential component of resuscitation of the trauma victim. In 1984 a retrospective review of trauma deaths showed that up to 18% of patients died during prehospital transport either of exsanguination, airway obstruction, or ventilatory compromise, problems that could have been treated (Jacobs, Sinclair, Beiser, & D'Agostino, 1984). It has been reported that prehospital intubation was responsible for the documented improvement in patient outcome (O'Brien, Danzi, Sowers, & Hooker, 1988). All trauma patients with adequate ventilatory status should be given 100% FIO_2 through a nonrebreather mask at 10 to 15 liters. If a problem with oxygenation or ventilation has been identified or if the nurse anticipates a ventilatory problem due to the patient's condition, then endotracheal intubation should be instituted. Hypovolemic shock, trauma to the cervical spine, airway obstruction, a full stomach, elevated intracranial pressure, and limited equipment and poor lighting in the field may make intubation difficult (Ligier, Buchman, Breslow, & Deutschman, 1991). If the midface is stable, blind nasal intubation is the logical initial airway approach in trauma patients with potential cervical spine injury.

Multiple attempts at nasal intubation do not improve the success rate. Most successful nasal intubations are accomplished on the first or second attempt (Wraa, Osborn, & Rhee, 1993); therefore another approach should be considered after two unsuccessful attempts. The Endotrol tube* may be of assistance. Pulling the ring on the proximal end of the tube allows the caregiver to manipulate the tip of the tube toward the trachea. The patient should be prepared for nasal intubation with application of a vasoconstrictor, such as Afrin spray, to decrease tissue edema and epistaxis. Insertion of a nasopharyngeal airway (NPA) coated with xylocaine jelly dilates and desensitizes the naris

before insertion of the tube. If nasal intubation is unsuccessful, then either an unrelaxed oral or rapid sequence induction, as described in Chapter 6, should be used. During any intubation attempt, a second person must perform manual cervical spine immobilization. If oral intubation is unsuccessful, then the nurse should move to a surgical cricothyrotomy without delay. It has been shown that surgical cricothyrotomy in the field can be performed reliably by specially trained nurses. The majority of patients requiring cricothyrotomy are the most critically injured with unmanageable airways, so a significant complication rate can be expected. The most common complication noted was bleeding from around the operative site (Nugent, Rhee, & Wisner, 1991). Experience has shown that #6 Shiley tracheotomy tubes were at times difficult to insert in female patients due to the outer diameter being slightly larger than the cricothyroid membrane. Shiley makes a #6 tube without an inner cannula (Shiley #6 SCT), which works well for cricothyrotomies because it has a smaller outer diameter but the same inner diameter as a regular #6. Needle cricothyrotomies may be made for pediatric patients using the Acutronic Transtracheal Catheter* and a jet insufflator, such as the low-frequency jet vent by Anesthesia Medical Specialties.* All tube placements should be confirmed by auscultation after completion of the procedure and after every significant move. Tools helpful in determining tube placement and effectiveness of ventilations are the Easy-cap† end-tidal CO_2 detector, which changes colors from purple to yellow during exhalation to indicate the presence of CO_2, and the use of pulse oximetry to determine oxygen saturation.

Securing the endotracheal tube can be difficult on the trauma patient. Many times the patient has blood or vomit about the face, render-

---

*Mallinckrodt, Inc., St. Louis, MO 63134.

*Anesthesia Medical Specialties, Inc., Sante Fe Springs, CA 90670.
†Nellcor, Inc., Hayward, CA 94545.

ing tape ineffective. Use of premade securing devices, such as the Endo-lok,* which does not need to adhere to the skin, are useful for oral intubation. The Endo-lok also has a built-in bite block that protects the tube. Nasal tubes are easily secured with twill tape by making a half-hitch knot, placing it over the tube and tightening, securing, and tying the tape around the patient's head.

During transport, monitoring of EKG, non-invasive blood pressure, pulse oximetry, temperature, and if possible, captometry is important for the continual reassessment of the patient. Use of captometry is particularly helpful with the evaluation of hyperventilation of the head-injured patient because it gives a readout of the CO_2 level and allows the caregiver to adjust the respiratory rate to keep the level in a therapeutic range. There are several compact transport monitors, such as the Propaq,† that provide monitoring and documentation of these parameters.

If the patient develops a tension pneumothorax or appears to have a significant pneumothorax and is going to be transported by air with a significant altitude change, a pleural decompression should be done. This can be accomplished by insertion of a chest tube or a needle decompression. Needle decompression with a regular catheter over the needle tends to become kinked and therefore is ineffective. Parr‡ has developed a kit called the Nightengale pneumothorax set that contains a betadine swab, xylocaine 1%, small #11 blade, 13-gauge Cook catheter, and extension tubing with a Heimlich valve attached. Insertion on the affected side should be at the second intercostal space, midclavicular line, or fourth intercostal space, anterior-axillary line. In the trauma pa-

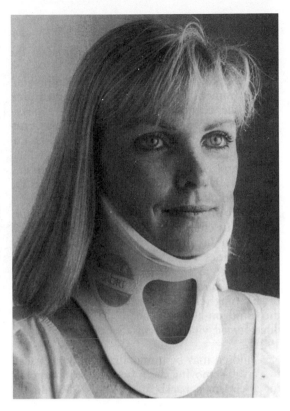

Fig. 7-6 Adult Stifneck collar. (Courtesy California Medical Products, Inc., Long Beach, CA.)

tient, where time is critical, the fourth intercostal space is easily identifiable by using the nipple line on a man and the curve of the breast on a woman.

Cervical spine immobilization should be maintained using a rigid cervical collar, such as the Stifneck,* which comes in multiple sizes for pediatric and adult patients (Figure 7-6). The patient should then be placed on a long board or scoop stretcher and secured to prevent movement during transport. The head should be secured to the board last, since adjustment of the

---

*Respironics, Inc., Monroeville, PA 15146.
†Protocol Systems, Inc., Beaverton, OR 97006.
‡Parr Emergency Medical Product Sales, Inc., Galloway, OH 43119.

---

*California Medical Products, Long Beach, CA 90804.

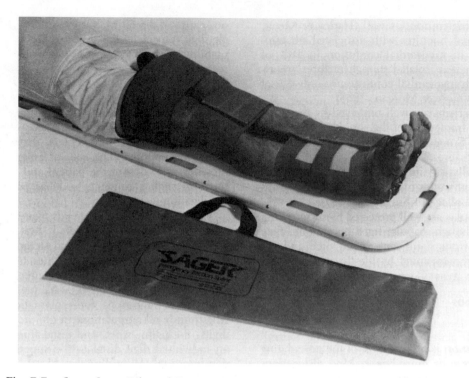

Fig. 7-7   Sager Super Bilateral Emergency Traction Splint. (Courtesy Minto Research and Developmental, Inc., Redding, CA.)

straps across the body may cause movement. The head should be secured to prevent lateral movement using devices such as the Head Bed* or the Ferno-Washington head immobilizer.† A small amount of padding should be placed under the adult's head and under a child's shoulder to maintain neutral alignment. Cervical alignment should be maintained manually at all times during the immobilization process.

Severe hemorrhage should be controlled by applying direct pressure. Moderate bleeding may be controlled by securing bulky dressings with an elastic bandage or gauze.

Fractures of the extremities are easily immobilized with cardboard splints or pillows circumferentially taped around the affected extremity. Midshaft femur fractures should be placed in a traction splint. The Sager splint* is easily applied and can be used for bilateral fractures (Figure 7-7).

Maintaining the patient's body temperature is an important aspect of the treatment of shock. Heat can be conserved by placing a solar blanket between two sheets or a sheet and blanket and placing this on the stretcher, lying the backboard on top and cocooning the patient. This allows easy access to patients and the

*California Medical Products, Long Beach, CA 90804.
†Ferno-Washington, Inc., Wilmington, OH 45177.

*Minto R & D, Inc., Redding, CA 96002.

CASE STUDY

A 15-year-old male has jumped from an overcrossing approximately 20 feet onto the road. The roadway has been secured by the police, and the scene is safe. On arrival, the fire personnel informed the nurse that the patient had been found in a prone position. They have logrolled the patient onto a backboard, placed a rigid cervical collar, and are administering O_2 at 15 liters through a nonrebreathing mask (NRBM). At primary assessment the patient has sonorous respirations at a rate of 26, is in trismus, and is responsive to pain by flexor posturing. His skin is warm and dry and has good color. He has a strong radial pulse, and capillary refill is 2 seconds. A large laceration to the right parietal region with moderate bleeding is noted. A deformity of the right shoulder is noted with distal pulses intact. The chest is intact, the abdomen is soft to palpation, the pelvis is stable, and no deformities to the lower extremities are noted.

While the patient is being placed on pulse oximetry, the nares are prepared with Afrin spray, and a nasopharygeal airway with lidocaine jelly is inserted in the right nares without difficulty; O_2 through a NRBM is reapplied. With fire personnel maintaining manual cervical alignment, the nurse nasally intubates the patient. Clear and equal breath sounds are noted with no sounds over the epigastrium; an Easycap is applied and shows a positive color change from purple to yellow signifying proper placement. The nasoendotracheal tube is secured, and the patient is hyperventilated with 100% FIO_2. Pulse oximetry shows a saturation of 100%. During the intubation fire personnel have secured the patient to the backboard. The head is secured with a head bed, and transport is begun to an appropriate trauma center.

During transport the patient is placed on the monitor with EKG, NIBP, and pulse oximetry. Vitals are 160/90, 68, spontaneous 5/ assisted 24, saturation 100%. Secondary survey shows the patient to have a disconjugate gaze, pupils at 3 mm, equal and nonreactive, and a GCS score of 5 (E-1, V-1, M-3). The rest of the secondary survey findings were negative. A large-bore peripheral IV was started and run at an open rate. Transport time was 10 minutes.

What were the priorities of care at the scene?
1. *Scene safety.* The nurse needs to check with the scene commander to ensure that the roadway

has been secured. If not, the patient needs to be moved.
2. *Secure a patent airway while maintaining cervical immobilization.* Because of the patient's level of consciousness his airway needs to be protected and ventilations should be assisted. With an apparent closed head injury it will be important to hyperventilate the patient to decrease his PCO_2.
3. *Rapid transport to an appropriate facility.* In the urban environment, if transport time by ground is more than 15 minutes, consider helicopter transport if available. In the rural environment, if transport time to the local hospital by ground is greater than the time to the trauma center by air, consider helicopter transport.

---

ability to vent patients should they become too warm.

Intravenous solutions should be kept warm before transport. If the environment at the scene has caused the intravenous (IV) solutions to chill, coiling the tubing around a chemical heat pack is helpful. Peripheral IV access should be gained by using a 14- or 16-gauge catheter for optimal infusion. Crystalloid solutions such as lactated Ringer's solution or normal saline should be used.

SUMMARY

Trauma is a surgical disease, and maintaining a focus on priorities is essential to the successful management of the trauma patient in the prehospital setting. Scene time and transport to an appropriate facility are imperative to a favorable patient outcome. The nurse in the prehospital setting gathers clues from the scene to help anticipate injury patterns while evaluating safety and scene situation. The primary survey determines any life-threatening conditions, which are managed simultaneously. It is at this time that the patient is identified as a critical or noncritical patient. If critical, then transport

Table 7-1   Nursing Diagnoses, Interventions, and Evaluative Criteria for Transport of the Trauma Patient

Diagnosis	Interventions	Evaluative Criteria
Ineffective airway clearance.	Provide chin-lift or jaw-thrust maneuver. Remove blood and secretions with suction. Intubate and ventilate if needed, maintaining cervical spine immobilization.	Airway will be patent.
Ineffective breathing pattern.	Provide supplemental oxygen. Intubate and ventilate if needed, maintaining cervical spine immobilization.	Respiratory effort will be non-labored or supported.
Impaired gas exchange.	Administer oxygen. Monitor patient with pulse oximeter. Monitor patient for signs and symptoms of hypoxia. Intubate and ventilate if needed, maintaining cervical spine immobilization. Use CO_2 detector if intubated.	O_2 saturations will be above 94%. Patient will demonstrate no changes in mental status, agitation, or lethargy. CO_2 detector readings will indicate proper placement of the tube.
Actual or potential fluid volume deficit.	Provide IV access with large-bore catheter (14-16 gauge). Administer crystalloid fluid as needed.	Blood pressure and heart rate will be within normal limits. Capillary refill will be ≤2 seconds.
High risk for cervical, thoracic, and/or lumbar spine injury.	Place patient in a rigid cervical collar. Secure patient to a long spine board.	Patient's spine will be maintained in neutral position. No further injury will occur during transport.
Potential altered body temperature.	Preserve body heat. Warm IV fluids.	Patient will be normothermic.
Pain.	If blood pressure is stable, administer analgesics as needed. Provide reassurance.	Pain will decrease.
Fear.	Provide information regarding care and transport. If family is present, provide directions to receiving facility. Provide reassurance.	Patient will verbalize less fear regarding care and transport. Family will be able to locate the patient.

should begin as soon as possible with the secondary survey being completed during transport. During transport the nurse continually monitors and reassesses the patient. See Table 7-1 for nursing care of the trauma patient during transport.

Research has shown that deaths from trauma occurring during the second peak can be significantly reduced by rapid assessment, recognition and intervention of life-threatening conditions, and rapid transport. Responding to trauma requires teamwork. Cooperation and clear communication between the multiple agencies involved in the prehospital setting help to expedite transport and continuity of care. The nurse in the prehospital environment adds a new dimension of knowledge, experience, and skills that enhances the delivery of safe and effective care to the trauma patient.

RESOURCES

Association	Course
American College of Surgeons Committee on Trauma 55 East Erie St. Chicago, IL 60611-2797 (312) 664-4050	Advanced Trauma Life Support Course (ATLS)
Emergency Nurses Association Trauma Nursing Committee 230 E. Ohio St., Suite 600 Chicago, IL 60611 (312) 649-0297	Trauma Nurse Core Curriculum (TNCC)
National Flight Nurses Association 6900 Grove Rd. Thorofare, NJ 08086 (609) 384-6725	Flight Nurse Advanced Trauma Course (FNATC)
National Association of Emergency Medical Technicians 9140 Ward Parkway Kansas City, MO 64114 (816) 444-3500	Prehospital Trauma Life Support (PHTLS)

REFERENCES

American College of Surgeons Committee on Trauma. (1989). *Advanced trauma life support: Student manual.* Chicago: American College of Surgeons.

Boyd, C., Odom, J., Campbell, R., & Martin, M. (1991). Penetrating abdominal trauma and the basics of ballistics. *The Journal of Air Medical Transport, 10*(1), 6-8.

Jacobs, L., Sinclair, A., Beiser, D., & D'Agostino, R. (1984). Prehospital advanced life support: Benefits in trauma. *The Journal of Trauma, 24*(1), 8-13.

Lee, G. (1991). *Flight nursing principles and practice.* St. Louis: Mosby.

Ligier, B., Buchman, T., Breslow, M., & Deutschman, C., (1991). The role of anesthetic induction agents and neuromuscular blockade in the endotracheal intubation of trauma victims. *Surgery, Gynecology & Obstetrics, 173,* 477-481.

National Association of Emergency Medical Technicians. (1990). *Prehospital trauma life support: Student manual.* Akron, OH: Emergency Training.

Neff, J., & Kidd, P. (1993). *Trauma nursing—The art and science.* St. Louis: Mosby.

Nugent, W., Rhee, K., & Wisner, D. (1991). Can nurses perform surgical cricothyrotomy with acceptable success and complication rates? *Annals of Emergency Medicine, 20*(4), 367-370.

O'Brien, D., Danzi, D., Sowers, M., & Hooker, E. (1988). Airway management of aeromedically transported trauma patients. *The Journal of Emergency Medicine, 6,* 49-54.

Sheehy, S. (1992). *Emergency nursing—Principles and practice.* St. Louis: Mosby.

Snyder, J. (1993). Evaluation of trauma care. In J. Neff & P. Kidd (Eds.), *Trauma nursing: The art and science* (pp. 3-20). St. Louis: Mosby.

Wraa, C., Osborn, M., & Rhee, K., (1993). Analysis of emergent nasotracheal intubation by an air medical program. Manuscript submitted for publication.

CHAPTER 8

Transport of Patients with Environmental Illness or Injury

OBJECTIVES

1. Discuss the general interventions for the patient who is experiencing an environmental emergency before and during transport
2. Describe the care of patients with selected environmental emergencies before and during transport
3. Identify potential safety risks for the prehospital nurse caring for the patient experiencing an environmental emergency before and during transport

COMPETENCIES

1. Perform an environmental scene assessment
2. Demonstrate methods to keep a patient warm during transport
3. Identify specific antidotes for insect and snake bites

The environment in which we live and are a part is both beautiful and potentially hazardous. The area of the country or the service area in which the nurse works contributes to the type of environmental emergencies the nurse working in the prehospital environment will experience.

Over the past several decades more and more people have ventured out into the wilderness in search of its beauty and peace (Houston, 1989). Young and old, individuals and families now routinely venture beyond their common surroundings. As men and women expand their habitats, environments once undisturbed are now being explored and developed, exposing women, men, and children to potential hazards, as well as upsetting nature's balance. One recent example of the results of these changes appeared in an article in the *Journal of Wilder-*

ness Medicine that described the care of patients who sustain an attack from a cougar (Conrad, 1992)!

Although climates, terrains, inhabitants, and creatures vary, nurses encounter similar environmental emergencies including heat and cold emergencies, submersion injuries, and bites. These emergencies do not occur only in the wilderness but can easily happen in the home or backyard.

Preparation for rendering care in specific emergencies, as well as having appropriate equipment and supplies (Figures 8-1 and 8-2), is mandatory. If one of the roles of the nurse is search and rescue, then appropriate knowledge and training should be acquired. If nurses have not learned these skills, they need to work with those that have. The Wilderness Medical Society published recommendations for per-

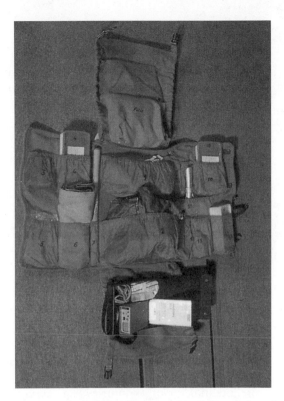

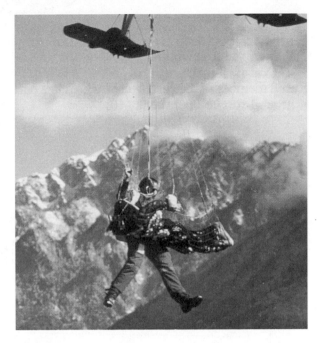

Fig. 8-2   Special equipment has been developed for mountain rescue. Pictured here is the horizontal net, used where the victim has trauma to the vertebral column. (From *Color Atlas of Mountain Medicine* by J. Vallotton and F. Dubas, 1991, St. Louis: Mosby.)

Fig. 8-1   Rescue packs must be fully equipped, lightweight, and comfortable to carry on the back. Pictured here is the GRIMM action pack. (From *Color Atlas of Mountain Medicine* by J. Vallotton and F. Dubas, 1991, St. Louis: Mosby.)

forming prehospital emergency care in the wilderness (Box 8-1) (Otten, Bowman, Hackett, Spadafora, & Tauber, 1991).

This chapter discusses the care of the patient who has sustained an environmental illness or injury and describes the specific care required for some selected environmental emergencies.

GENERAL ASSESSMENT OF THE PATIENT WITH AN ENVIRONMENTAL ILLNESS OR INJURY

The assessment of the patient with an environmental emergency begins with an evaluation of the environment in which the patient was found. The initial evaluation should include the safety of the environment for both the nurse and the patient, the potential mechanisms of injury, and the possibility of other sources of illness or injury. Unlike other patient care situations, the nurse must be sure that it is safe to approach the patient and provide care. If the environment remains unsafe, the nurse may become ill or injured and be unable to provide patient care.

History

The history obtained from the patient or others who may have information about the environmental illness or injury provides clues about the type of environmental illness or injury the patient may have incurred. General historical

---

Box 8-1
SUMMARY OF WILDERNESS PREHOSPITAL EMERGENCY CARE CURRICULUM

1. Review of basic principles of anatomy, physiology, and emergency care, emphasizing the differences and unique problems within the wilderness environment
2. Review of common illnesses and injuries emphasizing the differences and unique problems within the wilderness environment
3. Instruction about the causes, assessment, and treatment of unique wilderness illnesses and injuries not usually seen in the urban environment
4. Instruction about extended care in the environment until evacuation and transport can occur
5. Instruction in the principles of wilderness survival, search and rescue, and victim extrication, packaging, and transportation
6. Offer suggestions for survival kits
7. Instruction about the prevention of wilderness injuries and illnesses

Note. From "Wilderness Prehospital Emergency Care (WPHEC) Curriculum" by E. Otten, W. Bowman, M. Hackett, M. Spadafora, and D. Tauber, *Journal of Wilderness Medicine,* 1991, 2, pp. 80-87.

---

information that should be obtained includes the following:
1. Description of the environment in which the patient was found
   a. Altitude
   b. Type of water (fresh or salt)
   c. Depth of water
   d. Temperature
2. Age of the patient
3. History of other medical problems (e.g., diabetes, cardiovascular disease)
4. History of drug abuse

5. Allergies
6. Current medications
7. History of anaphylaxis
8. History of treatment for similar problem (e.g., snake envenomation treated with antivenin)
9. Onset of symptoms
10. Type of animal, insect, reptile that may be suspect
11. Length of time in the environment
12. Type of clothing patient was wearing
13. Witnesses' accounts
14. Symptoms before the nurse's arrival
    a. Respiratory distress
    b. Altered mental status
    c. Vital signs
    d. Body temperature
    e. Nausea, vomiting
    f. Skin lesions
    g. Edema
    h. Seizures
15. Type of water patient found in (fresh, salt)
16. Potential for other injuries (e.g., cervical spine injury)
17. Social situation
18. Potential for child abuse

Physical Assessment

I. Inspection
   A. Environment
      1. Animals, insects, reptiles
      2. Temperature
      3. Type of water (e.g., fresh, salt)
      4. Altitude
      5. Depth of water
   B. Airway: patent, maintainable, nonmaintainable
      1. Edema
      2. Frothy sputum
   C. Respiratory rate and effort
      1. Hyperventilation
      2. Hypoventilation
      3. Tachypnea

D. Skin color
  1. Pale
  2. Mottled
  3. Cyanotic
  4. Flushed
E. Skin appearance
  1. Presence of fang marks
  2. Rashes
  3. Vesicles
  4. Patterns of injury
  5. Edema
  6. Ulcerations
  7. Rashes
  8. Hives
  9. Cutis marmorata (skin marbling)
F. Wounds
  1. Location
  2. Size
  3. Shape
  4. Depth
II. Palpation
  A. Peripheral and central pulses
  B. Pulse rate, rhythm, quality
  C. Skin temperature
  D. Core temperature
  E. Crepitus, deformities
  F. Sensory
  G. Reflexes
III. Percussion
  A. Chest
  B. Abdomen
IV. Auscultation
  A. Breath sounds
  B. Blood pressure
  C. Bowel sounds

As with any other emergency, as problems are identified during the initial assessment appropriate interventions are performed. For example, if patients are unable to maintain their airway, immediate interventions are executed. The assessment of the patient with an environmental illness or injury helps the nurse provide specific interventions based on the type of environmental illness or injury and the effects it is having on the patient.

GENERAL INTERVENTIONS FOR THE PATIENT WITH AN ENVIRONMENTAL ILLNESS OR INJURY

Each environmental illness or injury requires specific interventions and care. However, the following general interventions are applicable in most situations:

1. Transport the patient to a safer environment
   a. Hot environment to a cooler environment
   b. Cold environment to a warmer environment
   c. Away from snakes, insects, and animals
   d. Descend from altitude
   e. Ascend from depth
2. Establish a patent airway, anticipate the need for more definitive airway management during transport related to the potential complications from the specific environmental illness or injury
3. Provide supplemental oxygen during transport
4. Immobilize the patient's cervical spine if trauma is suspected
5. Establish intravenous access with a large-bore peripheral catheter, intraosseous needle, central line
6. Provide fluid resuscitation as indicated with an isotonic solution (normal saline, lactated Ringer's)
7. Place patient on a cardiac monitor
8. Monitor patient's body temperature
9. Provide appropriate environment for transport depending on the environmental illness or injury (e.g., warmth for the hypothermic patient)
10. Remove any constricting jewelry or clothing from affected body parts
11. Remove any wet clothing
12. Transport patient in the appropriate position

13. Transport patient at the appropriate altitude
14. Administer appropriate medications when indicated (e.g., antivenin)

ASSESSMENT AND INTERVENTIONS RELATED TO SPECIFIC ENVIRONMENTAL ILLNESSES AND INJURIES

Temperature Regulation

Numerous thermosensitive end organs exist in the skin, spinal cord, and limb muscles (Danzl, Pozos, & Hamlet, 1989; Yarbrough & Hubbard, 1989). When body temperature is altered, temperature-sensitive hypothalamic neurons react (Danzl, Pozos, & Hamlet, 1989). The body attempts to keep itself at a temperature around 98.6° F, or 37.1° C.

The body generates heat through basal metabolism, which is fueled by food and exercise (Stewart, 1990). The body may also attempt to conserve heat through conduction, convection, and radiation (Stewart, 1990). The body loses heat through evaporation, conduction, convection, radiation, and transpiration (Stewart, 1990; Hofstrand, 1992).

When the body is exposed to cold, mechanisms of temperature regulation are triggered that cause the patient to shiver to conserve heat. Vasoconstriction is also initiated for heat conservation. The lower the patient's temperature falls, the less able the body is to respond. Mechanisms of heat conservation no longer work at temperatures below 24° C (75° F) (Danzl, Pozos, & Hamlet, 1989). Core temperature is lowered by three specific mechanisms: dilation of cutaneous blood vessels, sweating, and inhibition of heat production from shivering and chemical thermogenesis (Mellor, 1992).

Cold-Related Emergencies

Predisposing Factors

Many factors predispose both adults and children to developing emergencies related to the cold. Both the young and old are particularly susceptible to becoming victims of hypothermia. The young are at risk because of their large surface area to body weight ratio, minimal amounts of subcutaneous fat, thinner skin, and delayed ability to shiver, particularly in the neonate (Hofstrand, 1992). Outside (deliveries during transport) and precipitous deliveries can leave the newborn at risk for hypothermia.

The elderly are susceptible to hypothermia because of an impaired ability to perceive the cold, decreased resting peripheral blood flow, and less capability to produce heat (Danzl, Pozos, & Hamlet, 1989).

The trauma patient is uniquely susceptible to developing hypothermia during transport because of the removal of clothing for injury identification, administration of unwarmed fluids, and administration of anesthetic agents (Luna, Maier, Pavlin, Anardi, Copass, & Oreskovich, 1987). Also, evaluation and resuscitation may compound heat loss, and many serious injuries are related to alcohol intoxication. Immobility due to injury decreases the patient's ability to maintain a protected environment. CNS injuries may impair thermoregulation.

Burn victims with extensive tissue damage resulting in impaired skin integrity are at a serious risk of becoming hypothermic during transport. The chance of this occurring increases when the patient has been treated with wet dressings.

Patients rescued after submersion may be hypothermic. Heat is conducted from the body 20 to 30 times faster in cold water (Stewart, 1989).

Medications that are used before and during transport place the patient at risk of becoming hypothermic. Drugs used for sedation alter the patient's ability to perceive cold. Chemical paralyzation places the patient at risk of becoming hypothermic (Semonin-Holleran, Johnston, & Storer, 1992).

Other risk factors for the development of hypothermia that the prehospital nurse must be aware of include the following:

- Hiking
- Medications (barbiturates, phenothiazine)
- Hypothyroidism
- Malnutrition
- Sepsis

Frostbite

Frostbite is defined as "true tissue freezing" (Mills, 1991). When the tissue freezes, it actually forms ice crystals. In addition to this, vascular stasis and decreased blood flow contribute to the development of tissue damage (Figure 8-3) (Hofstrand, 1992). Frostbite has been classified as either superficial (first degree, second superficial degree) or deep (second deep degree, third degree).

Mixed injuries may also occur with frostbite. The person may suffer an immersion and frostbite injury, a freezing-thawing-refreezing hypoxic injury, compartment syndrome with frostbite, a fracture and frostbite, and hypothermia with frostbite (Mills, 1991).

Risk Factors

1. Age
2. Duration of exposure
3. Improper clothing
   a. Constricting
   b. Not covering high-risk areas such as the ears, nose, feet, hands, fingers
4. Alcohol intoxication
5. Drug intoxication (reported cases of deep frostbite of the nose from cocaine abuse)
6. Drugs that cause vasoconstriction such as nicotine
7. Malnutrition
8. History of previous cold injury

Signs and Symptoms

The signs and symptoms of frostbite depend on the amount of injury that has occurred. It is important to not only focus on the obvious injury from frostbite, but also to assess the patient for the possibility of hypothermia. The signs and symptoms of frostbite are classified

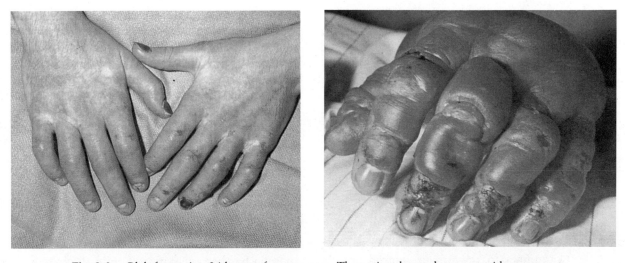

Fig. 8-3   Bleb formation 24 hours after exposure. The patient has undergone rapid rewarming in warm water for approximately 30 minutes, until the fingertips flushed. It should be noted that the blebs are large, pink, and extend right to the fingertips—an excellent prognostic sign. Until the blebs developed, following the rapid rewarming, this patient still had feeling in his fingertips, which disappeared as the blebs separated the superficial from the deep structures. (From *Color Atlas of Mountain Medicine* by J. Vallotton and F. Dubas, 1991, St. Louis: Mosby.)

the same as burns—first, second, and third degree (Mills, 1991).

1. First degree
   a. Paleness
   b. Cyanosis
   c. Edema
   d. Decreased sensation to injured area
2. Second superficial degree
   a. Cyanosis
   b. Edema
   c. Blisters
   d. Decreased sensation to injured area
   e. Anesthesia at injured area
3. Second deep degree
   a. Paleness, significant cyanosis
   b. Edema
   c. Anesthesia
4. Third degree
   a. Paleness, cyanosis, necrosis
   b. Edema
   c. Anesthesia

Treatment

BEFORE TRANSPORT. Once frostbite has been recognized, the amount and type of care needed are dictated by the amount of time it will take to transport the patient to a hospital. One of the most dangerous complications of frostbite is thawing and then refreezing (Mills, 1991; Smith, Robson, & Heggers, 1989). The following important points made by Mills (1991, p. 91) apply to providing prehospital care for the patient with frostbite:

1. Thawing should not be attempted when there is danger of the injured area refreezing.
2. Frostbite may be a sign of hypothermia.
3. Use of excessive heat such as steam or campfires to rewarm an injured area is very dangerous and may cause unnecessary damage.

If the patient is less than 2 hours from the hospital the nurse should perform the following interventions:

1. Assess and stabilize the patient's airway, breathing, and circulation
2. Monitor the vital signs
3. Obtain a core temperature
4. Place patient in a warm environment
5. Remove any wet clothing or constricting clothing and place with dry, loose-fitting clothing
6. Identify the area of injury
7. Perform a brief motor sensory evaluation of injured area
8. Immobilize the extremity with a padded splint
9. Provide pain management as needed

If the patient is more than two hours from the hospital, the nurse should perform the following interventions (Smith, Robson, & Heggers, 1989):

1. Rapidly rewarm the injured extremities in warm water, 38 to 41° C (100.4 to 105.8° F)
2. Place the rewarmed extremities in dressings
3. Place patient in a warm environment so that freezing does not recur
4. Leave blisters intact

DURING TRANSPORT

1. Monitor airway, breathing, and circulation
2. Provide supplemental oxygen when indicated by the method of transport
3. Monitor temperature
4. Dress and immobilize injured area
5. Provide pain management as needed by the patient

Hypothermia

Hypothermia has been defined as a core body temperature of less than 35° C (95° F). Hypothermia has been classified as mild (body temperatures between 32 to 35° C, or 90 to 95° F) moderate (body temperature 28 to 32° C, or 82 to 90° F) and severe hypothermia (body temperature below 28° C, or 82° F) (Jolly & Ghezzi, 1992). The predisposing factors for the development of hypothermia have been previously discussed.

Signs and Symptoms

1. Feeling cold, shivering (stops at around 31° C, or 88° F) (Paton, 1991)
2. Core body temperature below 35° C (95.0° F)
3. Inability to protect airway
4. Tachypnea
5. Bradypnea—rate of 4 to 6
6. Pulmonary edema
7. Exhaustion
8. Altered mental status
9. Irritable
10. Coma
11. Absence of reflexes
12. Fixed and dilated pupils
13. Cardiac dysrhythmia
    a. Tachycardia
    b. Bradycardia
    c. Atrial fibrillation
    d. Ventricular fibrillation
14. Presence of a J or Osborne wave on the EKG monitor
15. Nonpalpable pulses
16. Skin pallor
17. Cyanotic
18. Paradoxical undressing

Treatment

MILD AND MODERATE HYPOTHERMIA. As with frostbite, the amount and type of care that the patient requires and receives are determined by the degree of hypothermia and the duration of the transport. Rescue teams operating in areas of the country where severe hypothermia occurs generally have advanced equipment and supplies including low-reading thermometers, portable oxygen heaters, and cardiac monitors (Stewart, 1991). Rossman (1992, p. 46) points out that "the idea in initial stabilization is not to rewarm the patient or to treat nonurgent conditions. The goal is simply to reduce heat loss." The initial care of the patient with mild and moderate hypothermia includes:

1. Recognizing the severity of the hypothermia
2. Placing the patient in a warm environment
3. Establishing a patent airway
4. Placing the patient on heated, humidified oxygen, airway warming increases the rate of rewarming and will improve cardiac rhythm and cardiovascular, cerebral, and pulmonary functions (Lloyd, 1991).
   a. Electrical-powered humidifier
   b. Warming rod
5. Removing any wet clothing and replacing with warm protective covering
6. Obtaining intravenous access and administering warm fluids
7. Placing the patient on a cardiac monitor
8. Monitoring vital signs
9. Obtaining a temperature

SEVERE HYPOTHERMIA. The patient with severe hypothermia needs to be transported carefully and rapidly to the hospital (Figures 8-4 and 8-5). If the patient is in cardiopulmonary arrest, the Wilderness Medical Society recommends initiation of CPR with the following exceptions (Danzl, Pozos, & Hamlet, 1989; Iserson, 1989):

1. The patient has a specified do-not-resuscitate status
2. The patient has suffered a lethal injury
3. Initiation of CPR will leave the nurse and others at risk (in the rescue situation)
4. Chest wall compression is impossible
5. Any evidence of spontaneous respirations or movement

The previous interventions should be initiated and include any of the following if indicated:

1. Establish a patent airway
   a. Intubation
   b. Cricothyrotomy
2. Do not defibrillate until the patient is warm

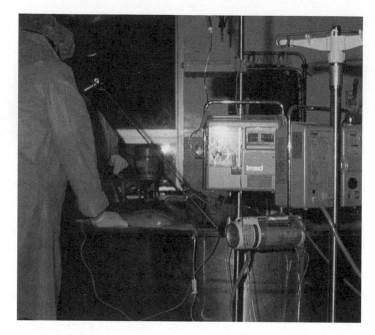

Fig. 8-4 Peritoneal dialysis is continued as the patient is placed in a warm tub for rapid rewarming of the extremities, when his core temperature reaches 27° C. The patient's deep hypothermia and multiple episodes of freezing and thawing resulted in marked, overwhelming sepsis that required emergency bimalleolar amputation of the feet; the hands fared better with minimal phalangeal loss. (From *Color Atlas of Mountain Medicine* by J. Vallotton and F. Dubas, 1991, St. Louis: Mosby.)

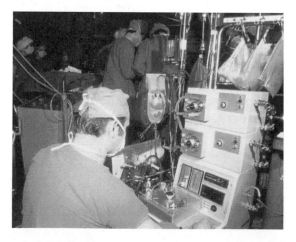

Fig. 8-5 Extracorporeal circulation is the best rewarming method for deep accidental hypothermia. (Courtesy of P. Segantini.)

3. Ventricular fibrillation may be treated with bretylium

DURING TRANSPORT

1. Monitor the patient's airway, breathing, and circulation
2. Monitor patient's temperature
3. Keep patient warm and dry
4. Continuously monitor for cardiac dysrhythmia

Heat-Related Emergencies

Heat-related emergencies range from simple illnesses such as heat cramps to the potentially fatal illness of heat stroke. The early recognition and appropriate care provided by the prehospital nurse will help decrease the potential consequences of heat-related emergencies.

Predisposing Factors

Heat-related illnesses occur because of increased heat production, decreased dissipation of heat, and depletion of salt and water. Predisposing factors for the development of heat-related illnesses include the following (Mellor, 1992; Tek & Olshaker, 1992; Yarbrough, Hubbard, 1989):

- Cardiovascular disease
- Diabetes
- Cystic fibrosis
- Quadriplegia
- Fever
- Psychosis
- History of prior heat-related illness
- Drugs
  - Anticholinergics
  - Phenothiazine
  - Cyclic antidepressants
  - Lithium
  - Hallucinogens
  - Diuretics
- Ethanol
- Dehydration from exercise
- Inappropriate clothing for the heat
- Poor fluid intake
- Lack of supervision of the elderly or the young
- Athletes
- Military recruits

Heat Cramps

Heat cramps result from strenuous work in a hot environment. Individuals with heat cramps may or may not be acclimated to the warmer environment. Cramps develop in the muscles that are being stressed. This may occur as a result of salt loss from sweating.

Signs and Symptoms
- Cramping in muscles used during exertion
- Normal mental status
- May or may not have an elevated temperature

Treatment
BEFORE TRANSPORT
1. Assess and stabilize the patient's airway, breathing, and circulation
2. Place patient in a cool environment
3. Assess the level of the patient's dehydration
4. Mild dehydration is treated with oral fluids such as Gatorade
5. Severe hydration is treated with intravenous normal saline

DURING TRANSPORT
1. Continuous monitoring of airway, breathing, and circulation
2. Continue rehydration through oral or intravenous fluids

Heat Exhaustion

Heat exhaustion occurs because of excessive loss of salt and water. Individuals working in a hot environment without adequate fluid replacement are at greatest risk.

Signs and Symptoms
- Fatigue
- Headache
- Nausea
- Profuse sweating
- Dizziness
- Postural hypotension
- Dehydration
- Elevated temperature (to 40° C)

Treatment
BEFORE TRANSPORT
1. Assess and stabilize the patient's airway, breathing, and circulation
2. Place patient in a cool environment
3. Obtain intravenous access and administer normal saline

DURING TRANSPORT
1. Monitor the patient's airway, breathing, and circulation
2. Continue intravenous normal saline administration
3. Keep patient in a cool environment

Heat Stroke

Heat stroke is a serious and sometimes fatal heat-related illness. It results from the body's inability to regulate its thermoregulatory mechanisms to meet the demands of heat stress (Yarbrough & Hubbard, 1989). The clinical hallmark of heat stroke is an altered mental status and a body temperature above 40.6° C.

Signs and Symptoms
- Neurological findings
  □ Severe headache
  □ Ataxia
  □ Bizarre behavior
  □ Seizures
  □ Coma
- Body temperature greater than 40° C
- Sweating is often absent
- Tachypnea
- Tachycardia

Treatment
BEFORE TRANSPORT
1. Assess and stabilize the patient's airway, breathing, and circulation
2. Consider intubation because aspiration and seizures are common
3. Assist ventilations as indicated
4. Administer supplemental oxygen
5. Establish intravenous access with normal saline
6. Closely monitor patient's response to fluid resuscitation
7. Place patient in a cool environment immediately
8. Remove all clothing
9. Place wet blankets and provide air circulation around the patient
10. Alternative cooling method: apply ice packs to patient's neck, groin, and axilla
11. Open windows and doors during transport
DURING TRANSPORT
1. Monitor airway, breathing, and circulation
2. Monitor patient for signs and symptoms of pulmonary edema
3. Place patient on cardiac monitor and pulse oximeter
4. If patient begins shivering:
   a. Chlorpromazine may be administered intravenously
   b. Diazepam may be administered intravenously
5. Observe for and treat seizure activity
   a. Administer diazepam or lorazepam intravenously for seizure activity
6. Continue rapid cooling interventions

Altitude Emergencies

Increased access to high-altitude environments over the years has led to more cases of altitude emergencies (Tso, 1992). Altitude emergencies occur because of changes in altitude that result in hypoxia. As the altitude increases, both the barometric pressure and partial pressure of oxygen decrease (Hackett, Roach, & Sutton, 1989). High altitude begins at 8000 feet. Very high altitude ranges from 14,000 to 18,000 feet, and extreme altitude is from 18,000 to 29,000 feet (Stewart, 1990).

Prevention is the best treatment for altitude emergencies (Iserson, 1989). Procedures to prevent altitude emergencies include staged ascent, high carbohydrate diet, appropriate exercise level, and drug prophylaxis. Drugs that are currently being used include acetazolamide and dexamethasone (Iserson, 1989; Rabold, 1992; Tso, 1992). The most important treatment for the patient who is suffering from an altitude emergency is to descend. However, this may not always be possible because of weather or rescue problems. Nurses involved in the care of these patients need to be educated so that they do not become victims.

Acute Mountain Sickness

Acute mountain sickness (AMS) generally occurs in healthy individuals between the ages of 1 to 20 years of age who rapidly ascend to altitudes of 3000 meters (approximately 9800 feet). Cold, amount of exertion at altitude, and a previous history of AMS can contribute to the development of this illness (Oelz, 1991). Its onset is usually sudden and occurs within 24 to 72 hours of the ascent.

Signs and Symptoms
AMS is divided into mild and serious.
MILD
- Headache
- Anorexia
- Insomnia
- Dyspnea on exertion

SERIOUS
- Vomiting
- Severe headaches
- Dizziness
- Ataxia
- Tachypnea
- Rales
- Vivid hallucinations
- Retinal hemorrhage

Treatment
The patient with mild AMS should rest before further ascent. If there is no improvement with rest, headache analgesia, or nausea medication, the patient must be transported from altitude.

BEFORE TRANSPORT
1. Assess and stabilize the patient's airway, breathing, and circulation
2. Perform baseline neurological assessment
3. Descend
4. Administer oxygen
5. During descent, if patients are being carried, be sure that they are in a position to prevent aspiration
6. Give aspirin or acetaminophen with codeine for headache
7. Give prochlorperazine 10 mg parentally or orally every 6 hours, or 25 mg rectally every 12 hours; or promethazine 25 mg parentally, or 25 to 50 mg rectally every 8 hours for nausea
8. Give dexamethasone 4 mg orally or parentally every 6 hours

DURING TRANSPORT
1. Monitor the patient's airway, breathing, and circulation
2. If patient is being transported by air, monitor for altitude effects on patient and descend if indicated
3. Continue supplemental oxygen during transport
4. Continue monitoring neurological status
5. Keep patient warm during transport

High Altitude Cerebral Edema
High altitude cerebral edema (HACE) usually occurs at elevations above 12,000 feet and is the result of chronic hypoxia (Clarke, 1991; Tso, 1992).

Signs and Symptoms
- Headache
- Unsteadiness of gait
- Disorientation
- Hallucinations
- Nystagmus
- Hemiparesis
- Coma

Treatment
BEFORE TRANSPORT
1. Assess and stabilize the patient's airway, breathing, and circulation
2. Descend to lower altitude
3. Administer supplemental oxygen
4. Perform a baseline neurological assessment
5. Give dexamethasone 4 to 8 mg orally or parentally every 6 hours
6. Keep the patient warm

DURING TRANSPORT
1. Monitor the patient's airway, breathing, and circulation
2. Continue supplemental oxygen
3. Place patient on cardiac monitor and pulse oximeter
4. Obtain intravenous access for medication administration if patient has an altered mental status

5. If patient is to be transported by air, monitor for effects of altitude on patient and descend as indicated

High Altitude Pulmonary Edema

High altitude pulmonary edema (HAPE) occurs in individuals who rapidly ascend to altitudes of 3000 meters. Most patients who develop HAPE are generally young, healthy, and male. Symptoms begin about 2 to 4 days after ascent.

Signs and Symptoms
- Initially a nonproductive cough becoming productive with bloody, frothy sputum
- Shortness of breath
- Weakness
- Rales
- Tachypnea
- Tachycardia
- Cyanosis
- Hallucinations
- Coma
- Chest x-ray study shows patchy, fluffy infiltrates (Figure 8-6)

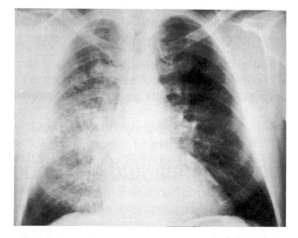

Fig. 8-6 Typical chest X ray of high altitude pulmonary edema (HAPE) at Capanna Margherita (4554 meters). (From *Color Atlas of Mountain Medicine* by J. Vallotton and F. Dubas, 1991, St. Louis: Mosby.)

Treatment
BEFORE TRANSPORT
1. Assess and stabilize the patient's airway, breathing, and circulation
2. Administer supplemental oxygen
3. Severe respiratory distress may require intubation; positive end-expiratory pressure (PEEP) may be useful for oxygenation
4. Place patient on a cardiac monitor and pulse oximeter
5. Descend promptly to a lower altitude, usually 2000 to 4000 feet
6. Administer medication, which may include:
   a. Nifedipine (10 to 20 mg) sublingually followed by 20 mg of slow-release preparation every 6 hours
   b. Acetazolamide
7. If the patient is in extremis:
   a. Morphine sulfate 5 to 15 mg intravenously
   b. Furosemide 40 mg intravenously
8. Keep patient warm to decrease metabolic needs
DURING TRANSPORT
1. Monitor the patient's airway, breathing, and circulation
2. Provide supplemental oxygen by mask or bag-valve if patient is intubated
3. Suction to keep airway clear
4. Monitor oxygen saturation
5. Administer medications as patient's condition dictates
6. Keep patient warm

Diving and Submersion Emergencies
Diving Emergencies

Just as there has been an increase in people traveling to higher altitudes, diving has also increased in popularity. Diving places individuals at risk for injury from pressure changes that can result in decompression sickness, gas toxicities, and barotrauma (Smith, 1992).

Large changes in pressure occur with relatively small changes in water depth (Figure 8-7). When a person descends into the water, the

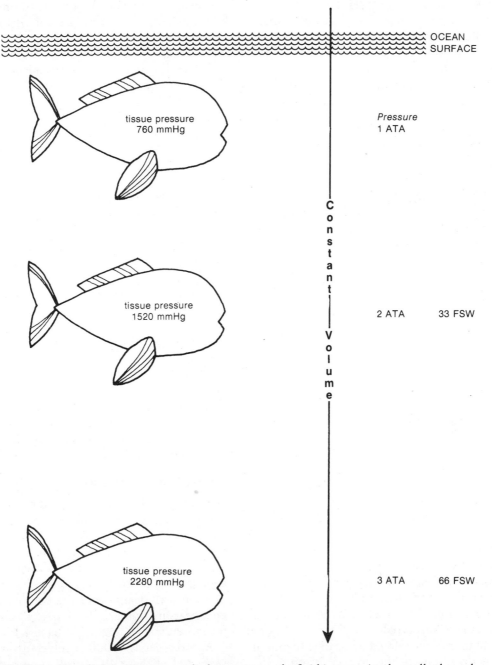

Fig. 8-7   Pascal's law. Pressure applied to any part of a fluid is transmitted equally throughout the fluid. (From *Management of Wilderness and Environmental Emergencies* by P.S. Auerbach and E.C. Geehr, 1989, St. Louis: Mosby.)

barometric pressure increases. Increased barometric pressure can cause mechanical damage to gas-filled organs such as the lungs and bowl and alter the solubility of gases in body tissues (Stewart, 1990).

The care of the patient who has sustained a diving emergency is based on the particular type of illness or injury incurred. As with altitude emergencies, if prehospital nurses are involved in the direct rescue of the patient, they need to be educated and capable.

Decompression Sickness

Decompression sickness is also known as *the bends*. It is caused by the formation of gas bubbles in tissues and venous blood. Gas bubbles are more likely to occur in the brain, spinal cord, pulmonary system, inner ear, and joints. Symptoms of decompression sickness usually appear within 1 to 2 hours after diving (Jerrard, 1992).

Signs and Symptoms
- Pain in shoulders and elbows
- Pruritis
- Rashes
- Cutis marmorata (skin marbling)
- Seizures
- Hemiplegia
- Blurred vision
- Tunnel vision
- Nausea and vomiting
- "Chokes," substernal pain, cough, dyspnea

Treatment
BEFORE TRANSPORT
1. Assess and stabilize the patient's airway, breathing, and circulation
2. Immobilize the patient's cervical spine if trauma is suspected
3. Obtain history related to the dive (depth of the dive, time of the dive, violation of decompression procedures)
4. Prepare for transport to a decompression chamber
5. Administer 100% oxygen

6. Evaluate for possible pneumothorax
7. If pneumothorax is present, insert chest tube(s) before transport
8. Obtain intravenous access and administer normal saline or lactated Ringer's for hypotension
9. Place patient on a cardiac monitor and pulse oximeter
10. If patient is in a referral center, insert Foley catheter to maintain urinary output at 1 to 2 ml/hr
11. Keep patient warm

DURING TRANSPORT
1. Monitor airway, breathing, and circulation
2. Administer 100% oxygen and use a tight-fitting mask
3. If the patient is cold, administer warm, humidified oxygen
4. Monitor the patient's oxygen saturation
5. Administer fluids to keep the patient normotensive
6. Insert chest tube before transport when indicated
7. Keep patient warm
8. Place patient in left lateral decubitus and supine position for transport
9. Monitor the patient's neurological status
10. If transporting the patient by air, monitor patient for additional stresses from altitude

Submersion Emergencies

A submersion emergency is the result of an injury or injuries from submersion in water or other substances (e.g., grain) (Olshaker, 1992; Stewart, 1992). Additional definitions of submersion emergencies include drowning, which is defined as death from asphyxia due to submersion with death occurring before 24 hours, and near-drowning, which describes survival for more than 24 hours (Olshaker, 1992).

Approximately 8000 people drown each year, and of these 40% are younger than age 4. Drowning is the second leading cause of accidental death (Anderson, Roy, & Danzl, 1991; Haley, 1993).

Stewart (1989) described the pathophysiology of a submersion as an initial panic followed by breath-holding hyperventilation that can result in aspiration and swallowing of a large amount of water. Swallowing a lot of fluid may induce vomiting and aspiration of gastric contents. There may be struggling before consciousness is lost, and the patient becomes hypoxic. The end result of submersion is aspiration of a fluid or materials such as sand, gravel, or mud. Aspiration leads to pulmonary injury, the further development of hypoxia, and finally, cerebral injury. Outcomes from submersion incidents range from no sequelae to severe neurological deficits and death (Stewart, 1989).

Factors associated with near-drowning include the inability to swim, use of alcohol or illicit drugs, seizures, trauma, hyperventilation, hypothermia, cerebrovascular accidents, myocardial infarctions, and child abuse and neglect (Olshaker, 1992).

Over the years researchers have attempted to identify specific prognostic factors that may help predict the potential outcome of a submersion incident. Boxes 8-2 and 8-3 contain examples of scoring systems (Anderson, Roy, & Danzl, 1991; Orlowski, 1979).

If victim rescue is required, it is important that only professionally educated individuals perform the rescue. It is tempting to be a hero, but may make one an additional victim.

The care of the patient who has suffered a submersion emergency is based on history of the incident, initial assessment, and stabilization of airway, breathing, and circulation. The cervical spine should be immobilized if there is any history of trauma.

Many patients who suffer from a submersion incident are also hypothermic. All wet clothing should be removed before transport and the patient wrapped in warm, dry blankets. If the patient has severe hypothermia, active warming measures may need to be instituted during transport.

Conn (1980) and Modell (1980) have developed a classification of near-drowning that provides a method of evaluating the neurological status of the patient (Table 8-1).

Box 8-2
ORLOWSKI SCORE: PROGNOSTIC FACTORS IN PEDIATRIC CASES OF DROWNING AND NEAR-DROWNING

1. Age < 3 years
2. Estimated maximum submersion > 5 minutes
3. No attempt at resuscitation for at least 10 minutes after rescue
4. Patient in a coma on admission to the emergency department
5. Arterial blood gas pH ≤ 7.10

1 point awarded for each unfavorable prognostic factor.
Score ≤ 2 = 90% chance of recovery
Score of ≥ 3 = 5% chance of recovery

Note. From "Prognostic Factors in Pediatric Cases of Drowning and Near-Drowning" by J. Orlowski, 1979, *Journal of the American College of Emergency Physicians, 8,* pp. 176-179.

Box 8-3
SUBMERSION OUTCOME SCORE

1. Arterial pH ≤ 7.10
2. Pao_2/PAo_2 ≤ 0.35
3. Anion gap ≥ 15

One point awarded for each variable present.
Score of ≥ 2 predicted poor outcome, i.e., death or permanent neurological sequelae

Note. From "Submersion Incidents: A Review of 39 Cases and Development of the Submersion Outcome Score" by K. Anderson, T. Roy, and D. Danzl, 1991, *Journal of Wilderness Medicine, 2,* pp. 27-36.

Table 8-1 Conn and Modell's Classification of Near-Drowning

Category	Description
A. (Awake)	Alert, fully conscious
B. (Blunted)	Obtunded, stuporous but arousable.
	Purposeful response to pain.
	Normal respirations.
C. (Comatose)	Comatose, not arousable.
	Abnormal response to pain.
	Abnormal respirations.
C.1 (Decorticate)	Flexor response.
	Cheyne-Stokes respirations.
C.2 (Decerebrate)	Extensor response.
	Central hyperventilation.
C.3 (Flaccid)	No response to pain.
	Apneustic or "cluster" breathing.
C.4 (Deceased)	Flaccid, apneic, no detectable circulation.

Note. From "Cerebral Salvage in Near-Drowning following Neurologic Classification by Triage" by A. Conn, J. Montes, G. Barker, and J. Edmonds, 1980, *Canadian Anaesthesia Society Journal, 27,* pp. 201-210; and from "Near-Drowning: Correlation of Level of Consciousness and Survival" by J. Modell, S. Graves, and E. Kuck, 1980, *Canadian Anaesthesia Society Journal, 27,* pp. 215-221.

Treatment

BEFORE TRANSPORT

1. Obtain a history about the incident
   a. Time the incident occurred
   b. Amount of time patient was submerged
   c. Description of the incident
      - Type of water (fresh or salt), fluid, or material submerged in
         □ Possible contaminants
         □ Fluid temperature
   d. Age of the patient
   e. Past medical history
   f. Initial appearance of the patient at the scene of the incident

2. Assess and stabilize the patient's airway, breathing, and circulation
   a. Immobilize cervical spine
   b. Administer high-flow oxygen
   c. If the patient is cold, use warm humidified oxygen
   d. Assess breath sounds
   e. Place patient on pulse oximeter
   f. Place patient on a cardiac monitor
   g. Initiate intravenous access
3. Remove all wet clothing and place patient in warm, dry blankets
4. If patient is hypothermic, initiate rewarming
5. Perform baseline neurological assessment

DURING TRANSPORT

1. Monitor the patient's airway, breathing, and circulation
2. Use PEEP when patient has been intubated to help decrease degree of intrapulmonary shunting, diminish the ventilation-perfusion mismatch, and increase the functional residual capacity (Olshaker, 1992)
3. Use measures to control increases in the patient's intracranial pressure
   a. Hyperventilation to maintain $Paco_2$ between 25 and 30
   b. Monitor for and control seizure activity
   c. Elevate head of bed 30% if cervical spine has been cleared
   d. Use sedation and neuromuscular blocking agents as ordered or per protocol
   e. Osmotic diuretics as ordered or per protocol

Bites and Stings

Many creatures can inflict injury by biting and stinging. To provide the best care for the victim that has sustained an injury from a bite or sting, the nurse practicing in the prehospital care environment needs to be familiar with some general principles in the management of bites and stings. The nurse also needs to be aware of what type of animals, insects, or reptiles live in the practice environment that may be a source of potential injury.

Insects, reptiles, and animals may bite or sting for defense or to inject venom that is used to prepare particular victims for consumption. The effects of envenomation on the human victim is determined by the size and health of the patient, the amount of venom injected, the location of the venom injection, the amount of exertion or activity the patient engaged in after the bite or sting, and whether the patient has been previously exposed to the particular venom (Arendt & Arendt, 1992).

The effects of venoms can range from a local reaction at the site of envenomation, such as a painful wheal, to a systemic reaction, such as nausea, vomiting, and seizures. The effects of the venom depend on its composition.

Bite wounds are complicated because they are both a crush injury and involve contamination. Bacteria that may contaminate bite wounds are listed in Box 8-4. Bite injuries may also result in transmission of specific diseases

from vectors such as those carried by insects, for example, Lyme's disease.

One life-threatening complication of a bite or sting is anaphylactic shock. Unfortunately, about 50 to 100 people die each year of insect stings, and the majority of these deaths are from anaphylaxis (Stewart, 1990). Rapid identification and treatment of anaphylaxis are needed to prevent death. Signs and symptoms of anaphylaxis include shortness of breath, bright red rash, hives, edema of the face, wheezing, hypotension, and cardiovascular collapse. Box 8-5 contains a summary of treatment for anaphylaxis.

Although there are multiple sources of stings

Box 8-4
POTENTIAL BACTERIAL CONTAMINANTS IN BITE WOUNDS

Aerobic Bacteria

Staphylococcus aureus
Streptococcus
Eikenella corrodens

Anaerobic Bacteria

Bacteroides
Enterobacter
Proteus mirabilis

Other Pathogens

Hepatitis virus
Clostridium tetani
Herpes virus
Rabies virus

Note. From *Wounds and Lacerations* by A. Trott, 1991, St. Louis: Mosby.

Box 8-5
TREATMENT OF ANAPHYLAXIS

1. Assess and stabilize the patient's airway, breathing, and circulation
2. Obtain vascular access
3. Epinephrine subcutaneously, intramuscularly, or intravenously (0.3-0.5 ml for adults; 0.01 ml/kg not to exceed 0.3 ml in children under 12 years of age) (Epinephrine infusion 0.1 μg/kg/min to a maximum dose of 1.5 μ/kg/min)
4. Diphenhydramine 25-30 mg intramuscularly or intravenously
5. Hydrocortisone 4-8 mg/kg intravenously
6. Cimetidine 5 to 10 mg/kg
7. Bronchodilator for wheezing
8. Fluid resuscitation for profound hypotension

Note. From *Emergency Drug Therapy* by W. Barsan, M. Jastremski, and S. Syverud, 1991, Philadelphia: W.B. Saunders; from "Allergic and Immunologic Diseases" by G. Farles and C. Johnston in *Pediatric Emergency Medicine* by R. Barkin (Ed.), 1992, St. Louis: Mosby; and from "Arthropod Envenomation and Parasitism" by S. Minton and H. Bechtel in *Management of Wilderness and Environmental Emergencies* by P. Auerbach and E. Geehr (Eds.), 1989, St. Louis: Mosby.

and bites, a brief summary of the identification and care of bites and stings from some specific insects and reptiles are included in the following sections.

Snake Bites

About 45,000 people in the United States are bitten by snakes each year. In 1991 4000 people sought treatment in a health-care facility (Arendt & Arendt, 1992; Tully & Wingert, 1992). There are four types of venomous snakes in the United States with at least one species of poisonous snake in every state except Alaska, Maine, and Hawaii. The Crotalidae family contains three of these snakes—the rattlesnake, copperhead, and moccasin (Gold & Barish, 1992). These snakes are also known as pit vipers and account for 60% of the venomous bites. Figure 8-8 demonstrates how to distinguish poisonous from nonpoisonous snakes.

The venom of Crotalidae is potent and can cause paralysis, respiratory depression, and death.

Another family of venomous snakes in the United States are the Elapidae, which includes coral snakes. These snakes have round pupils, black snouts, and a distinctive color pattern. The venom of the coral snake is neurotoxic.

Envenomation is graded either by description or a number system depending on which reference is used. Table 8-2 contains a grading system of envenomation (Tully & Wingert, 1992).

Signs and Symptoms of Envenomation
PIT VIPER ENVENOMATION
- Fang punctures
- Pain
- Edema
- Erythema

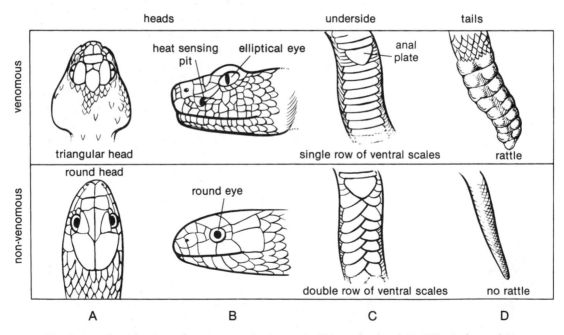

Fig. 8-8 Identification of venomous pit vipers. **A,** Triangular head. **B,** Elliptical eye; heat-sensing facial pits on sides of head near nostrils. **C,** Single row of ventral scales leading up to anal plate. **D,** Rattles on tail (baby rattlers only have "buttons" but are still quite venomous). (From *Management of Wilderness and Environmental Emergencies* by P.S. Auerbach and E.C. Geehr, 1989, St. Louis: Mosby.)

Table 8-2   Grade of Envenomation

Severity	Findings
None	Fang marks only, no local or systemic signs or symptoms
Minimal	Fang marks with slowly progressive local swelling, no systemic symptoms
Moderate	History of multiple or provoked bites or bite of a large venomous snake or highly toxic species; fang marks with rapid progression of edema that goes beyond the bite site; systemic symptoms of nausea and vomiting; metallic taste; paresthesia
Severe	History of bite from a toxic snake; prolonged imbedding of the fangs; multiple bites; rapid progressive swelling; subcutaneous hemorrhage; severe systemic signs and symptoms including muscle fasciculation, and shock

Note. From "Venomous Animal Bites and Stings" by S. Tully and W. Wingert in *Pediatric Emergency Medicine.* by R. Barkin (Ed.), (pp. 403-411), St. Louis: Mosby.

CORAL SNAKE ENVENOMATION
- Small puncture sites
- Little or no pain at the bite site
- Local edema
- Paresthesia at the bite site

SYSTEMIC SIGNS AND SYMPTOMS OF PIT VIPER ENVENOMATION
- Diaphoresis
- Chills
- Weakness
- Nausea and vomiting
- Tingling sensation
- Metallic taste
- Shock

SYSTEMIC SIGNS AND SYMPTOMS OF CORAL SNAKE ENVENOMATION
- Nausea and vomiting
- Dizziness

Table 8-3   Antivenin Dosages

Grade of Envenomation	Initial Treatment
None	No antivenin, local care, tetanus immunization
Mild	3-5 vials of antivenin
Moderate	6-10 vials of antivenin
Severe	15+ vials of antivenin

Note. From "Rescue Operations for Snakebite" by D. Arendt and D. Arendt, 1992, *American Journal of Nursing, 92*(7), pp. 26-30.

- Weakness
- Respiratory paralysis
- Fasciculation

Treatment

The following sections present a summary of information from multiple sources regarding treatment of the patient who has been bitten by a snake. When in doubt about the management of these patients before and during transport, the nurse should always consult an expert to prevent further injury and complications.

Antivenin Administration

Administration of antivenin before the patient is transported to definitive care is usually contraindicated. However, if (1) the patient's life is threatened owing to the poison of snake venom, (2) the duration of transport to the definitive facility is long, (3) the nurse is able to manage anaphylaxis during transport, and (4) the antivenin is available in the appropriate dose, then antivenin may be initiated (Iserson, 1989). Table 8-3 summarizes antivenin dosages based on the grade of envenomation (Arendt & Arendt, 1992). The dosage of antivenin is based on the severity of envenomation; the adequate dosage is imperative. According to Sullivan and Wingert (1989, p. 498), "children receive more milligrams of venom per kilogram of body weight than do adults, have less body water with which to dilute the venom, and have less inherent resistance to its effects. Children may require larger doses per unit of body weight than do adults."

BEFORE TRANSPORT (Arendt & Arendt, 1992; Burgess, Dart, Egen, & Mayersohn, 1992; Davidson, Schafer, & Jones, 1992; Gold & Barish, 1992; Iserson, 1989)

1. Move patient to a safe environment
2. Keep the patient calm
3. Assess and stabilize the patient's airway, breathing, and circulation
4. Identify signs and symptoms of envenomation
5. If bite has just occurred, a Sawyer extractor may be used to remove venom
6. Place the patient in a supine or prone position for transport
7. Remove any constricting clothing or jewelry from the injured limb
8. Apply a constricting band around the extremity proximal to the site of injury. The band *should not* obstruct arterial or deep venous flow
9. Evaluate peripheral pulses and sensation of the injured limb
10. Place cotton or gauze between immobilized digits to decrease injury from swelling
11. Obtain baseline circumferential measurement of the injured limb
12. Establish intravenous access
13. Administer supplemental oxygen
14. Place patient on a cardiac monitor
15. Place patient on a pulse oximeter
16. Morphine is contraindicated for pain management because it causes vasodilation
17. Contact local Poison Control or snake expert for additional advice
18. If snake is to be transported with the patient, be sure it is in a safe container, such as a bucket with a lid

DURING TRANSPORT

1. Monitor the patient's airway, breathing, and circulation
2. Monitor the patient for signs and symptoms of systemic envenomation
3. If antivenin has been initiated before transport, monitor for signs and symptoms of anaphylaxis and treat per order or protocol

Arthropod Envenomation

Each year in the United States more people die of the effects of arthropod envenomation than any other type of venomous source (Iserson, 1989; Tully & Wingert, 1992). These arthropods include scorpions, spiders, and Hymenoptera (honeybee, hornets, yellow jackets, and fire ants).

Scorpion Stings

There are about 50 species of scorpions that can cause serious problems in humans. Dangerous scorpions in the United States belong to the genus *Centruroides,* family Buthidae. These scorpions inhabit Arizona, New Mexico, Texas, and California. The venom of the scorpion is neurotoxic. Children bitten by scorpions may develop life-threatening signs and symptoms (Allen, 1992; Bond, 1992; Banner, 1989).

Signs and Symptoms of Envenomation
- Signs and symptoms of anaphylaxis
- At the site of the sting
  - Burning pain
  - Minimal swelling
  - Redness
  - Numbness and tingling
- Tachycardia
- Hypertension
- Pulmonary edema
- Seizures
- Perspiration
- Piloerection
- Hyperglycemia
- SLUDGE phenomenon
  - Salivation
  - Lacrimation

❑ Relaxation of the sphincters (urination and defecation)
❑ Gastric hyperdistention
❑ Bradycardia and hypotension

Treatment

BEFORE TRANSPORT

1. Assess and stabilize the patient's airway, breathing, and circulation
2. If sting has just occurred, a Sawyer Extractor may be used to remove the venom
3. Identify the grade of envenomation
4. Apply local cold compresses
5. Give analgesics for pain relief
6. Establish an intravenous line
7. Place patient on a cardiac monitor
8. Place patient on a pulse oximeter
9. Treat specific symptoms:
   a. Tachyarrhythmias may be treated with propranolol
   b. Hypertension may be treated with labetalol or esmolol infusions
   c. Seizures are treated with diazepam or lorazepam
10. Atropine may need to be administered if cholinergic effects are profound

DURING TRANSPORT

1. Monitor the patient's airway, breathing, and circulation
2. Monitor the patient for signs and symptoms of systemic envenomation
3. Continue pain management

Spider Bites

There are 30,000 species of spiders with only about 50 that may cause envenomation problems in humans. In the United States the black widow *(Latrodectus mactans)* and the brown recluse *(Loxosceles reclusa)* can cause local and systemic problems (Allen, 1992; Clark, Wethern-Kestner, Vance, & Genkin, 1992; Rees & Campbell, 1989). Black widow venom is highly potent and is a neurotoxin. There is an antivenin available.

These spiders are located all over the United States. They like dark places such as barns, woodpiles, and hikers' sleeping bags.

Signs and Symptoms of Envenomation

BLACK WIDOW

■ Limb pain
■ Local adenopathy
■ Redness, swelling, urticaria
■ Cramping pain generally starts in the thighs, abdomen, chest
■ Tonic contractions
■ Tremors
■ Flushed face
■ Facial sweating
■ Fear of death

BROWN RECLUSE

■ Initial bite not painful
■ In hours or days after bite, a lesion develops that
   ❑ initially is edematous, red, or blanched
   ❑ later becomes a blue-gray macular halo
■ Systemic signs and symptoms
   ❑ Fever
   ❑ Malaise
   ❑ Scarlatiniform rash
   ❑ Leukocytosis
   ❑ Vomiting
   ❑ Diarrhea
   ❑ Disseminated intravascular coagulopathy
   ❑ Shock

Treatment

BEFORE TRANSPORT

1. Assess and stabilize the patient's airway, breathing, and circulation
2. Keep the patient calm
3. Immobilize the injured limb
4. Use the Sawyer's Extractor if the bite has occurred within 3 minutes
5. Apply cool compresses to the bitten limb
6. Assess peripheral circulation and sensation of the injured limb
7. Manage pain as needed

8. Benzodiazepines and opiates may help relieve cramping from black widow envenomation

DURING TRANSPORT
1. Monitor the patient's airway, breathing, and circulation
2. Monitor patient for signs and symptoms of systemic envenomation

Stinging Insects

Insects usually sting because their habitats have been disturbed. The most common stinging insects belong to the order Hymenoptera and include bees, wasps, and ants (Minton & Bechtel, 1989). The major complication of envenomation from stinging insects is the potential for anaphylactic shock.

Signs and Symptoms of Envenomation
- Local pain, swelling, redness
- Pruritus
- Hives
- Angioedema
- Respiratory distress

Treatment
BEFORE TRANSPORT
1. Assess and stabilize the patient's airway, breathing, and circulation
2. Treat anaphylaxis (see Box 8-5)
3. If sting has just occurred, use Sawyer's Extractor to remove venom
4. Apply cool compresses for local comfort
5. Provide pain management

DURING TRANSPORT
1. Continue to monitor the patient's airway, breathing, and circulation
2. Monitor the patient for signs and symptoms of systemic envenomation

SUMMARY

The care of the patient with an environmental illness or injury is based on recognizing the

Table 8-4 Nursing Diagnoses, Interventions, and Evaluative Criteria for the Patient with an Environmental Illness or Injury

Diagnosis	Interventions	Evaluative Criteria
Ineffective thermoregulation.	Identify patient's risk for developing hypothermia/hyperthermia. Provide specific interventions for either hypothermia or hyperthermia. Monitor patient's temperature during transport.	Patient's body temperature will be as close to normal as possible during transport. Each intervention will be evaluated for effectiveness. The patient will state they are comfortable.
Ineffective breathing pattern related to anaphylaxis as evidenced by shortness of breath, wheezing, and upper airway edema.	Treat anaphylaxis as listed in Box 8-5.	Patient's airway will be clear. Respiratory rate and effort will be within normal limits.
High risk for injury related to the injection of venom from a bite or sting.	Keep patient calm. Use Sawyer's Extractor to remove venom if bite or sting occurred within 3 minutes. Immobilize injured limb.	Patient will be calm. Venom will be contained.

source of the illness or injury, removing the patient to a safe, controlled environment, and providing assessment and interventions related to the specific illness or injury. Table 8-4 contains examples of specific nursing diagnoses that may be used in the care of the patient with an environmental emergency including alterations in thermoregulation, high risk for injury, and ineffective breathing patterns.

RESOURCES

Wilderness Medical Society
    Post Office Box 2463
    Indianapolis, IN 46206

REFERENCES

Allen, C. (1992). Arachnoid envenomation. *Emergency Medicine Clinics of North America, 10,* 269-298.

Anderson, K., Roy, T., & Danzl, D. (1991). Submersion incidents: A review of 39 cases and development of the submersion outcome score. *Journal of Wilderness, 2,* 27-36.

Arendt, D., & Arendt, D. (1992). Rescue operations for snakebite. *American Journal of Nursing, 92*(7), 26-30.

Banner, W. (1989). Scorpion envenomation. In P. Auerbach & E. Geehr (Eds.), *Management of wilderness and environmental emergencies.* St. Louis: Mosby.

Bond, G. (1992). Antivenin administration for *Centruroides* scorpion sting: Risks and benefits. *Annals of Emergency Medicine, 21*(7), 788-791.

Burgess, J., Dart, R., Egen, N., & Mayersohn, M. (1992). Effects of constriction bands on rattlesnake venom absorption: A pharmacokinetic study. *Annals of Emergency Medicine, 21*(9), 1086-1093.

Clark, R., Wethern-Kestner, S., Vance, M., Genkin, R. (1992). Clinical presentation and treatment of black widow spider envenomation: A review of 163 cases. *Annals of Emergency Medicine, 21*(7), 782-787.

Clarke, C. (1991). High-altitude cerebral edema. In J. Vallotton & F. Dubas (Eds.), *Mountain medicine.* St. Louis: Mosby.

Conn, A., Montes, J., Barker, G., & Edmonds, J. (1980). Cerebral salvage in near-drowning following neurologic classification by triage. *Canadian Anaesthesia Society Journal, 27,* 201-210.

Conrad, L. (1992). Cougar attack: Case report of a fatality. *Journal of Wilderness Medicine, 3*(4), 387-396.

Danzl, D., Pozos, R., & Hamlet, M. (1989). Accidental hypothermia. In P. Auerbach & E. Geehr (Eds.), *Management of wilderness and environmental emergencies.* St. Louis: Mosby.

Davidson, T., Schafer, S., & Jones, J. (1992). North American pit vipers. *Journal of Wilderness Medicine, 3*(4), 397-421.

Gold, B., & Barish, R. (1992). Venomous snakes. *Emergency Medicine Clinics of North America, 10,* 249-267.

Hackett, P., Roach, R., & Sutton, J. (1989). High altitude medicine. In P. Auerbach & E. Geehr (Eds.), *Management of wilderness and environmental emergencies.* St. Louis: Mosby.

Haley, K. (1993). *Emergency nursing pediatric course.* Park Ridge, IL: Emergency Nurses Association.

Hofstrand, H. (1992). Accidental hypothermia and frostbite. In R. Barkin (Ed.), *Pediatric emergency medicine.* St. Louis: Mosby.

Houston, C. (1989). Introduction. In P. Auerbach & C. Geehr (Eds.), *Management of wilderness and environmental emergencies.* St. Louis: Mosby.

Iserson, K. (1989). *Wilderness medical society position statements.* Port Reyes Station, CA: Wilderness Medical Society.

Jerrard, D. (1992). Diving medicine. *Emergency Medicine Clinics of North America, 10,* 329-338.

Jolly, B., & Ghezzi, K. (1992). Accidental hypothermia. *Emergency Medicine Clinics of North America, 10,* 311-327.

Lloyd, E. (1991). Equipment for airway warming in the treatment of accidental hypothermia. *Journal of Wilderness Medicine, 2,* 330-350.

Luna, G., Maier, R., Pavlin, E., Anardi, D., Copass, M., & Oreskovich, M. (1987). Incidence and effect of hypothermia in seriously injured patients. *Journal of Trauma, 27,* 1014-1018.

Mellor, M. (1992). Heat-induced illnesses. In R. Barkin (Ed.), *Pediatric emergency medicine.* St. Louis: Mosby.

Mills, W. (1991). Frostbite. In J. Vallotton & F. Dubas (Eds.), *Mountain medicine.* St. Louis: Mosby.

Minton, S., & Bechtel, H. (1989). Arthropod envenomation and parasitism. In P. Auerbach & E. Geehr (Eds.), *Management of wilderness and environmental emergencies.* St. Louis: Mosby.

Modell, J., Graves, S., & Kuck, E. (1980). Near-drowning: Correlation of level of consciousness and survival. *Canadian Anaesthesia Society Journal, 27,* 211-221.

Oelz, O. (1991). Acute mountain sickness. In J. Vallotton & F. Dubas (Eds.), *Mountain medicine.* St. Louis: Mosby.

Olshaker, J. (1992). Near-drowning. *Emergency Medicine Clinics of North America, 10,* 339-350.

Orlowski, J. (1979). Prognostic factors in pediatric cases of drowning and near-drowning. *Journal of the American College of Emergency Physicians, 8,* 176-179.

Otten, E., Bowman, W., Hackett, M., Spadafora, M., & Tauber, D. (1991). Wilderness prehospital emergency care (WPHEC) curriculum. *Journal of Wilderness Medicine, 2,* 80-87.

Paton, B. (1991). Hypothermia. In J. Vallotton & F. Dubas (Eds.), *Mountain medicine.* St. Louis: Mosby.

Rabold, M. (1992). Dexamethasone for prophylaxis and

treatment of acute mountain sickness. *Journal of Wilderness Medicine, 3,* 54-60.

Rees, R., & Campbell, D. (1989). Spider bites. In P. Auerbach & E. Geehr (Eds.), *Management of wilderness and environmental emergencies.* St. Louis: Mosby.

Rossman, L. (1992). Handling disasters in cold environments. *Journal of Emergency Medical Services, 17*(11), 38-47.

Semonin-Holleran, R., Johnston, D., & Storer, D. (1992). Chemical paralyzation as a potential risk factor for the development of hypothermia in the trauma patient transported from the scene by helicopter. *Paper presented at the Association of Air Medical Services,* Salt Lake City, Utah.

Smith, D., Robson, M., & Heggers, J. (1989). Frostbite and other cold-induced injuries. In P. Auerbach & E. Geehr (Eds.), *Management of wilderness and environmental emergencies.* St. Louis: Mosby.

Smith, K. (1992). High-altitude illness and dysbarism. In R. Barkin (Ed.), *Pediatric emergency medicine.* St. Louis: Mosby.

Stewart, C. (1990). *Environmental emergencies.* Baltimore: Williams & Wilkins.

Stewart, R. (1989). Submersion incidents: Drowning and near-drowning. In P. Auerbach & E. Geehr (Eds.), *Management of wilderness and environmental emergencies.* St. Louis: Mosby.

Sullivan, J., & Wingert, W. (1989). Reptile bites. In P. Auerbach & E. Geehr (Eds.), *Management of wilderness and environmental emergencies.* St. Louis: Mosby.

Tek, D., & Olshaker, J. (1992). Heat illness. *Emergency Medicine Clinics of North America, 10,* 299-310.

Tso, E. (1992). High-altitude illness. *Emergency Medicine Clinics of North America, 10,* 231-247.

Tully, S., & Wingert, W. (1992). Venomous animal bites and stings. In R. Barkin (Ed.), *Pediatric emergency medicine* St. Louis: Mosby.

Yarbrough, B., & Hubbard, R. (1989). Heat-related illnesses. In P. Auerbach & E. Geehr (Eds.), *Management of wilderness and environmental emergencies.* St. Louis: Mosby.

CHAPTER 9

Transport Considerations for Patients with Selected Medical Emergencies

OBJECTIVES

1. Discuss the general assessment of the patient with a medical emergency
2. Identify the equipment needed to transport the patient with selected medical emergencies
3. Discuss the implications related to patient and caregiver safety when performing CPR during transport
4. Describe the care before and during transport for the patient with a cardiac, respiratory, or neurological emergency

COMPETENCIES

1. Perform a patient assessment for each of the selected medical emergencies
2. Identify potential equipment problems
3. Safely perform CPR during transport
4. Administer specific medications for selected medical emergencies

One of the initial focuses of prehospital care and transport was to decrease the morbidity and mortality related to cardiac disease (O'Rourke, 1987). It has been shown that early identification of risk factors, rapid initiation of both basic and advanced life support, and transport by skilled, educated, and experienced personnel may make the difference between life and death for the patient with a cardiovascular illness (JAMA, 1992). During the past 30 years technological and pharmacological advances have further emphasized the need for early intervention before hospital admission. In addition, not all hospitals have the resources available for all patients, so patients need to be moved to other facilities for definitive care. Transport of the patient with a medical emergency presents unique challenges for the nurse providing care before and during this process.

The advent of new technological and pharmacological methods of managing such problems as acute myocardial infarction, respiratory failure, and cerebrovascular accident, the need for early identification of patient problems and early intervention, and the need for critical care during transport have pointed to the need for nursing to play a key role in the care of these patients before and during the transport process (Garza 1993; Hagley, 1993; Solomon & Hart, 1993; Sternbach & Sumchai, 1989). Administration of thrombolytic agents, monitoring of invasive lines, and operation of specific pieces of equipment such as an intraaortic balloon pump are only some of the interventions being performed by nurses during transport. This chapter focuses on the care of the patient with cardiovascular, respiratory, and neurological emergencies.

GENERAL ASSESSMENT

The assessment of the patient with a medical emergency begins with evaluation of the patient's airway, breathing, circulation, and neurological status. Not unlike the approach to the trauma patient, immediate interventions should be initiated during the primary assessment as soon as problems are identified.

History

When obtaining history related to a medical emergency, the nurse should question whether the patient has a history of cardiovascular, pulmonary, or neurological disease. Potential risk factors should be elicited. Risk factors related to cardiovascular, respiratory, and neurological emergencies include the following:
- Hypertension
- Diabetes
- Cigarette smoking
- Age
- Family history of disease (e.g., cardiovascular, diabetes, neurological)

Other pieces of history that should be gathered include the following:
- Onset of symptoms
- Signs and symptoms the patient had before the arrival of the nurse
- Treatments initiated and their results (e.g., pain medications, ceasing activities)
- History of this disease process (e.g., previous myocardial infarction, cerebral vascular accident)
- Medications that the patient is taking

Risk Factors for Cardiovascular Emergency
- Family history of premature cardiovascular disease
- Diabetes mellitus
- Hypertension
- Postmenopausal women
- Prior myocardial infarction
- Hyperlipidemia
- Lack of exercise
- Excessive weight

Risk Factors for Respiratory Emergency
- Recent surgery
- History of smoking cigarettes or toxic substances (crack, marijuana)
- Recent childbirth
- Multiple orthopedic injuries
- History of prolonged bedrest
- History of pulmonary diseases (asthma, chronic obstructive pulmonary disease, pulmonary emboli)
- Involvement in a closed-space fire
- History of need to be intubated or mechanically ventilated

Risk Factors for a Neurological Emergency
- Previous neurological disease (stroke, intracerebral bleeds)
- History of seizures (partial or generalized)
- Cardiovascular disease
- History of carotid bruits
- History of carotid endarterectomy

Description of Pain Patterns

Headaches, chest pain, and abdominal pain are common complaints of patients in a medical emergency. Obtaining a description of the patient's pain pattern helps to determine the potential source of the pain and to evaluate the

---

Box 9-1

EXAMPLE OF A PAIN PATTERN: ACUTE MYOCARDIAL INFARCTION

Pain Quality	Radiation of Pain
Crushing, squeezing, stabbing, heaviness, burning	Usually on the left side of the anterior chest; radiates to left arm, back, neck, and jaw

---

Note. From *Clinical Nursing* by J. Thompson, G. McFarland, J. Hirsch, & S. Tucker, 1993, St. Louis: Mosby.

effectiveness of treatment both before and during transport.

A frequently used mnemonic that helps facilitate pain description is *PQRST:*

P — Provoking factors related to the pain

Q — Quality of the pain

R — Region and radiation of the pain

S — Severity of the pain

T — Time

The components of this mnemonic were explained in detail in Chapter 5. An example of a pain pattern is listed in Box 9-1.

Physical Examination

I. Inspection
   A. Airway
      1. Patent
      2. Maintainable
      3. Nonmaintainable
   B. Respiratory effort
   C. Respiratory patterns
      1. Labored
      2. Irregular
   D. Respiratory rate
   E. Frothy sputum
   F. Size and shape of the chest
   G. Patient's position of comfort
      1. Lying
      2. Sitting
   H. Level of consciousness
   I. Skin color
      1. Pallor
      2. Cyanosis

   J. Diaphoresis
   K. Neck vein distention
   L. Cardiac rhythm
   M. Behavior
   N. Facial expressions
      1. Grimacing
      2. Fear
   O. Body language
      1. Clenching fist
      2. Restlessness
      3. Equality of movement
         a. Upper and lower extremities
         b. Chest wall
   P. Inability to lie flat
   Q. Obvious edema
   R. Bleeding from intravenous sites, nasotracheal or nasogastric tube particularly in patients receiving thrombolytic therapy

II. Palpation
   A. Peripheral and central pulses
   B. Pulse rate, rhythm, quality, location
   C. Pulses paradox ($\geq$ 12 mm Hg fall in systolic blood pressure during inspiration)
   D. Skin temperature
   E. Central and peripheral edema
   F. Crepitus
   G. Tracheal position
   H. Reflexes
      1. Deep tendon
      2. Plantar
      3. Corneal
   I. Areas of tenderness (e.g., patient's legs)

J. Thrills
K. Right upper quadrant pain and tenderness
L. Liver engorgement
III. Auscultation
   A. Breath sounds
      1. Presence
      2. Equality
   B. Adventitious sounds
      1. Crackles
      2. Wheezing
   C. Heart sounds
   D. Bruits
      1. Carotid
      2. Aortic
   E. Bowel sounds
   F. Blood pressure

During the primary assessment the nurse should intervene as soon as life-threatening problems are identified. Interventions are planned and initiated based on the potential for problems during transport.

GENERAL INTERVENTIONS

Although each medical emergency requires its own specific interventions, some general interventions need to be initiated before transport. These include the following:

1. Establish a patent airway, anticipating the need for more definitive airway management during transport related to the potential complications of the specific medical emergency
2. Provide supplemental oxygen as tolerated by the patient
3. Attach pulse oximeter to patient
4. Establish intravenous access with a large-bore peripheral catheter or central line
5. If intravenous lines are already in place, assess and ensure that they are patent and secure before transport
6. If invasive lines are present and will be attached to monitors for transport, evaluate their patency by attaching a transport monitor and obtain an initial reading
   a. Label all lines
   b. Secure all connections
   c. Place sterile caps on all open ports
   d. Maintain line patency
7. Immobilize or splint the affected limb(s) where any invasive lines are with a blanket or similiar covering to restrict mobility and decrease the possibility of pulling any lines out
8. If invasive lines are not going to be used during transport, ensure patency by capping, flushing, or placing pressure bags
9. Attach cardiac monitor
10. Obtain an EKG or a rhythm strip and transfer results to the receiving facility
11. Anticipate need for further interventions during transport by intervening before transport, for example:
   a. Placing external pacing pads
   b. Placing defibrillator pads
12. Calculate appropriate drug dosages and place medications on infusion devices
13. Transport patient in the appropriate position
   a. Head of bed elevated for cerebral vascular accident, chest pain, orthopnea
14. Monitor patient for potential complications from treatments (e.g., thrombolytic therapy)
15. Consider sedation to help decrease patient anxiety during transport
16. Consider neuromuscular blocking agents along with sedation or analgesia if the patient is combative, resists mechanical ventilation, or increases the risk of self-injury or injury of the transport team
17. Provide documentation
   a. Initial assessment
   b. Assessment during transport
   c. Response to medications and treatments
   d. Any complications that occur during transport

Transport Equipment

Perhaps no other type of patient (except the neonate) may require such a variety of equipment during transport than the patient with a medical emergency. Examples of equipment that may be used include the following:

- Cardiac monitor
- Defibrillator
- Hemodynamic monitor
- External pacer
- Pulse generator
- Intraaortic balloon pump
- Ventricular assist devices
- Ventilator
- Pulse oximeter
- CO_2 monitor
- Intravenous infusion pumps and monitors
- Cardiac thumper

Over the years improvements have been made to decrease equipment size and weight, and a variety of equipment can be operated by an electrical source or by batteries. Current equipment is modular and multifunctional, so one unit can be used as a cardiac monitor, defibrillator, external pacer, pulse oximeter, and CO_2 monitor (Figure 9-1).

The prehospital nurse needs to be able not only to operate the equipment, but also to "trouble shoot" problems when they occur. Sometimes other team members such as perfusionists and respiratory therapists are needed.

Previously, particularly during air transport,

safety concerns were related to the use of specific types of equipment. Defibrillation and pacing during air transport have recently been evaluated and found to be safe for both the patient and the transport team (Dedrick, Darga, Landis, & Burney, 1989; Gordon & O'Dell, 1991; Waggoner, Landis, Nelson, & Dedrick, 1991). The development of hands-off defibrillation has improved safety during transport by either ground or air (Figure 9-2).

Wedge-Stecher (1990) has emphasized the importance of planning and organization when multiple pieces of equipment are used for patient care during transport. Equipment requires adequate space and should be stored where it can be viewed during transport. Power sources must also be appropriate and sufficient for the duration of the transport. Finally, safety should always be of primary concern. Connectors and equipment need to be secured for the safety of both the patient and the crew.

Cardiopulmonary Resuscitation during Transport

Cardiopulmonary resuscitation (CPR) during transport may present unique problems and difficulties for the nurse. In addition, administration of CPR during transport can potentially put the prehospital care team at risk for injury

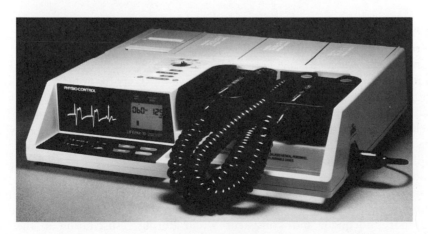

Fig. 9-1   Multifunctional monitor. (Courtesy of Physio-Control, Redmond, Washington.)

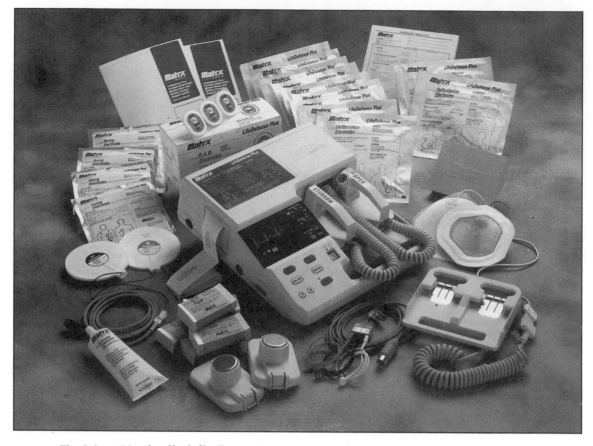

Fig. 9-2 "Hands-off" defibrillator. (Courtesy of Matrix Medical, Inc., Orchard Park, NY.)

(Stapleton, 1991). Depending on the number of people in the transport team, each member may have to perform several functions during resuscitation including compressions, ventilations, and medication administration. Several factors may influence the effectiveness of CPR during transport, including chest compression, ventilation, and the size of the transport vehicle. A study by Stapleton (1991) that evaluated CPR during ground transport found that compression rates varied when performed by a team member. He noted that gas-powered compressors ensured more adequate and consistent compressions. Manually triggered resuscitators maintained an adequate ventilation volume throughout transport as compared with bag-valve-mask ventilations. Finally, the size of the transport vehicle and the positioning of the patient and crew members during transport and resuscitation influence the effectiveness of CPR.

Safety

Safety needs to be the primary concern of the nurse when resuscitation is being performed during transport. Many needlestick injuries occur during resuscitation in the hospital. The smaller work space in both ground and air ambulances increases that risk greatly. When nurses and other members of the team are performing resuscitation, they are usually out of their seats and restraints and may sustain injuries due to sudden stops or changes in altitude. Although defibrillation has been demonstrated to be generally a safe procedure during transport, injury is always a possibility because of limited space.

Drug Therapy

Drug therapy and other procedures such as defibrillation and pacing should be in accord with the protocols for advanced cardiac life support (ACLS) and pediatric advanced life support (PALS). Although adherence to protocols varies widely, protocols provide a foundation and framework for providing ALS to the patient in cardiopulmonary arrest (Miller & Wilson, 1992).

Summary

Performing CPR during transport requires an organized plan that prioritizes the safety of crew and patient. Appropriately restraining the patient and nurse, delivering effective resuscitation, and using safe systems to deliver drugs (such as a needleless system) will help decrease the possibility of injury to both the nurse and the patient.

ASSESSMENT AND INTERVENTIONS FOR SPECIFIC MEDICAL EMERGENCIES
Cardiovascular Emergencies

Over the past 30 years a concerted public effort has been made toward the prevention and treatment of cardiovascular diseases. However, cardiovascular disease still accounts for 1 million deaths each year, and many of these are sudden cardiac deaths (JAMA, 1992).

One of the major strategies identified by the American Heart Association to decrease the mortality and morbidity from cardiovascular disease is referred to as the *chain of survival* (JAMA, 1992). The chain of survival consists of early recognition of signs and symptoms of cardiac disease, rapid activation of the EMS system, basic cardiac life support (BCLS), automatic defibrillation, and ACLS including intubation and medication administration (JAMA, 1992).

Since 1966, when the National Academy of Sciences–National Research Council recommended that health-care providers be taught CPR, one of the chief focuses of prehospital care has been the management of patients with a cardiovascular emergency (Gabram, Piacentini, & Jacobs, 1990; JAMA, 1992; O'Rourke, 1987). The first mobile intensive care units contained monitors, defibrillators, pacers, and antidysrhythmic drugs. Today, automatic defibrillators are used in the field by various professionals, including fire, police, and civilian, to improve patient outcome from cardiovascular emergencies.

The advances in pharmacological and technological care of patients with cardiac disease have demonstrated the need for rapid transport of these patients whether by ground or air for definitive care that may not be available in the referring hospital. For example, cardiac catheterization, insertion of an intraaortic balloon pump, or a heart transplant are only a few examples of the need to transfer a patient from one institution to another.

These patients are usually in critical condition, may have multiple invasive lines, and are receiving advanced pharmacological therapy. In addition, some institutions or teams may elect to insert such devices as intraaortic balloon pumps before transport to improve patient outcome. The care of these patients is challenging and many times extremely complicated. Nurses who have experience with critically ill patients are required to not only provide the best care during transport, but also to be ready to manage any untoward events that may occur (Gore,

Haffajee, Goldberg, Ostroff, Shustak, Cahill, Howe, & Dalen, 1983; Schneider, Borok, Heller, Paris, & Stewart, 1988; Wynn, 1991).

Myocardial Infarction

About 1.5 million people are diagnosed with an acute myocardial infarction each year; approximately 500,000 die, and one half of these deaths occur before arrival at the hospital (Hagar & Kloner, 1990). The advent of thrombolytic therapy and advanced technological treatments such as angioplasty have changed the focus of care of patients with myocardial infarctions. The "heart" of cardiovascular care is now to prevent any further additional injury to muscle. One of the ways this may be accomplished is by the timely transfer of patients to tertiary care centers. The earlier thrombolytic therapy is administered and reperfusion occurs, the better the patient outcome will be (Atkins & Wainscott, 1991; Hagley, 1993).

Although thrombolytic therapy has become available in most institutions throughout the United States, other therapies may not be. For example, cardiac catheterization, intraaortic balloon pumping, left ventricular assist devices, and heart transplants may be accessible in limited places.

The care and transport of the patient who is having a myocardial infarction requires an or-ganized and skilled approach. Anticipatory planning for potential complications from thrombolytic therapy and management of the medications and equipment the patient may require are a couple of the challenges that the nurse may face.

Signs and Symptoms

Approximately 80% of patients having a myocardial infarction complain of chest pain (Hagley, 1993). Other signs and symptoms include the following:
- Nausea and vomiting
- Diaphoresis
- Anxiety
- Voiced fear of death
- Electrocardiograph changes (Table 9-1)
- Cardiac dysrhythmia
- Elevation in cardiac enzymes

Treatment

BEFORE TRANSPORT. Once the diagnosis of myocardial infarction has been made, definitive care should be initiated. Currently, one of the most common treatments for an acute myocardial infarction is administration of thrombolytic therapy. Four thrombolytic agents are available in the United States. These drugs and their dosages are listed in Table 9-2. These drugs are usually administered within 6 hours

Table 9-1 Location of Myocardial Infarctions and Associated ST-Segment Changes

Location of Infarct	Leads with ST-Segment Elevation	Leads with ST-Segment Depression and/or Reciprocal Changes
Inferior	2, 3, aVF	I, aVL, V_1-V_4
Anterior (extensive)	I, aVL, V_1-V_6	2, 3, aVF, aVR
Anteroseptal	V_1-V_4	
Anterolateral	I, aVL, V_3-V_6	
Lateral	I, aVL, V_5-V_6	2, 3, aVF
High anterolateral	I, aVL	
Posterior	V_6	V_1-V_2

Note. From *Flight Nursing: Principles and Practice* by G. Lee (Ed.), 1991, St. Louis: Mosby.

Table 9-2 Thrombolytic Agents and Their Dosages Used in the Management of Acute Myocardial Infarctions

Agent	Dosage
Streptokinase	1.5 million U intravenously over 60 minutes
Anisoylated plasminogen-streptokinase activator complex	30 U over 5 minutes
Tissue plasminogen activator	100 mg intravenously over 3 hours: administration times may vary
Urokinase	Variable

Note. From "Emergency Intervention for Acute Myocardial Infarction: Thrombolytic Agents and Adjuvant Therapy" by M. Hagley, 1993, *Emergency Medicine Reports, 14*(2), 9-16.

of the onset of pain. However, protocols vary throughout the United States, and some patients have benefited from thrombolytic therapy if administered more than 6 hours after pain onset (Hagley, 1993).

Because of protocol and treatment variance, the nurse needs to know the protocols being used in the area of service or by the referring hospitals. The nurse should also be familiar and comfortable with administering any medications that the patient may require both before and during transport. Table 9-3 contains a list of some of these medications, with dosages, routes of administration, and benefits, currently being used to treat the patient with an acute myocardial infarction.

If nurses initiate thrombolytic therapy, they need to be aware of the potential contraindications for the use of these agents. These include but are not limited to the following:
- Major trauma or surgery within 2 weeks of the onset of the myocardial infarction
- Pregnancy or less than 4 weeks postpartum
- Known intracranial tumor
- Prior neurosurgery

Table 9-3 Medications That May Be Used in the Treatment of the Patient with Acute Myocardial Infarction

Medication	Dose	Benefit
Morphine sulfate	4-8 mg	Decreases and relieves chest pain
Heparin	5000 U intravenous bolus followed by 1000 U/hr infusion	Improves patency in patients treated with tissue plasminogen activator
Aspirin	160 or 325 mg daily; give one when diagnosis made	Improves survival
Atenolol	5 mg intravenously over 5 minutes; repeat in 10 minutes	Improves survival
Metoprolol	5 mg intravenously three times at 2-minute intervals	Improves survival
Nitroglycerin	50 mg in 250 ml of 5% dextrose in water at 10 μg/min; increase as needed	Improvement of symptoms; improves survival

Note. From "Emergency Intervention for Acute Myocardial Infarction: Thrombolytic Agents and Adjuvant Therapy" by M. Hagley, 1993, *Emergency Medicine Reports, 14*(2), 9-16.

- Cerebral vascular accident within the past 6 months
- Head trauma within 1 month
- Diabetic hemorrhagic retinopathy
- Severe hypertension (uncontrolled or difficult to control with medication)
- Recent transient ischemia attack
- Current menstruation
- Bleeding disorders
- Significant liver dysfunction
- Active internal bleeding
- Ongoing anticoagulant

Some protocols specify minimum age requirements for the patient receiving the drug. Once again, this varies throughout the country and

from expert to expert. Box 9-2 contains an example of a transport protocol for the patient receiving thrombolytic therapy.

A general assessment of the patient should be completed as previously discussed. A baseline evaluation of the patient's chest pain should be performed. Many nurses find using a number scale from 0 to 10 or 1 to 10 helpful in estimating the effects of treatments, such as morphine sulfate and nitroglycerin administration.

Additional nursing care for the patient with an acute myocardial infarction should include the following:

1. Ensuring that the airway is patent and maintainable

Box 9-2
CARE OF THE PATIENT RECEIVING THROMBOLYTIC THERAPY DURING TRANSPORT

1. Determine if thrombolytic therapy has been initiated and what type of drug the referring facility has started. If a particular protocol is being used, be sure that information is available.
2. Be sure all equipment that may be needed during transport (e.g., monitor, defibrillator, pacemaker, hemodynamic monitor) is on board either the air or ground ambulance.
3. On arrival at the referring facility:
   a. Obtain patient history/report
   b. Perform patient assessment
   c. Determine the amount and time of the initial treatment with thrombolytic agent
   d. Calculate current drug dosages and rates (sometimes this can be done before arrival if the information is available)
   e. Place medications on infusion pumps or intravenous monitors
   f. Determine the time for any changes in the rate of thrombolytic therapy
   g. Determine the level of the patient's pain
   h. Obtain appropriate specimens and documents from the referring facility
4. During transport:
   a. Monitor the patient for any complications related to thrombolytic therapy:
      - Excessive bleeding, oozing from intravenous sites
      - Blood in emesis
      - Bleeding from invasive line sites, around or through endotracheal or nasotracheal tube
      - Intracranial hemorrhage
      - Anaphylaxis
      - Hypotension
   b. Medicate for nausea and vomiting
   c. Monitor and treat as *needed* any reperfusion dysrhythmia
   d. Manage patient's chest pain as needed and prescribed
   e. Provide sedation as necessary for patient anxiety

2. Providing supplemental oxygen
3. Placing patient on the cardiac monitor
4. Applying pacer or defibrillation pads when indicated
5. Securing all intravenous lines
6. Corroborating drug dosages and placing medications on intravenous pumps or monitors
7. Obtaining documentation of previously administered medications

8. Checking that all equipment is functioning

DURING TRANSPORT
1. Assess and maintain the patient's airway, breathing, and circulation
2. Continuously assess and manage the patient's chest pain as directed
3. Monitor for cardiac dysrhythmia
4. Treat cardiac dysrhythmia based on ACLS protocols (Box 9-3)

Box 9-3
SUMMARY OF PROTOCOL CHANGES IN ADVANCED CARDIAC LIFE SUPPORT

1. It is imperative to access EMS care as soon as possible, as the first step in BCLS protocol.
2. The unresponsive victim with spontaneous respirations should be placed in the recovery position if no cervical spine trauma is suspected.
3. Esophageal obturator airway, esophageal gastric tube airway, combination esophageal-tracheal tube, and pharyngeal lumen airway are considered a therapeutic option that is not well established by evidence but may be helpful and probably is not harmful.
4. High-dose epinephrine is recommended for pediatric patients.
5. Sodium bicarbonate indications for use remain variable. It is recommended for treatment in hyperkalemia and some selected overdoses.
6. Calcium administration is recommended only in known overdoses of calcium channel blockers.
7. Adenosine is recommended as the drug of choice for paroxysmal supraventricular tachycardia.
8. New detailed protocols have been developed for bradycardia, tachycardia, pulseless electrical activity (PEA) (previously known as electromechanical dissociation [EMD]), hypotension, acute pulmonary edema, refractory ventricular fibrillation, hypothermia, and lightning injuries.
9. Endotracheal administration of drugs requires higher dosages followed by a flush.
10. Intravenous drugs should be followed by a flush.
11. Intraosseous access is recommended for children up to 6 years of age for emergency administration of medications.
12. Glucose-containing intravenous fluids are discouraged.
13. Thrombolytic agents are considered a therapeutic option that is always acceptable (except for accepted contraindications) and considered useful and effective.
14. Information about the early recognition of cerebrovascular accidents (CVA) and the need for intervention are emphasized.
15. The need to establish advanced directives and do-not-resuscitate orders is discussed.

Note. From "Guidelines for Cardiopulmonary Resuscitation and Emergency Cardiac Care" by JAMA, 1992, *Journal of the American Medical Association, 268*(16), 2180-2181.

5. Continuously monitor medications being infused and their effects
6. When thrombolytic therapy is being administered, monitor the patient for signs and symptoms of:
   a. Systemic bleeding
      - Vomiting blood
      - Blood in the Foley catheter
      - Bleeding from intravenous or invasive line sites
   b. Intracranial hemorrhage
      - Alteration in mental status
      - Unresponsiveness
      - Pupillary changes
      - Motor/sensory deficits
   c. Anaphylaxis
   d. Hypotension

Cardiogenic Shock

Cardiogenic shock occurs when damage to cardiac muscle causes severe cardiac dysfunction, rendering the heart incapable of meeting the body's demands. The most common cause is from myocardial infarction. Other causes include end-stage cardiomyopathy, valvular heart disease, cardiac tamponade, and open heart surgery (Thompson, McFarland, Hirsch, & Tucker, 1993). Criteria for the diagnosis of cardiogenic shock include a systolic blood pressure of less than 80 mm Hg, a cardiac index of less than 2.0 liters, changes in mental status, oliguria, cyanosis, and increased capillary refill time (Wedge-Stecher, 1990).

Patients sustaining cardiogenic shock may be transferred for several reasons including the need for intraaortic balloon pumping, placement of a ventricular assist device, and cardiac transplant. An intraaortic balloon pump provides support for a failing myocardium by using counterpulsation. The balloon pump inflates during diastole and deflates during systole, increasing the blood flow to the coronary circulation. The pump may also enhance cardiac output, decrease systolic pressure, increase diastolic pressure, decrease heart rate, and increase urinary output (Brister & Shragge,

1992). A ventricular assist device mechanically approximates normal hemodynamic states (Thompson, McFarland, Hirsch, & Tucker, 1993). How the device functions is based on the type of device in place. Sometimes these devices are already in place before the patient is transferred.

Treatment

BEFORE TRANSPORT
1. Assess and stabilize the patient's airway, breathing, and circulation
2. Calculate medication dosages and place on intravenous infusion or monitor pumps
3. If patient is awake, consider sedation to decrease anxiety during transport
4. Assess the patency of all invasive lines
5. Secure all lines
6. If an intraaortic balloon pump or ventricular assist device is in place, assess the functioning of these devices
7. Consider and plan for the effects of the mode of transport, particularly air transport, on the function of the intraaortic balloon pump or ventricular assist device

DURING TRANSPORT
1. Continue monitoring the patient's airway, breathing, and circulation
2. If intraaortic balloon pump or ventricular device is in place, monitor the patient for potential complications such as emboli, thrombosis, aortic rupture, impaired circulation, and bleeding
3. Place and secure equipment within view and reach so that appropriate interventions can be rapidly provided
4. Have emergency equipment available

Intraaortic Balloon Pump

Box 9-4 summarizes care of the patient before and during transport with an intraaortic balloon pump in place. Even though this particular protocol addresses air transport, the principles are also applicable to ground transport.

Box 9-4
DATA FOR INTRAAORTIC BALLOON PUMP

I. Indications

The intraaortic balloon pump (IABP) is indicated for the management of:
   A. Cardiogenic shock
   B. Severe congestive heart failure
   C. Refractory ischemia
   D. Ventricular septal defects

II. Contraindications

The IABP is contraindicated in patients with:
   A. Aortic valve stenosis
   B. Aortic dissection

III. Policy
   A. All IABP flights must be accompanied by a third flight crew member. There will be a minimal delay in liftoff to await the third team member. This will provide for a safe and efficient transfer of the critically ill cardiac patient.
   B. Equipment for IABP transfer:
      1. IABP console 90 T and power pack
      2. IABP extension tubing
      3. 50-ml Luer-Lok syringe
      4. One extra helium tank (200 psi)
      5. One EKG cable
      6. Arterial line cable
      7. Arterial line setup:
         a. Transducer
         b. Arterial flush solution (500 ml 0.9 normal saline with 1000 units of heparin or equivalent ratio).
   C. Loading with IABP
      1. Remove the secondary stretcher.
      2. Load the IABP into the right aft of the aircraft.
      3. Lock the IABP into the stretcher mounts of the aircraft.
      4. Plug IABP into the outlet aft of the bench seat.
      5. Place power pack aft of IABP and secure with Velcro straps.
   D. In flight to the referring hospital the following will be completed:
      1. Turn on the invertor switch.
      2. Assemble pressure cable and arterial line.
      3. Assemble EKG cable.
      4. Assemble IABP extension tubing.
      5. Set IABP augmentation to minimum and volume alarm to maximum.
   E. A portable chest x-ray is taken to determine the proper position of the balloon catheter.
   F. Attach patient to IABP 90 T console:
      1. Turn power on to trigger select EKG.
      2. Turn gas on (replace tank at 25 psi).

Note. From Loyola LIFESTAR, Loyola University Medical Center, Maywood, Illinois.   *Continued.*

Box 9-4, cont'd
DATA FOR INTRAAORTIC BALLOON PUMP

3. Put timing on "Auto" and keep alarm on.
4. Establish EKG signal and adjust size.
5. Establish arterial line and calibrate transducer.
6. Set initial counterpulsation on 1:2 and adjust glowworm.
7. Disconnect patient's IABP catheter from extension tubing and attach the Datascope extension tubing.
    a. For an Aries balloon pump, remove the Aries extension tubing distal from the white plastic triangle. Attach the 6-foot Datascope extension tubing to the white plastic triangle. Connect the tubing to the Datascope IABP.
    b. For a Kontron balloon pump, keep all of the tubing. Use the 14-inch Datascope connection tubing. Insert Datascope tubing into end of Kontron pump and connect to Datascope balloon pump.
    c. For a Datascope balloon pump disconnect extension tubing from the balloon pump and attach this tubing to the Datascope 90 T balloon pump.
8. Autofill IABP. When complete, it will read "autofill complete."
9. Hit "assist/standby."
10. Turn augment to maximum.
11. Adjust timing as needed.
G. Vital signs are to be recorded every 5 to 10 minutes.
H. Check the site of insertion for a dressing.
I. Splint the affected limb with a blanket or similar covering to restrict mobility of the affected extremity.
J. Pulses, sensation, capillary refill, and blanching should be assessed in all extremities before, during, and after flight.
K. Monitor EKG for arrhythmias and urine output for > 30 ml/hr.
L. Complications may occur, and the flight team is responsible to respond appropriately.
    1. Cardiopulmonary arrest
        a. Set trigger select to "internal."
    2. Disabled pump
        a. Disconnect the IABP from the extension tubing.
        b. Place a stopcock on the end of the IAB catheter.
        c. Deflate the IAB with a syringe.
        d. Manually reinflate IAB with one half volume—26 ml every 5 minutes.
    3. Ruptured IAB: This will be noted with sudden loss of augmentation on the arterial line waveform and blood in the balloon pumping. If this occurs, shut off the console to the patient, and notify LIFESTAR Center for medical control.
M. Document the following on the flight record:
    1. Patient aortic end-diastolic pressure.
    2. Peak systolic pressure.
    3. Augmented systolic pressure.
    4. Augmented diastolic pressure.
    5. Balloon aortic end diastolic pressure.
    6. Counter pulsation ratio of IABP (1:1, 1:2, 1:3).
    7. Pulses, sensation, capillary refill, and blanching of the extremity with the IABP.

Box 9-4, cont'd
DATA FOR INTRAAORTIC BALLOON PUMP

N. Loading patients into helicopter on 90 T IABP:

Procedure
1. Load patient into helicopter with one flight crew member holding onto IABP catheter tubings. Lock stretcher into the stretcher mounts.
2. Load IABP into right aft side of helicopter. Lock IABP into the mounts.
3. Plug power pack into IABP and into wall outlet aft bench seat.

Special considerations
1. Be careful not to pull on IABP catheter when loading patient to prevent displacement of catheter.
2. Be certain the clamps are locked into the floor to prevent movement of IABP during flight.
3. Use aircraft power whenever possible to save battery power.

O. Unloading patients from helicopter on the 90 T IABP:

Procedure
1. All IABP patients unloaded from the helicopter will be "cold" unloads.
2. Unplug IABP from outlet in aircraft.
3. Remove power pack.

4. Remove stretcher mounts from IABP and unload the IABP.
5. Unload the patient stretcher from the aircraft.

6. While holding onto the IABP catheter, unload the patient from the rear of the aircraft.
7. Transport patient quickly and efficiently to the appropriate department.
8. Assist in transferring patient to IABP in the unit and return IABP 90 T to equipment room
9. Restock IABP transfer bag and plug IABP into wall outlet to maintain a fully charged unit.

Special considerations

2. Must use battery power while moving patient to ICU.
3. Take the power pack out of the helicopter for unloading purposes. The power pack need not accompany the transport to the ICU.

5. Member must hold IABP catheter to prevent pulling on the catheter and possible dislodgement.
6. Again, to prevent any dislodgement of the catheter, hold the IABP catheter.

Continued.

Box 9-4, cont'd
DATA FOR INTRAAORTIC BALLOON PUMP

Loyola University Medical Center Aeromedical Transportation Services—LIFESTAR Cardiac Emergencies: Intraaortic Balloon Pump

1. RMC [specific to LIFESTAR]
2. Continue IABP timing of 1:1, 1:2, or 1:3.
3. If the heart rate is ≥ 120, change the timing of the IABP to 1:2; notify medical control physician of the change.
4. Monitor SBP, augmented BP, and afterload reduction.
5. If the augmented BP is ≤ 90 mm Hg on the IABP at 1:2, resume 1:1.
6. If the agumented BP is still ≤ 90 mm Hg, refer to the Cardiogenic Shock SMO, 1.14.
7. When assessing blood pressure, if Swan Ganz is in place, monitor PAS/PAD, CVP, and PCWP readings.
8. Obtain previous readings.
9. If CVP or PCWP is decreased, and/or augmented BP ≤ 90 mm Hg, and/or patient's clinical assessment is one of hypovolemia, give 0.9 normal saline or lactated Ringer's 250 ml IV bolus if there are no signs of CHF or pulmonary edema.
10. If the CVP and/or PCWP does not increase with the fluid bolus and there are no signs of CHF or pulmonary edema, give an additional 100 to 200 ml of 0.9 lactated Ringer's.
11. If the CVP and/or the PCWP does not increase, contact medical control physician.
12. If the CVP and/or PCWP is elevated and augmented BP is ≤ 90 mm Hg, refer to the Cardiogenic Shock SMO to initiate dopamine.
13. If the CVP and/or PCWP is elevated and/or the patient's clinical assessment reveals sign of CHF or pulmonary edema refer to the CHF/Pulmonary Edema SMO 1.15.

Note. From Loyola LIFESTAR, Loyola University Medical Center, Maywood, Illinois.

Respiratory Emergencies

Causes of respiratory emergencies include airway obstruction, adult respiratory distress syndrome (ARDS), allergic reactions, and pulmonary emboli. The major challenge in the care of the patient with a respiratory emergency is to prevent or improve hypoxia.

The initial assessment of the patient with a respiratory emergency guides the nurse in preparing the patient for transport. According to Koenig and Pratt (1987, p. 154), "the purpose of assessment is to determine the need for acute intervention and ventilatory assistance. Whenever in doubt, use the most aggressive therapy."

Signs and Symptoms

Signs and symptoms of respiratory distress and potential respiratory failure include (Koenig & Pratt, 1987; Lee & Bristol, 1991; Thompson, McFarland, Hirsch, & Tucker, 1993):

- Respiratory rate greater than 30
- Pulse rate less than 60 or greater than 120
- Use of accessory muscles
    - Supraclavicular
    - Abdominal muscles (in the adult patient)
- Nasal flaring
- Chest wall retractions
- Decreased chest wall movement

- Respiratory patterns
  - ❑ Labored
  - ❑ Irregular
- Breath sounds
  - ❑ Wheezes
  - ❑ Crackles
  - ❑ Absence of breath sounds
- Alterations in mental status
- Progressive exhaustion
- pH less than 7.2
- P_{CO_2} greater than 55 mm Hg
- P_{O_2} less than 60 mm Hg
- Decreased vital capacity

Treatment

Mechanical Ventilation

Over the past 10 years mechanical ventilators have been developed for use during transport (Rouse, Branson, & Semonin-Holleran, 1992). Transport ventilators can be used for both transport of patients from accident scenes and for the care of patients with complicated respiratory problems, such as adult respiratory distress.

Using a ventilator during transport offers both advantages and disadvantages for the nurse. The advantages of a transport ventilator include the constant maintenance of ventilation and oxygenation, as well as freeing an additional pair of hands that may allow the nurse to administer medications or perform other needed patient care tasks. The disadvantage of using a mechanical ventilator during transport is that the nurse or other team member loses the ability to evaluate the patient's lung compliance. Some ventilators may have limited alarms, and if the patient should develop such complications as a pneumothorax, displaced endotracheal tube, or obstruction, it may not be easily recognized by the nurse until the patient is in severe distress (Nolan & Baskett, 1992). Other potential complications associated with mechanical ventilation include equipment malfunction, inappropriate use of equipment, and an exaggerated physiological response to

changes in intrathoracic pressure (Ingenito & Drazen, 1992).

When using a mechanical ventilator during transport, the nurse needs to pay attention to several things. Understanding the concepts related to mechanical ventilation is important for the successful use of mechanical ventilators so that tidal volumes, respiratory rates, and oxygenation requirements can be appropriately calculated and evaluated. Box 9-5 summarizes mechanical ventilation concepts. Figure 9-4 shows a ventilator mounted in a transport vehicle.

When patients are intubated and being ventilated, they lose the ability to provide humidity for the upper airway and also are at risk of developing infection (Rouse, Branson, & Semonin-Holleran, 1992). To compensate for the lack of humidity, an artificial nose may be attached between the endotracheal tube and ventilator connector.

To prevent the potential for infection, disposable connectors should be used. These are placed between the patient's endotracheal tube and ventilator connection. When disposable connectors are not used, the connection between the ventilator and the patient should be cleaned in warm, soapy water, soaked in a bacteriostatic solution, rinsed, and dried (Hill & Dolan, 1982).

When possible and available, specialists in respiratory therapy should be consulted. In some cases, a respiratory therapist is able to accompany the nurse. Before transport, a respiratory therapist can help the nurse better prepare for problems that may occur with mechanical ventilation during transport. Patient movement, vibration, altitude, and oxygen flow may affect the type of machine being used and need to be considered during the planning process. Several types of transport ventilators are available (Table 9-4).

BEFORE TRANSPORT

1. Determine if there are any indications for intubation including (American College of Emergency Physicians, 1993; Department

Box 9-5
MECHANICAL VENTILATION CONCEPTS

Concept	Definition
Tidal volume (V_T)	The volume inspired or expired during a normal breath. During mechanical ventilation, tidal volume is calculated as 10 to 15 ml/kg.
Inspiratory time (T_I)	The time from the beginning of inspiratory flow until the beginning of expiratory flow. During mechanical ventilation of adults, T_I is 1 to 2 seconds. In infants, T_I is 0.5 to 1 second.
Expiratory time (T_E)	The time from start of expiratory flow to start of inspiratory flow.
Inspiratory flow (V_I)	The flow of gas measured at the airway opening during inspiration. Normal inspiratory flow during mechanical ventilation is 60 to 100 L/minute.
Respiratory frequency	Breathing cycles or breaths per minute delivered by a ventilator.
I:E ratio	The ratio of inspiratory time to expiratory time. Normal I:E ratio is 1:3. During mechanical ventilation I:E should be 1:2 or greater to prevent air trapping.
Positive end-expiratory pressure (PEEP)	Positive pressure applied during the expiratory phase following delivery of a mandatory breath or spontaneous breath.
Peak inspiratory pressure (PIP)	The highest proximal airway pressure produced in the patient circuit during the inspiratory phase. The stiffer the patient's lungs, the greater the PIP.
Control variable	Which variable the ventilator will control. Ventilators normally control either flow (tidal volume) or pressure (peak pressure).
Trigger variable	The initiation of a breath is known as a trigger. Breaths can be triggered by the ventilator (time triggered) or by the patient (pressure triggered).
CPAP	Continuous positive airway pressure.

Note. From "Mechanical Ventilation during Air Medical Transport: Techniques and Devices" by M. Rouse, R. Branson, & R. Semonin-Holleran, 1992, *Journal of Air Medical Transport, 11*(4), 5-8.

of Transportation, 1988):
a. Pathologic hypotension
b. Significant facial trauma
c. Known spinal cord injuries
d. Significant chest injuries
e. Pao_2 < 60 torr on 40% to 60% supplemental oxygen
f. Pco_2 exceeds 50 mm Hg
g. Singed nasal hair
h. Erythematous posterior pharynx
i. Overt respiratory stridor
j. Need to use neuromuscular blocking agents for transport
k. Decreased level of consciousness and inability to maintain an airway
2. If patient is intubated, evaluate tube placement
   a. Auscultate breath sounds
   b. View chest X ray if available
   c. Place CO_2 detector on tube to assess placement
   d. Place patient on CO_2 monitor

Table 9-4 Transport Ventilators

Ventilator Name and Manufacturer	Power Source	Weight (kg)	Size (cm)	Alarms	Gas Consumption	Ventilator Modes
IC-2A, Bio-Med Devices, Stanford, Calif.	Pneumatic	3.9	8.6 × 15.6 × 26	No alarms	12 L/minute	CMV,* IMV,† CPAP,‡ PEEP§
MVP-10, Bio-Med Devices	Pneumatic	2.3	20 × 23 × 7	No alarms	3 L/minute	IMV, CPAP, PEEP
MAX, Hamilton Medical Corp., Reno, Nev.	Battery	5.0	30 × 8 × 16.5	Low-battery alarm, oxygen alarm for low supply and disconnection	Does not use gas	IMV
Uni-Vent 706, Impact Medical Corp., West Caldwell, N.J.	Battery, but can run off AC in aircraft	1.4	20 × 13 × 5.5	Low battery, PIP limited to 80 cm H_2O	Does not use gas	CMV
Uni-Vent 750, Impact Medical Corp.	Battery, but can run off AC in aircraft	4.3	23 × 11.4 × 29.2	High and low gas pressure, apnea, external power, battery	Does not use gas	CMV, AMV, IMV, PEEP
AutoVent 2000 and 3000, Life Support Products, Irvine, Calif.	Pneumatic	0.68	15 × 9 × 4.5	Pressure	0.5 L/minute	IMV
Hope Automatic Resuscitator, Matrix Medical, Orchard Park, N.Y.	Pneumatic	1.3	18 × 9 × 6	Pressure	0.5 L/minute	CMV
Omni-Vent, Columbian Medical Marketing, Topeka, Kan.	Pneumatic	2.5	10 × 13 × 15	No alarms	Not specified	CMV
Ambumatic, Ambu Inc, Linthicum, Md.	Pneumatic	725 grams	16 × 9 × 4	Pressure	25 mL/cycle	CMV

Note. From "Mechanical Ventilation during Air Medical Transport: Techniques and Devices" by M. Rouse, R. Branson, & R. Semonin-Holleran, 1992, *Journal of Air Medical Transport, 11*(4), 5–8.
*Control mode.
†Intermittent mandatory ventilation.
‡Continuous positive airway pressure.
§Positive end-expiratory pressure.

3. Evaluate intravenous line placement and need for hydration
4. Consider sedation and/or neuromuscular blocking agents for transport to decrease patient anxiety and for safety and to protect the airway
5. Attach pulse oximeter to patient
6. Attach cardiac monitor to patient
7. Obtain baseline vital signs
8. Check security of all lines
9. Administer bronchodilators as prescribed by inhalation, intravenously, or endotracheally (see Table 9-5 for a list of suggested medications and their dosages)
10. Consider administration of corticosteroids

for patients who do not respond to bronchodilators as prescribed at a dosage intravenously of methylprednisolone 60 to 80 mg intravenous bolus every 6 to 8 hours or hydrocortisone 2.0 mg/kg bolus every 4 hours or hydrocortisone 2.0 mg/kg intravenous bolus, then 0.5 mg/kg/hr continuous infusion

DURING TRANSPORT
1. Continuous assessment and appropriate intervention of the patient's airway, breathing, and circulation
2. Continuous assessment of patient's respiratory function
   a. Physical assessment of breath sounds

Table 9-5 Bronchodilators Used for Inhalation Therapy

Drug	Available Form	Dosage
Albuterol		
Metered-dose inhaler	90 µg/puff	Two inhalations every 5 minutes for total of 12 puffs
Nebulizer solution	0.5% (5 mg/ml)	0.1 to 0.15 mg/kg/dose up to 5 mg every 20 minutes for 1 to 2 hours
Metaproterenol		
Metered-dose inhaler	650 µg/puff	Two inhalations
Nebulizer solution	5% (50 mg/ml)	0.1 to 0.3 ml (5 to 15 mg)
	0.6% unit dose vial of 2.5 ml (15 mg)	As above (5 to 15 mg); do not exceed 15 mg
Terbutaline		
Metered-dose inhaler	200 µg/puff	Two inhalations every 5 minutes for a total of 12 puffs
Injectable solution used in nebulizer		0.1% (1 mg/1 ml) solution in 0.9% NaCl solution for injection Not FDA approved for inhalation
Epinephrine	1:1000 (1 mg/ml)	0.01 mg/kg up to 0.3 mg subcutaneously every 20 minutes for three doses
Terbutaline	(0.1%) 1 mg/ml solution for injection in 0.9% NaCl	Subcutaneous 0.1 mg/kg up to 0.3 every 2 to 6 hours as needed. IV 10 µg/kg over 10 minutes loading dose. Maintenance: 0.4 µg/kg/minute; increase as necessary by 0.2 µg/kg/minute and expect to use 3 to 6 µg/kg/minute

Note. From "Acute Exacerbations of Asthma Care in Hospital-Based Emergency Departments" by American College of Emergency Physicians, 1993, Dallas: The Author.

when possible, chest wall rise and fall, and pulses

   b. End-tidal CO_2 detectors/monitors

   c. Pulse oximeter

   d. Cardiac monitor

3. Continuous assessment and monitoring of any equipment that is being used during transport (e.g., ventilator)
4. Continuously monitor and evaluate the patient's response to any treatment given during transport
5. Provide sedation as prescribed or as needed
6. Confirm tube placement each time after patient is moved (e.g., from ambulance stretcher to bed)

Neurological Emergencies

Each year approximately 500,000 people sustain a cerebrovascular accident (CVA) (Garza, 1993). One third of these people will recover, one third will have a permanent disability, and one third will die (Garza, 1993). Generally 30% of these CFAs are hemorrhagic, and the remaining 70% are thrombotic or embolic in origin (Garza, 1993).

Recent advances in the care of the CVA patient include administration of thrombolytic agents for nonhemorrhagic events, use of free radical scavengers, and emergent surgeries. The care of the patient with a CVA has been refocused to provide rapid identification and intervention (Solomon & Hart, 1993). As pointed out by Solomon and Hart (1993, p. 30), "research related to the treatment of the stroke patient is now focusing on "reperfusion with a thrombolytic agent(s); stopping the propagation and preventing recurrent embolism with anticoagulation or antiplatelet agents; and neuron protection with agents such as nimodipine." Similar to the care of the patient with an acute myocardial infarction, the need for CVA patients to receive definitive care has created a role for the critical care nurse involved in transport.

Neurological Assessment

The baseline neurological assessment provides baseline data about the patient and helps to uncover the potential source of the neurological emergency. A neurological assessment comprises five components: level of consciousness (mental status), pupillary response, motor responses, sensory responses, and vital signs.

Level of Consciousness

Evaluating the patient's level of consciousness includes ruling out the potential for other causes of altered mental status. For example, medications, metabolic disturbances, alterations in body temperature, infections, hypoxia, diabetes, multiple organ failure, and encephalopathies may cause alterations in the patient's level of consciousness (Henry & Stapleton, 1992).

A mnemonic described by Nevill, Adelstein, and Loos (1991, p. 253) offers another technique to evaluate potential causes of an altered level of consciousness. This is *UNCONSCIOUS,* which represents the following:

   U—Units of insulin
   N—Narcotics
   C—Convulsions
   O—Oxygen
   N—Nonorganic
   S—Stroke
   C—Cocktail
   I—Intracranial pressure
   O—Organism
   U—Urea
   S—Shock

If the patient is awake, carrying on a brief conversation focusing on why the patient is having problems and what is going to happen will furnish the nurse with an idea of the patient's mental status (Sullivan, 1990). Both the Glasgow coma scale and the AVPU method discussed in Chapter 5 offer other methods to evaluate the patient's level of consciousness.

Description	Clinical significance
Ipsilateral miosis (Horner's syndrome): one pupil is smaller. Ptosis of the eyelid occurs, as well as anhidrosis of the face ipsilateral to the small pupil.	Occurs with downward displacement of the hypothalamus with herniation. May also occur with internal carotid artery occlusion.

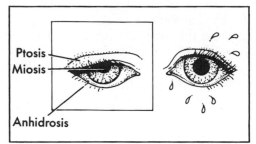

Description	Clinical significance
Bilateral miosis: light reaction may be seen with magnifying glass. Pupils are both small or "pinpoint" (2 mm).	Continued herniation or hemorrhage into the pons. Other causes include ophthalmic miotic drugs (acetylcholine, pilocarpine, physostigmine, and edrophonium), opiates, and metabolic encephalopathies.

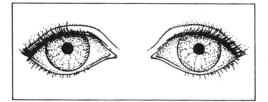

Ipsilateral mydriasis (hutchinsonian pupil): one pupil is larger than the other. The larger pupil is unreactive to light (often referred to as a *blown pupil*).	Occurs in rapidly progressing intracranial hypertension as the result of compression of the third cranial nerve.

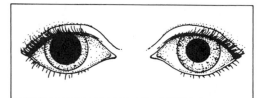

Bilateral midposition: both pupils (4-5 mm) are unreactive to light (referred to as *fixed and dilated*).	Occurs with midbrain compression from transtentorial/central herniation. Other causes include high doses of dopamine (30 mcg/kg/min) in the presence of shock; drugs (amphetamines, cocaine, atropine, and scopolamine); severe anoxia; and brain death.

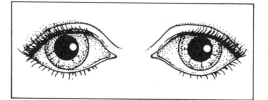

Bilateral mydriasis: both pupils are >6 mm and unreactive to light.	Terminal stages of herniation. Other causes include atropine, hypothermia, and severe barbiturate intoxication.

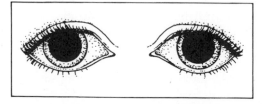

Fig. 9-3 Pupillary abnormalities. *Miosis,* Constricted; *mydriasis,* dilated; *ptosis,* dropping upper eyelid; *anhidrosis,* lack of sweat. (Adapted from "Pathologic Pupillary Signs: Self-Learning Module (Part 2)" by B.S. Bishop, 1991, *Critical Care Nurse,* 11(7), pp. 58-67. In *Trauma Nursing: The Art and Science* by J.A. Neff and P.S. Kidd, 1992, St. Louis: Mosby.)

Pupillary Response

Pupils are assessed for three parameters: size, reactivity to light, and equality (Henry & Stapleton, 1992). Charts are available that demonstrate pupil size in millimeters, which helps to estimate and document pupil size.

Abnormal findings include the following (Figure 9-3):

- Constricted pupils
- Fixed dilated pupils
- Irregular pupillary shape and size
- Unilateral pupillary changes

Motor and Sensory Response

Motor and sensory response begins with an observation of the patient's movement. If patients are awake and cooperative, they may be asked to raise arms or legs. The nurse should observe for any weakness or drifting.

If the patient does not respond to verbal stimuli, a noxious stimulus such as rubbing the patient's sternum may be applied and motor response observed. Abnormal findings include the following:

- Lack of movement
- Flaccid posture
- Unilateral weakness or absence of movement
- Decorticate posturing (unilateral or bilateral)
- Decerebrate posturing (unilateral or bilateral)
- Rigidity

A brief cranial nerve assessment may provide some additional information about the patient's motor/sensory status. Table 9-6 contains a cranial nerve assessment.

In the unconscious patient, several cranial nerve reflexes assume prognostic significance and are specifically evaluated (Sullivan, 1990). These include the oculocephalic reflex (doll's eyes) and oculovestibular (caloric) reflexes. These reflexes when present indicate functioning of cranial nerves III, IV, VI, and VIII and the brain stem (Sullivan, 1990).

Table 9-6   Cranial Nerve Assessment

Cranial Nerve	Assessment
I	Smell
II	Vision, Snellen chart
III	Pupillary constriction, eyelid elevation
III, IV, VI	Extraocular eye movements
V	Facial sensation, jaw clenching
VII	Facial movements, taste
VIII	Hearing
IX, X	Gag, swallowing
XI	Shoulder shrug
XII	Elevation of uvula

Note. From "Neurological Assessment" by J. Sullivan, 1990, *Nursing Clinics of North America, 25*(4), 802.

Vital Signs

Changes in intracranial pressure affect vital signs. Vital signs obtained should include blood pressure, pulse, respirations, and, when possible, a temperature. Hypertension, bradycardia, and ataxic respirations are ominous indications of increasing intracranial pressure and impending herniation. Both hypothermia and hyperthermia complicate neurological evaluation and need to be considered when evaluating the patient.

Signs and Symptoms of CVA

Signs and symptoms of CVA or CVA in process including the following:

1. Alterations in airway and respiratory function
2. Alterations in mental status
   a. Restlessness
   b. Difficulty in communicating (slurred speech, aphasia)
   c. Lethargy
   d. Unresponsiveness
3. Headache
4. Alterations in vital signs
   a. Hypertension

b. Bradycardia
c. Ataxic respirations
5. Nausea and vomiting
6. Alterations in motor/sensory response
   a. Weakness
   b. Unilateral motor deficits
   c. Unilateral sensory deficits
   d. No response to stimuli

Treatment

Before Transport

1. Perform primary assessment and intervene as indicated
2. Determine the need for intubation to protect patient's airway or control the patient's intracranial pressure
3. If patient is intubated, evaluate tube placement by physical assessment, chest X-ray study if available, end-tidal CO_2 detector
4. Monitor patient's end-tidal CO_2 when hyperventilating the patient
5. Attach pulse oximeter to the patient
6. Perform a baseline neurological assessment

7. Obtain baseline vital signs
8. If patient is hypertensive, administer medications as prescribed (Table 9-7)
9. Calculate appropriate dosages for intravenous medications and place on intravenous infusion pumps or monitors
10. Attach a cardiac monitor to the patient
11. If patient is anxious, agitated, or combative, consider sedation or neuromuscular blocking agents
12. Elevate head of the bed to facilitate cerebral venous blood outflow (Morris, 1992)

During Transport

1. Continuously monitor the patient's airway, breathing, and circulation and intervene as needed
2. Monitor and evaluate any equipment used during transport
3. Continue sedation or neuromuscular blocking agents as indicated during transport
4. Decrease excessive stimulation during transport (e.g., provide hearing protection)

Table 9-7   Medications That May Be Used To Manage Hypertension for the Patient with a Cerebral Vascular Accident

Medications	Dosage	Adverse Reactions
Esmolol	Intravenous loading, 500 µg/kg/minute; 50 µg/kg/minute for 4 minutes; may repeat every 5 minutes increasing maintenance infusion by 50 µg/kg/minute (maximum of 200 µg/kg/minute)	Induration, inflammation at the insertion site, nausea and vomiting, hypotension, congestive heart failure, dyspnea, cough
Labetalol	Intravenous 200 mg/160 ml of 5% dextrose in water, run at 2 ml/minute; intravenous bolus 20 mg over 2 mintues; may repeat 40 to 80 mg every 10 minutes, not to exceed 300 mg	Orthostatic hypotension, nausea and vomiting, rash, dyspnea, ventricular dysrhythmia
Nitroprusside sodium	Intravenous infusion of 50 mg in 2 to 3 ml of 5% dextrose in water, then dilute in 250 5% dextrose in water, run at 0.5 to 0.8 µg/kg/minute	Dizziness, headache, nausea and vomiting

Please note that these are only some of the drugs used in the management of hypertension related to cerebral vascular accidents.

Note. From *Nursing Drug Reference* by L. Skidmore-Roth, 1993, St. Louis: Mosby.

Table 9-8   Medications Used for Treatment of Seizures

Medications	Dosage	Adverse Reactions
Diazepam	Intravenous bolus 5 to 20 mg 2 mg/minute; may repeat every 5 to 10 minutes; not to exceed 60 mg	Respiratory depression, drowsiness
Lorazepam	2 to 4 mg intravenously	Orthostatic hypotension, tachycardia, dizziness, drowsiness
Phenobarbital	Intravenous infusion 10 mg/kg; run no faster than 50 mg/minute; may give up to 20 mg/kg	Drowsiness, nausea and vomiting, hallucinations
Phenytoin	Intravenous loading dose of 900 mg; 1.5 g run at 50 mg/minute	Hypotension, ventricular fibrillation, nausea and vomiting, pain at the IV site

Note. From *Nursing Drug Reference* by L. Skidmore-Roth, 1993, St. Louis: Mosby.

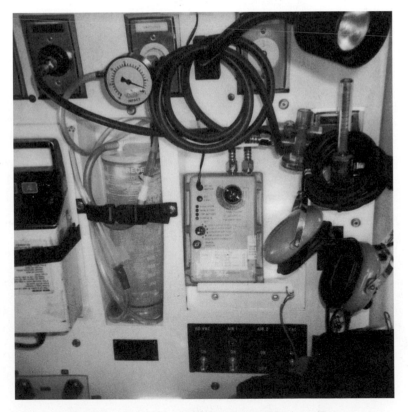

Fig. 9-4   Transport ventilator mounted in a vehicle.

Table 9-9   Nursing Diagnoses, Interventions, and Evaluative Criteria for Patients with a Medical Emergency

Diagnosis	Interventions	Evaluative Criteria
Pain related to damage to the myocardium from acute myocardial infarction as evidenced by the patient's verbalizing the presence of pain.	Evaluate patient's level of pain using a selected numbering scale (e.g., pain level 0 to 10 or 1 to 10). Administer pain medication as prescribed; increase nitroglycerin as prescribed. Reevaluate patient's pain after each intervention. Inform the patient of the need to tell the nurse about pain during transport. Monitor and treat the patient for any adverse effects from medications (e.g., respiratory depression, hypotension).	Patient is able to describe pain using a numbering system. Patient feels comfortable verbalizing level of pain. Patient describes some relief from the pain. Adverse side effects are recognized early and are appropriately treated.
Gas exchange impaired related to impending respiratory failure as evidenced by a $Po_2 > 60$, nasal flaring, use of accessory muscles of breathing, cyanosis, and presence of adventitious breath sounds.	Determine the need for intubation before transport. Assess for proper tube placement by auscultating breath sounds, using a CO_2 detector, watching for improvement in the patient's condition. Place patient on a transport ventilator using appropriate settings (e.g., tidal volume, rate). Attach pulse oximeter to the patient.	Patient will have the following: A patent airway. Breath sounds present and equal bilaterally. Appropriate change in CO_2 detector. Appropriate ventilator settings based on patient's age, tidal volume and respiratory problem. Pulse oximeter readings will be with 93% to 100%.
High risk for injury related to the pharmacological interventions that may be required for treatment of the patient with a medical emergency as evidenced by bleeding from thrombolytic therapy, severe hypotension from antihypertensive agents	Monitor for any adverse reactions by observing the patient for any obvious or occult bleeding when receiving thrombolytics. Treat as prescribed: Direct pressure. Avoid intramuscular injections. Avoid invasive procedures once drugs are started as much as possible. Measure blood pressure every 5 minutes when administering antihypertensive agents.	Early recognition of bleeding sites. Any bleeding brought under control. Decreased incidence of hypotension.

5. Monitor and treat any seizure activity as prescribed (Table 9-8)

SUMMARY

The care and transport of the patient with a medical emergency challenge the prehospital nurse. These patients usually are critically ill, receive both pharmacological and technological treatments, and require complete and competent care during transport. Preplanning and organization can not only decrease the time needed for patient preparation, but also help prevent the development of untoward complications during transport. Table 9-9 contains some specific nursing diagnoses, collaborative interventions, and expected outcomes for the care of the patient with a medical emergency (Kim, McFarland, & McLane, 1993).

REFERENCES

American College of Emergency Physicians (ACEP). (1993). *Acute exacerbations of care in hospital-based emergency departments.* Dallas: American College of Emergency Physicians.

Atkins, J., & Wainscott, M. (1991). Role of emergency medical services. *Heart & Lung, 20*(5), 576-581.

Brister, S., & Shragge, W. (1992). Mechanical assistance of the failing heart. In J. Hall, G. Schmidt, & L. Wood (Eds.), *Principles of critical care* (pp. 366-373). New York: McGraw-Hill.

Dedrick, D., Darga, A., Landis, D., & Burney, R. (1989). Defibrillation safety in emergency helicopter transport. *Annals of Emergency Medicine, 18*(1), 69-71.

Department of Transportation. (1988). *Air medical crew national standard curriculum* (pp. 103-110). Pasadena, CA: Association of Air Medical Services.

Gabram, S., Piancentini, L., & Jacobs, L. (1990). The risk of aeromedical transport for the cardiac patient. *Emergency Care Quarterly, 72*, 81.

Garza, M. (1993). Brain attack. *Journal of Emergency Medical Services, 18*(4), 60-62.

Gordon, R., & O'Dell, K. (1991). Permanent internal pacemaker safety in air medical transport. *Journal of Air Medical Transport, 10*(2), 22-23.

Gore, J., Haffajee, C., Goldberg, R., Ostroff, M., Shustak, C., Cahill, N., Howe, J., & Dalen, J. (1983). Evaluation of an emergency cardiac transport team. *Annals of Emergency Medicine, 12*(11), 675-678.

Hagar, J., & Kloner, R. (1990). Acute myocardial infarction. *Cardiovascular Reviews Reports, 11*, 39-67.

Hagley, M. (1993). Emergency intervention for acute myocardial infarction: Thrombolytic agents and adjuvant therapy. *Emergency Medicine Reports, 14*(2), 9-16.

Henry, M., & Stapleton, E. (1992). *EMT prehospital care.* Philadelphia: W.B. Saunders.

Hill, D., & Dolan, A. (1982). *Intensive care instrumentation.* London: Academic Press.

Ingenito, E., & Drazen, J. (1992). Mechanical ventilators. In J. Hall, G. Schmidt, & L. Wood (Eds.), *Principles of critical care* (pp. 142-154). New York: McGraw-Hill.

JAMA. (1992). Guidelines for cardiopulmonary resuscitation and emergency cardiac care. *Journal of the American Medical Association, 268*(16), 2171-2302.

Kim, M., McFarland, G., & McLane, A. (1993). *Pocket guide to nursing diagnoses.* St. Louis: Mosby.

Koenig, W., & Pratt, F. (1987). Medical emergencies. In V. Cleary, P. Wilson, & G. Super (Eds.), *Prehospital care* (pp. 153-161). Rockville, MD: Aspen Publications.

Lee, G., & Bristol, C. (1991). Pulmonary system. In G. Lee (Ed.), *Flight nursing: Principles and practice* (pp. 315-329). St. Louis: Mosby.

Miller, R., & Wilson, J. (1992). *Manual of prehospital emergency medicine.* St. Louis: Mosby.

Morris, M. (1992). Transport considerations for the head-injured patient: Are we contributing to secondary injury? *Journal of Air Medical Transport, 11*(7), 9-13.

National Heart, Lung, and Blood Institute. (1990). Morbidity and mortality chartbook on cardiovascular, lung, and blood diseases, 1990. Bethesda, MD: The Author.

Neville, S., Anderson, W., & Loos, L. (1991). Neurologic trauma emergencies. In Lee, G. (Ed.), *Flight nursing: Principles and practice* (pp. 101-122). St. Louis: Mosby.

Nolan, J., & Baskett, P. (1992). Gas-powered and portable ventilators: An evaluation of six models. *Prehospital and Disaster Medicine, 7*, 25-34.

O'Rourke, B. (1987). Emergency Medical Services system legislation. In V. Cleary, P. Wilson, & G. Super (Eds.), *Prehospital care* (pp. 3-8). Rockville, MD: Aspen Publications.

Rouse, M., Branson, R., Semonin-Holleran, R. (1992). Mechanical ventilation during air medical transport: Techniques and devices. *Journal of Air Medical Transport, 11*(4), 5-8.

Schneider, S., Borok, Z., Heller, M., Paris, P., & Stewart, R. (1988). Critical cardiac transport. *American Journal of Emergency Medicine. 6*(5), 449-452.

Skidmore-Roth, L. (1993). *Nursing drug reference.* St. Louis: Mosby.

Solomon, D., & Hart, R. (1993). Advances in stroke management. *Emergency Medicine, 2*(28), 25-37.

Stapleton, E. (1991). Comparing CPR during ambulance transport. *Journal of Emergency Medical Services, 16*(9), 63-72.

Sternbach, G., & Sumchai, A. (1989). Is aeromedical transport of patients during acute myocardial infarction safe? *Journal of Emergency Medicine, 7,* 73-77.

Sullivan, J. (1990). Neurologic assessment. *Nursing Clinics of North America, 25*(4), 795-809.

Thompson, J., McFarland, G., Hirsch, J., & Tucker, S. (1993). *Clinical nursing.* St. Louis: Mosby.

Waggoner, R., Landis, D., Nelson, K., & Dedrick, D. (1991). Airborne defibrillation . . . The sequel. *Journal of Air Medical Transport, 10*(2), 19-21.

Wedge-Stecher, T. (1990). Fixed-wing transport of a patient requiring intra-aortic balloon pump and left ventricular assist device, *Journal of Air Medical Transport, 9*(2), 6-8.

Wynn, J. (1991). The role of hospital delivery systems in the treatment of patients with acute myocardial infarction: Rural hospital setting. *Heart & Lung, 20*(5), 581-583.

CHAPTER 10

Transport Considerations for Intoxicated Patients and Patients with Psychiatric Emergencies

OBJECTIVES

1. Describe the assessment of a patient with a psychiatric emergency.
2. Discuss the care of the intoxicated patient during transport
3. Identify the signs and symptoms of potential physical abuse.

COMPETENCIES

The transporting team should be able to:

1. Restate the decision-making process and demonstrate the assessment and interventional skills necessary to manage airway, breathing, and circulation.
2. Assess the environment for evidence of intoxicating substances.
3. Employ external resources to gather patient care information such as material safety data sheets (MSDS) or local drug and poison information centers.
4. Organize the materials necessary to decontaminate a patient externally.
5. Allow the patient to participate in care through decision making when appropriate.
6. Practice the art of listening as a method of emotional support for patients.
7. Choose the appropriate method of restraint (physical vs. chemical) for the patient with actual or high risk of out-of-control behavior.

Transport of the intoxicated patient and the patient with a psychiatric emergency can pose special and unpredictable challenges for the nurse. One patient's reaction to a particular substance may be totally different from another's reaction. For example, an overdose of propanolol in an otherwise healthy female may not cause the same complications as the same overdose in a female of equal age and body weight who concomitantly takes digoxin on a daily basis. Likewise the psychological reaction of an individual may be totally unpredictable in response to a given stressor.

The first section of this chapter discusses the issues involved in the transportation of the intoxicated patient. Care of the patient with a psychiatric emergency is discussed later. In both situations careful history taking and physical examination can alert the nurse to potential complications. Appropriate stabilization provides a calm and safe transport.

TRANSPORT OF THE INTOXICATED PATIENT
History

Intoxication means "the state of being intoxicated, especially of being poisoned by a drug or toxic substance" (Thomas, 1977). Almost any substance has the potential to intoxicate. This chapter discusses some of the more common substances seen in the emergency setting.

Intoxication may be accidental, purposeful, or iatrogenic (i.e., due to drug interactions). It is important to distinguish if the poisoning was purposeful, since the transporting nurse may need to take additional precautions to ensure safety.

History taking may prove to be difficult or unreliable because of the patient's altered mental status or embarrassment. All facts should be verified by family or friends if possible. If acting as a first responder at a scene, the nurse should look for any clues such as pill bottles or other containers to verify the patient's statements. Questions to be asked include what the patient took, when, why, how much, and how (route). Also important is the patient's medical history, history of prescribed drug usage, and allergies. If acting as a second responder, the nurse needs to elicit from the staff of the referring facility a history of signs and symptoms observed and treatment rendered to that point. Information gained can clue the nurse into the expected signs and symptoms to be observed during physical examination and the anticipated treatment.

Physical Examination

The physical assessment begins with the primary survey: a rapid assessment of the airway, breathing, circulation, and neurological deficits, and exposure *(ABCDE)* and the initiation of lifesaving interventions. Of these, airway is the most important. Basic questions to be answered include: does the patient have a patent airway? and will the patient be able to maintain the airway throughout transfer? Depending on the intoxicant involved and amount consumed, the patient's level of consciousness may decline rapidly, leading to airway compromise. Also, the transporting vehicle, for example, some helicopters, may make management of the airway en route virtually impossible. Therefore it is imperative that the airway be aggressively managed based on the standards of care and protocols of the team's medical control.

Breathing is assessed quickly by looking for the presence of respirations and the rate and quality of the respiratory effort. Auscultation may reveal absent or adventitious breath sounds in the young patients, who, for example, have been abusing crack cocaine.

Assessment of circulation can be quickly accomplished by palpating peripheral pulses for rate, regularity, and quality. The measurement of blood pressure and capillary refill reflects the adequacy of perfusion. Continuous cardiac monitoring is essential to detect arrhythmias. At least one intravenous line should be started in all intoxicated patients before transport in case pharmacological intervention becomes necessary during transport. Two intravenous lines should be started if the intoxicating substance has the potential to produce hypotension so that fluid boluses can also be given effectively.

Neurological deficits may be quickly assessed by judging the level of consciousness, observing pupils for size, equality, reactivity, and nystagmus, and evaluating the patient's sensorimotor functions. The level of consciousness can be determined by using the *AVPU* method:

A—Alert
V—Responds to verbal stimuli
P—Responds to painful stimuli

U—Unresponsive

The pupils should be equally affected by any intoxicating substance. If they are unequal in size or reactivity, the nurse should consider the possibility of concomitant head trauma or a chronic eye condition. Nystagmus, an involuntary eye movement, is characteristic of several toxins.

Intoxicants should affect sensory and motor functions bilaterally. If any unilateral gross deficits are uncovered during the rapid assessment, concomitant head or spinal cord injury should be considered. The unconscious patient should be observed for responses to stimuli. As evaluated by the Glasgow coma scale, does the patient localize or withdraw from painful stimuli? Does the patient demonstrate abnormal flexion or extension of the extremities? Is there no response to the stimuli at all? A finger-stick blood sugar should be completed on all patients with an altered level of consciousness. The administration of glucose in lieu of the results of the finger-stick blood sugar, naloxone, and oxygen may be a standard of care for any patient with a change in mental status.

Also, it is imperative to assess for and question any seizure activity. New-onset seizures are the hallmark of many toxins, and the early administration of diazepam or lorazepam may be appropriate.

Exposure of the trauma patient is completed to reveal hidden injuries. Similarly, exposure of the intoxicated patient may reveal hidden injuries, as well as hidden drugs or weapons. Exposure also may serve to stop the poisoning process by removing contaminated clothes. Warmth and privacy should be provided when undressing the patient. Any illicit items should be either transported with the patient or disposed of according to protocol. Measurement of the patient's temperature, if possible, may reveal additional and valuable information. Some toxins produce hypothermia or hyperthermia. Interventions may be necessary to prevent further complications.

The secondary survey involves a head-to-toe assessment looking for subtle signs and symptoms of potential complications and general information concerning the patient. The general appearance can provide a wealth of information in a short period of time. What is the patient's dress and personal hygiene? Is the clothing appropriate for the environment? Is the client clean or does the client appear or smell unkempt? What is the patient's mood, for example, angry or depressed over a failed suicide attempt? Is the patient indifferent to what is happening? Fear is a common emotion of any client requiring emergency transport to a hospital, but is the fear that the patient is exhibiting out of proportion for the event? It is helpful if family or friends can verify that the patient is either exhibiting normal coping mechanisms or is acting in a completely abnormal manner. What is the patient's apparent state of health? Does the patient appear healthy or frail and cachexic? Are there any peculiar odors about the patient? For example, with arsenic ingestion, a garlic odor may be noted.

A general assessment of the skin is completed to note color and detect rashes, burns, signs of needle tracks or lesions due to skin popping, as well as other signs of trauma. Palpation of the skin may reveal moisture and provide a general evaluation of temperature.

The head should be carefully inspected and palpated for signs of trauma in any patient with a change in mental status. The eyes are to be evaluated for redness of the conjuctiva, watering, and pain. Extraocular eye movements may be compromised by a neurological toxin. The patient should be questioned about changes in visual acuity. Blurred vision is characteristic of digitalis toxicity.

Observation of the mucous membranes of the nose may reveal redness, swelling, and irritation if the patient has been snorting illicit drugs or exposed to ammonia vapors. Dryness of the nasal and oral mucous membranes occurs with the ingestion of anticholinergics. The mouth should be observed for cyanosis and burns. Evaluation of the gag reflex is essential before transport. The loss of this reflex indicates that the airway needs protection throughout transport.

The lungs and heart require careful and persistent assessment throughout contact with the patient. The respiratory system can be evaluated by reassessing the patient's level of consciousness. A change in mental status is the earliest sign of hypoxia and must receive prompt attention. Observing the rate, depth, and effort of respirations, as well as the use of accessory muscles, is necessary for detection of early pulmonary edema, as seen in organophosphate exposure. Is there any abnormal respiratory pattern? Rapid, deep respirations are seen with salicylate poisoning. Use of the pulse oximeter and the skills of auscultation can assist in evaluation of effectiveness of gas exchange.

The cardiovascular system is assessed by measuring the heart rate and blood pressure. The rhythm and regularity of the pulse and the strength of peripheral pulses should be monitored on an ongoing basis. The patient's level of consciousness, color, capillary refill, and urinary output reflect the adequacy of perfusion. Most important is the continuous EKG monitoring, since dramatic arrhythmias occur with overdoses of tricyclic antidepressants, digoxins, beta-adrenergics, and calcium channel blockers.

The abdomen may be distended and firm if the ingested intoxicant is a gastrointestinal irritant. If vomiting is contraindicated, as in camphor ingestion, an antiemetic may be necessary.

The extremities are assessed for signs of trauma and sensorimotor function. Auscultation of bowel sounds may be slowed or absent with, for example, ingestion of anticholinergics.

Box 10-1
AIRWAY CLEARANCE: NURSING DIAGNOSIS, INTERVENTIONS, AND EVALUATIVE CRITERIA

Diagnosis	Interventions	Evaluative Criteria
Ineffective airway clearance related to mental status causing obstruction from the tongue, secretions, or potentially due to vomiting.	Perform basic cardiac life support. Perform Advanced cardiac life support. Perform Pediatric advanced life support. Monitor level of consciousness, respiratory rate, depth, and effort, and use of accessory muscles. Monitor heart rate and rhythm with electrocardiograph. Monitor skin temperature, moisture, and color. Monitor oxygen saturation with a pulse oximeter.	The patient will maintain a patent airway throughout transport as evidenced by the following conditions. ■ No decrease in mental status. ■ Respiratory rate, depth, and effort will not increase. ■ No use of accessory muscles. ■ No increase in heart rate. ■ No arrhythmias related to hypoxia. ■ Skin will remain warm and dry. ■ Color will remain natural. ■ Oxygen saturation will remain at 95% to 100%.

If it is possible to test the patient's stool for hemoccult blood, a positive result may be seen with an overdose of iron.

Additional Diagnostic Data

If the nurse is acting as a second responder, additional diagnostic data may be available at the referring facility that will aid in the assessment process. A chest X-ray study should be taken and evaluated for the presence of pulmonary edema, congestive heart failure, or pneumothorax. Arterial blood gases should be as-

sessed for the adequacy of gas exchange and for determining acid-base balance. A blood count should provide baseline information about the hemoglobin and hematocrit, which may prove valuable as a later comparison in the patient who develops gastrointestinal bleeding. The glucose level and electrolytes are important adjuncts when evaluating a patient with an altered level of consciousness, cardiac arrhythmias, or seizures. Blood levels of the intoxicating substance may provide valuable information to the transport team. For example, the patient with

---

Box 10-2
INEFFECTIVE BREATHING PATTERN: NURSING DIAGNOSIS, INTERVENTIONS, AND EVALUATIVE CRITERIA

Diagnosis

Ineffective breathing pattern due to toxin-induced hyperventilation, hyperthermia, presence of adventitious breath sounds (crackles, wheezes), absence of breath sounds (pneumothorax).

Interventions

Monitor vital signs.
Monitor respiratory rate, depth, and effort and use of accessory muscles.
Monitor oxygen saturation with a pulse oximeter.
Apply oxygen as necessary, progressing from simple to complex devices.
Treat temperature with cooling measures.
Treat adventitious breath sounds with bronchodilators, diuretics, preload reduction therapies, or with all three.
Perform needle decompression.
Insert chest tubes.

Evaluative Criteria

The patient will sustain an effective breathing pattern throughout transport as evidenced by the following conditions.
- Vital signs will remain within normal limits.
- Respiratory rate will decrease and remain within normal limits.
- No increase in depth and effort of respirations.
- Oxygen saturation will remain at 95% to 100%.
- Body temperature will not increase and will decrease during transport.
- Adventitious breath sounds will diminish.
- Bilateral breath sounds will be present.
- The level of consciousness will not deteriorate during transport.

a severe level of carboxyhemoglobin should be transported to the most immediate center with hyperbaric capabilities.

Nursing Diagnoses and Interventions

Nursing diagnoses, general interventions, and evaluation criteria related to the transport of the intoxicated patient are presented in Boxes 10-1 to 10-6. Specific interventions are addressed in Boxes 10-7 to 17. Dosages are not provided for antidote therapies. Antidotes should be administered according to the most recent research and the specifications of the transport team's medical control. For example, when administering atropine to the patient with organophosphate exposure, the drug is titrated

to eliminate bronchoconstriction and secretions in the airway. This may result in a dosage of 100 to 1000 mg of atropine during transport. Overdosing the patient with atropine may cause severe hyperthermia or cardiac dysrhythmias. Therefore protocols guiding this therapy should be reviewed and updated regularly.

Decontamination

It is important to decontaminate the intoxicated patient. The intoxicating substance should be eliminated as swiftly as possible to stop the poisoning process. The causative agent is eliminated either externally or internally. External decontamination begins with removing the patient from the poisonous environment.

Box 10-3

DECREASED CARDIAC OUTPUT: NURSING DIAGNOSIS, INTERVENTIONS, AND EVALUATIVE CRITERIA

Diagnosis	Interventions	Evaluative Criteria
Potential for decreased cardiac output related to cardiotoxic effects of ingested substances.	Monitor level of consciousness. Monitor vital signs. Monitor peripheral pulses. Monitor capillary refill. Monitor urinary output. Monitor skin color, temperature, and moisture. Monitor EKG continuously. Establish intravenous line. Provide advanced cardiac life support or pediatric advanced life support interventions for arrhythmias. Place external cardiac pacer on standby. Administer antidote therapy.	The patient will maintain an adequate cardiac output throughout transport as evidenced by the following conditions. ■ Level of consciousness will not decrease. ■ Vital signs will remain within normal limits. ■ Peripheral pulses will remain palpable. ■ Capillary refill will remain within normal limits. ■ Urinary output will remain adequate (1 ml/kg/hr). ■ Skin will remain warm and dry. ■ Color will remain natural. ■ Arrhythmias will be identified and treated promptly according to ACLS protocol.

This can be as simple as removing a patient from a garage or house filled with carbon monoxide or as complex as evacuating an industrial plant because of an arsine gas leak (California EMS Authority, 1990).

If acting as a first responder, several laws require employing agencies to provide extensive training in the recognition of hazardous materials, the use of protective gear, and the appropriate treatment for contaminated victims. Federal agencies providing legislation and guidelines in this area include the Occupational Safety and Health Administration (OSHA), the Department of Transportation (DOT), the Federal Emergency Management Agency (FEMA), the Environmental Protection Agency (EPA), the National Institutes of Health (NIH), and the Departments of Health and Human Services,

Labor and Commerce. Many states also have regulations regarding hazardous materials. Removing victims from the site of a hazardous material accident should be undertaken only by trained professionals. Additional information can be obtained by contacting one of the aforementioned agencies.

Eyes and skin need to be flushed if contaminated by an intoxicating substance. The eyes should be flushed with normal saline for 15 to 30 minutes while en route to the hospital. If the clothing and skin are contaminated, a more complex decontamination is involved. The patient should be positioned upwind from the site of exposure. All clothing should be removed, and the patient should be washed with soap and water, with the rescuer wearing protective gear. A warm environment and privacy are essential,

---

Box 10-4
CIRCULATION—FLUID VOLUME DEFICIT: NURSING DIAGNOSIS, INTERVENTIONS, AND EVALUATIVE CRITERIA

Diagnosis

Potential fluid volume deficit related to vomiting, diarrhea, and excessive urination, diaphoresis, or hyperventilation.

Interventions

Monitor level of consciousness.
Monitor vital signs.
Monitor peripheral pulses.
Monitor skin temperature and moisture.
Monitor urinary output.
Administer intravenous fluids.
Administer antiemetics.
Provide cooling measures.

Evaluative Criteria

The patient will not demonstrate signs and symptoms of fluid volume deficit throughout transport as evidenced by the following conditions.
- Level of consciousness will not decrease.
- Vital signs will remain within normal limits.
- Peripheral pulses will remain palpable.
- Skin will remain warm and dry.
- Urinary output will remain adequate (1 ml/kg/hr).
- Intravenous fluids and antiemetics will be administered according to protocol.

Box 10-5
NEUROLOGICAL DEFICIT: NURSING DIAGNOSIS, INTERVENTIONS, AND EVALUATIVE CRITERIA

Diagnosis

Potential for impaired thought process related to hypoxia, hypoglycemia, electrolyte imbalance, seizures, and potential trauma.

Interventions

Monitor level of consciousness.

Monitor vital signs.

Monitor oxygen saturation with pulse oximeter and administer oxygen accordingly.

Correct hypoglycemia.

Correct electrolyte imbalance.

Administer lorazepam or diazepam for seizures.

Prevent increased intracranial pressure due to trauma by hyperventilation, elevation of head of bed, administration of pharmacological therapies (mannitol, diuretics) per protocol.

Maintain safety of patient and transport team.

Evaluative Criteria

The patient will remain oriented (i.e., normal thought process) throughout transport as evidenced by the following conditions.

- Level of consciousness will not decrease.
- Vital signs will remain within normal limits.
- Seizure activity is treated promptly and according to protocol.
- no signs and symptoms of increasing intracranial pressure develop.

Box 10-6
THERMOREGULATION: NURSING DIAGNOSIS, INTERVENTIONS, AND EVALUATIVE CRITERIA

Diagnosis

Potential for alteration in thermoregulation related to toxin ingestion.

Interventions

Monitor level of consciousness.

Monitor vital signs.

Observe for shivering.

Provide cooling measures:
- Evaporative cooling with tepid water
- Ice packs to head, neck, axillae, and groin
- Suppress shivering
- Administer antipyretics

Provide warming measures:
- Warm intravenous fluids
- Preserve body heat with blankets

Control environment of transport vehicle as necessary.

Evaluative Criteria

The patient's temperature will return to or remain normal throughout transport as evidenced by the following conditions.

- Level of consciousness will not decrease.
- Vital signs will remain within normal limits.
- Skin temperature will remain within normal limits.
- The patient will not develop diaphoresis.

as is the need to properly dispose of the contaminated clothing and water. A strict protocol for decontamination should be developed and routinely reviewed.

If the intoxicating substance has been ingested, internal decontamination must be considered. Internal decontamination involves the induction of emesis, gastric lavage, administration of activated charcoal, or whole bowel irrigation. If uncertain which of these therapies should be used, the rescuer should consult with medical control or a local drug and poison information center.

Syrup of ipecac is used to induce emesis. Vomiting should not be induced in the patient with a decreased level of consciousness, if the ingested material is a strong caustic agent (acid or alkali), or if the ingested substance is likely to cause a rapid onset of neurological symptoms, as does camphor.

Gastric lavage, or pumping of the stomach, is unlikely to be performed in the prehospital

---

Box 10-7
OVER-THE-COUNTER ANALGESIC OVERDOSE

Analgesic	Signs and Symptoms	Interventions
Acetaminophen	Anorexia, nausea, vomiting, malaise, pallor, diaphoresis. Right upper quadrant pain and tenderness due to liver enlargement (usually 24 to 48 hours later). Jaundice, elevated liver enzymes, serum, and bilirubin, and prothrombin time.	Administer acetylcysteine (Mucomyst). May cause nausea and vomiting necessitating an antiemetic. Charcoal binds with 30% of the Mucomyst, necessitating an increased loading dose.
Salicylates Obtain a 4-hour postingestion level to predict range of severity	May be asymptomatic for hours if ingested sustained-release or enteric-coated preparations. Nausea, vomiting, tinnitus, confusion, lethargy, coma, seizures, hyperventilation, hyperthermia, hyperglycemia or hypoglycemia. Initial respiratory alkalosis followed by severe anion gap metabolic acidosis. Dehydration with loss of potassium. Seizures, elevated temperature, and coma as the toxicity becomes more severe. Hypoprothrombinemia.	Administer antiemetics. Intravenous fluid replacement. Treat seizures with lorazepam or diazepam. Correct hypoglycemia. Administer sodium bicarbonate 1 meq/kg/hr. Provide cooling measures. Maintain safety with restraints. Administer vitamin K.

Box 10-8
ALCOHOL OVERDOSE

Alcohol	Signs and Symptoms	Interventions
Ethanol	Ataxia, dysarthria, depressed sensorium, nystagmus, coma, respiratory suppression, hypoglycemia, hypovolemia, hypothermia, trauma, GI bleeding. Withdrawal seizures. Delirium tremens, elevated temperature, elevated heart rate, disorientation, and hallucinations.	Provide supportive care. Correct hypoglycemia. Administer thiamine and folate. Sedate according to medical protocol.
Methanol (found in pain strippers and windshield washer fluid)	Early signs similar to ethanol overdose. 6 to 12 hours after ingestion: visual disturbances, headache, vertigo, breathlessness. Seizures and coma in severe toxicity. Late signs: severe metabolic acidosis.	Provide supportive care. Administer sodium bicarbonate and folic acid. Give ethanol infusion to keep blood level between 100 and 200 mg/kl. Determine need for hemodialysis.
Ethylene glycol (found in deicers and antifreeze)	Nausea, vomiting, headache, stupor, seizures, coma, renal failure, and severe acidosis	Same as for methanol.

Box 10-9
ANTICHOLINERGIC OVERDOSE

Anticholinergic	Signs and Symptoms	Interventions
Antihistamines Atropine Antispasmodics Phenothiazines Plants: Nightshade and jimsonweed	Delirium, blurred vision, mychiasis, hallucinations, coma, dry mucous membranes, inhibition of sweating, hyperthermia, tachycardia, decreased gastric and bladder motility, and possible seizures.	Provide supportive care. Give physostigmine only for severe symptoms (hyperthermia or elevated heart rate). Monitor for side effects of bradycardia and seizures. Have atropine ready (contraindicated for patients with tricyclic antidepressant overdose).

Box 10-10
CARBON MONOXIDE POISONING

Carbon Monoxide	Signs and Symptoms	Interventions
	Headache, irritability, fatigue, dimness of vision, tachycardia, confusion, lethargy, coma, convulsions, metabolic acidosis. EKG rhythm may show ischemia or infarction.	Administer 100% oxygen. Provide supportive care. Administer hyperbaric therapy.

Box 10-11
DRUGS WITH CARDIOTOXIC EFFECTS

Drug	Signs and Symptoms	Interventions
Digoxin	Anorexia, nausea, vomiting, diarrhea, abdominal pain, blurred vision, color vision disturbance. Rhythm and conduction disturbances (three atrioventricular block, PVCs, bradycardia, atrial fibrillation). Hyperkalemia.	Provide supportive care. Treat arrhythmias according to ACLS or PALS protocols. Treat potassium imbalance. If countershock becomes necessary, use lowest voltage possible. Administer digibind-digitalis specific FAB fragment antibodies.
Beta-adrenergic blockers (Propranolol, atenolol, pindolol, and practolol)	Hypotension, bradycardia, bronchoconstriction, hypoglycemia, hyperkalemia. Arrhythmias (block). Death due to profound myocardial depression.	Provide supportive care. Give fluids and glucagon for hypotension. Treat arrhythmias according to ACES protocol.
Calcium channel blockers (Verapamil, nifedipine, diltiazem, and nitrendipine)	Hypotension. Decreased mental status. Metabolic acidosis. Bradycardia due to depression of the sinoatrial and atrioventricular nodes.	Provide supportive care. Administer calcium and dopamine. Sinoatrial node depression responds to atropine, isoproterenol, and external pacers. Atrioventricular node depression responds to calcium.

Box 10-12
HEAVY METAL INTOXICATION

Heavy Metal	Signs and Symptoms	Interventions
Iron	Four stages of intoxication: 1. 1 to 4 hours: nausea, vomiting, abdominal pain, hyperglycemia, hemorrhagic gastritis, shock, acidosis, and coma. 2. Next 6 to 24 hours: may appear improved. 3. 12 to 24 hours after ingestion: shock. 4. Later stage: pyloric stenosis, hepatic failure, and residual neurological damage.	Provide supportive care. Charcoal not effective. Perform whole bowel irrigation. Chelating agent: deferoxamine: ■ Side effect of hypotension with rapid intravenous administration. ■ Produces pink urine, which confirms the presence of free iron.
Lead (found in old paint glazes, fumes from welding and smeltering, and battery manufacturing)	Listlessness, headache, irritability, abdominal pain, constipation, and subtle behavioral changes. With severe toxicity: lethargy and peripheral neuropathy (extensor muscle weakness). Delirium and hallucinations.	Provide supportive care. Treatment depends on blood concentration. For the asymptomatic patient, give edetate calcium disodium (EDTA) intramuscularly or intravenously. For the symptomatic patient, give EDTA then dimercaprol (British antilewisite [BAL]) intramuscularly. ETDA side effects include reversible acute tubular necrosis and zinc and vitamin B_6 depletion. BAL side effects include hypertension, lacrimation, burning lips, nausea, and vomiting.
Arsenic (found in insecticides, rodenticides, wood preservatives, and shellfish)	Acute poisoning: crampy abdominal pain, vomiting, profuse watery diarrhea, burning mucous membranes, conjunctivitis, tremors, seizures, and garlic breath odor.	Provide supportive care. Administer dimercaprol and oral penicillamine. Side effects of penicillamine include nephrotic syndrome and loss of sense of taste. Give blood transfusion.

Box 10-12
HEAVY METAL INTOXICATION—cont'd

Heavy Metal	Signs and Symptoms	Interventions
	Chronic poisoning: peripheral sensory and motor neuropathy, malaise, anorexia, alopecia, anemia, and stomatitis.	Provide fluid therapy to prevent renal hemoglobin deposition.
	Arsine gas inhalation: rapid intravascular hemolysis and renal failure.	No chelation therapy indicated for acute gas exposure.
Mercury (produced during various manufacturing procedures; found in disinfectants, older cathartics and diuretics, and contaminated foods)	*Elemental mercury* due to inhaled mercury vapor causes encephalopathy, gingivitis, and pneumonitis. Chronic inhalation produces neuropsychiatric symptoms, tremors, anxiety, incapacitating shyness, and irritability.	Provide supportive care. Administer dimercaprol or penicillamine.
	Inorganic mercury causes gastritis with bloody emesis, diarrhea, acute tubular necrosis, gingivitis, salivation, dysarthria, intention tremor, nervousness, emotional outbursts, and memory loss.	
	Organic mercury causes tremor, neuropsychiatric symptoms, paresthesia, constriction of visual fields, loss of hearing, smell, and taste, incoordination, stupor, incontinence, and uncontrollable crying and laughter.	

---

setting. A gastric hose or Ewald tube is used to wash out the stomach contents. This method can be used only if the ingestion is recent (i.e., the intoxicating substance has not already passed into the intestines). Gastric lavage is contraindicated if hydrocarbons or a caustic agent (acid or alkali) is ingested, or if the patient has a decreased level of consciousness or other neurological symptoms (seizures) that may compromise the airway.

Activated charcoal is a binding agent that prevents absorption of the intoxicating substance. Several studies conducted by Rodgers and Matyunas (1986) have demonstrated the

Box 10-13
HYDROCARBON INTOXICATION

Hydrocarbon	Signs and Symptoms	Interventions
High-viscosity lubricants that are nontoxic (motor oil and white petrolatum)	Choking, gasping, coughing, delirium, and seizures.	No treatment.
Low-viscosity compounds with no known toxicity (furniture polish, mineral spirits, lighter fluid, kerosine, and gasoline)		Protect the airway and do not induce vomiting.
Low-viscosity compounds with unknown toxicity (pine oil and turpentine)		Induce emesis for large amount of ingestion (more than 1 ml/kg).
Low-viscosity compounds with established toxicity (benzene, toluene, camphor, phenol, and insecticides)		Induce emesis except for camphor, which causes rapid onset of seizures.

Box 10-14
ORGANOPHOSPHATE INTOXICATION

Organophosphates (found in insecticides)	Signs and Symptoms	Interventions
	Muscarinic: signs and symptoms due to increased parasympathetic stimulation include miosis, blurred vision, nausea, vomiting, diarrhea, salivation, lacrimation, bradycardia, abdominal pain, diaphoresis, wheezing, and urinary and fecal incontinence.	Decontaminate. Provide supportive care. Administer atropine for the onset of multiple signs and symptoms and titrate according to elimination of bronchoconstriction and secretions in the airway. Administer pralidoxime chloride (2-PAM) to relieve respiratory muscle weakness and paralysis. Administer diazepam to relieve seizures.
	Nicotinic: signs and symptoms due to increased sympathetic stimulation include paralysis, muscle weakness or fasciculation, hypertension, and tachycardia.	

Box 10-15
SEDATIVE/HYPNOTIC OVERDOSE

Sedative/Hypnotic	Signs and Symptoms	Interventions
Chloral hydrate Diazepam Placidyl Phenobarbital Pentobarbital	Nystagmus, ataxia, dysarthria, lethargy, somnolence, respiratory depression, hypotension, and hypothermia. With deep coma, may see negative oculocephalic reflexes, and pupils may become nonreactive.	Provide supportive care. Restore and maintain temperature. Treat hypotension with fluids or vasopressors. Administer flumazenil (Mazicon), which is contraindicated in known seizure disorders and tricyclic antidepressant overdoses.

Box 10-16
STREET DRUGS AND OVERDOSES

Drug	Signs and Symptoms	Interventions
Cocaine	Euphoria, excitement, restlessness, toxic psychosis, seizures in a temporal lobe, seizure pattern, hypertension, tachycardia, dysrhythmia, hyperthermia, myocardial ischemia or infarction, stroke, sudden cardiac death, and subdural hematoma.	Provide supportive care. Reduce hyperthermia. Suppress cardiac dysrhythmia. Decrease blood pressure. Perform BLS and ACLS interventions.
Phencyclidine (PCP; "angle dust" or "crystal")	Sympathomimetic. Hallucinogenic; bizarre paranoid behavior and extreme violence. Vertical and horizontal nystagmus, hypertension, tachycardia, hyperthermia, muscle rigidity, dystonias, and seizures. Rhabdomyolysis produces myoglobinuria and renal failure.	Provide supportive care. Sedation. Intravenous fluid and alkalization of the urine.
Opiates (Codeine, propoxyphene, and methadine)	Hypotension, bradycardia, hypothermia, respiratory depression, lethargy, coma, pinpoint pupils, and pulmonary edema.	Provide supportive care. Administer naloxone with intravenous push or infusion. Patient may develop acute withdrawal symptoms.
Amphetamines	CNS stimulation, vasoconstriction, hypertension, bradycardia, euphoria, mydriasis, restlessness, ventricular arrhythmias, seizures, hyperthermia, and stroke.	Provide supportive care. Sedate with diazepam, midazolam, haloperidol. Administer nitroprusside and phentolamine for hypertension. Administer propranolol for tachyarrhythmias.

Box 10-17
TRICYCLIC ANTIDEPRESSANT OVERDOSE

Antidepressant	Signs and Symptoms	Interventions
Amitriptyline	Mydriasis, dry mouth, tachycardia, agitation, hallucinations, rapid onset of coma, and seizures.	Provide supportive care.
Imipramine		Do not induce emesis because of risk of seizures.
Maprotiline	Cardiovascular effects include widened QRS, prolonged QT and PR intervals, atrioventricular block, ventricular tachycardia, hypotension.	Administer diazepam and phenytoin for seizures.
		Administer sodium bicarbonate, lidocaine, and phenytoin for arrhythmias and conduction defects.
	Hypoxemia and acidosis aggravate cardiac toxicity.	Administer intravenous fluids and sodium bicarbonate for acidosis.

---

superiority of charcoal alone versus the use of ipecac and charcoal in gastrointestinal decontamination. The taste of charcoal makes it difficult to drink, especially for children. Diluting it with water or providing water or juice may make the charcoal more palatable. Charcoal is contraindicated in the patient with a decreased level of consciousness or if the airway is compromised.

Whole bowel irrigation involves the use of cathartics or intestinal lavage. Laxatives or lavage are thought to decrease the absorption of the intoxicating substance by decreasing its time in the intestinal tract. Whole bowel irrigation is contraindicated for the patient who has ingested a caustic substance, has a recent history of bowel surgery, or has absent bowel sounds. This method of decontamination is unlikely to be used in the prehospital setting.

TRANSPORT OF THE PATIENT WITH A PSYCHIATRIC EMERGENCY

When asked to transport a patient with a psychiatric illness, health-care providers may have feelings of dread, fear, or disgust. The care of psychiatric patients is surrounded by many misperceptions. Probably the most spurious belief is that psychiatric patients are violent. A noted authority on psychiatric nursing, Ann Burgess (1990, p. 954), writes "it is important to note that violence is more prominent in persons who *are not* emotionally ill. In fact, less than 5% of all major crimes are committed by people with overt psychosis or mental retardation." Crimes committed by a mentally ill person, such as Jeffery Dahmer, are sensationalized by the media, adding to the stigma of mental illness. If a health-care provider is verbally or physically assaulted by a patient, more likely it was by someone who was intoxicated, hypoxic, hypoglycemic, or had a head injury rather than by a psychiatric patient.

The American Psychological Association defines a psychiatric emergency as "a situation that includes an acute disturbance of thought, behavior, mood, or social relationship as defined by the client or family or social unit" (Merker, 1986). A few of the more common psychiatric emergencies treated by prehospital care providers include abuse syndromes, depressive states, manic states, organically induced disorders, and thought disorders.

Abuse Syndromes

Probably nothing evokes more feelings than when providing emergency care for the victim of abuse. To observe the brutality and sympathize with the anguish of the victim of abuse elicit feelings of anger, concern, frustration, and fear. Domestic violence, child abuse, elderly abuse, and rape are on the rise. Many theories concerning abuse exist. Some believe abuse is a by-product of violence in American society, and others believe that the behavior is learned, passing from generation to generation.

The primary role of the prehospital care provider when treating the victim of abuse is to treat any life-threatening injuries and report suspicions to the appropriate authorities. In general, the signs of abuse of a spouse, a child, or an elderly person include injuries that are not congruent with the history of mechanism of injury, a hesitancy in providing detailed information about the injury, a delay in reporting symptoms, signs of depression or low self-esteem on the part of the victim, and increased anxiety in the presence of the possible batterer. Abuse can be difficult to confirm largely because the victims frequently have a relationship of intimidation with the abuser, and victims may actually be afraid for a variety of reasons to leave their assailant. For example, the life of a child, as well as the lives of family members, pets, and friends, may be threatened if others are told of the abuse. A battered woman may be fearful of leaving an abusive husband because of embarrassment, fear of retaliation, or fear of the uncertainty of daily living without an economical provider. Elderly persons may fear being placed in a nursing home if the truth about their social situations is revealed. Therefore the truth concerning injuries or an illness may be hidden. All the prehospital nurse can do is report suspicions. Specific signs and symptoms of child abuse, the battered spouse, and abuse of the elderly are listed in Boxes 10-18 to 10-20.

When the patient is a victim of rape, a wide range of emotions may be observed. The patient's demeanor may range from calmness to complete hysteria—and both of these emotions are considered normal. The one common emotion reported by rape victims is a sense of a complete loss of control. It is important that a sense of control be returned to the patient if possible. For example, if an intravenous line needs to be started, allow the patient to choose which arm will receive the infusion.

The signs and symptoms of rape vary. The patient may have no obvious physical injuries or may have sustained life-threatening trauma.

Box 10-18
SIGNS AND SYMPTOMS OF CHILD ABUSE

1. History of a "problem child" or accident proneness
2. Explanation of injury is inconsistent with the developmental ability of the child or with type and severity of injury
3. Caregiver appears overly concerned or shows a lack of concern
4. Child displays an inappropriate response to people or pain
5. Child displays inappropriate sexual behavior or mannerisms
6. Multiple lesions in various stages of healing; lesions characteristic of physical abuse such as cigarette-shaped burns, bruises in the shape of an instrument such as a belt buckle, bite marks, and immersion scalds
7. Deformity of long bones
8. Altered level of consciousness, seizure activity, signs of increased intracranial pressure
9. "Cauliflower ear"
10. Broken, loose, or missing teeth
11. Wears unseasonal clothing to cover injuries
12. General signs of poor hygiene

Box 10-19
SIGNS AND SYMPTOMS OF THE BATTERED SPOUSE

1. History of drug or child abuse in a previous or current marriage
2. Unequal power in decision making
3. Expressions of helplessness and powerlessness
4. Low self-esteem
5. Signs of depression
6. Hesitancy in providing detailed information about the injury
7. Inappropriate affect for the situation
8. Delayed reporting of symptoms
9. Types and sites of injuries
10. Inappropriate explanation of mechanism of injury
11. Increased anxiety in the presence of the possible batterer
12. Minimization of the frequency or seriousness of injuries

Box 10-20
SIGNS AND SYMPTOMS OF ELDERLY ABUSE

1. Dirty skin, hair, and nails, body odor, generally appears unkempt
2. Obviously needs, but refuses, medical treatment
3. Shows signs of poor judgment
4. Wanders and gets lost in own neighborhood
5. Sees and hears things that are not there
6. Older person or caregiver appears to misuse drugs or alcohol
7. Complains of abuse/neglect or misuse of money or property by a caregiver or family member
8. Appears confused and unable to manage daily activities
9. Appears physically frail and lacks support systems to maintain a safe environment
10. Recurring or unexplained injuries
11. Withdrawal or fearfulness

Questioning and examining the patient may be perceived as threatening and intrusive. Educate the patient as to which procedures are necessary and why. Ask the patient's permission to take vital signs. If the patient refuses, then use other assessment parameters to document the adequacy of oxygenation and perfusion. If procedures are required in the prehospital arena, such as starting intravenous lines, placing a cardiac monitor, or prophylactic use of military antishock trousers, then gentleness, privacy, and warmth are essential.

In all cases of abuse the preservation of evidence is a high priority and should begin at the scene. In cases of rape or child molestation, the victim should not be allowed to shower, bathe, drink, eat, brush teeth, gargle, urinate, or defecate if at all possible, since important evidence may be lost. If the patient insists on removing

"dirty" clothing or it is necessary to remove clothing for medical purposes, all items should be placed in separate paper bags with clear documentation of items collected. The chain of evidence must be preserved for legal purposes and should be turned over to the appropriate personnel with clear documentation. Any reported weapons at the scene should be investigated and handled by the police only.

Depression

Depression is an alteration in mood characterized by insomnia, weight loss, menstrual irregularity, loss of appetite, inability to concentrate or work normally, disinterest in sex, crying, restlessness, hyperactivity, or withdrawal from usual social contacts. The overwhelming characteristic in the patient with depression is a feeling of hopelessness. Objective signs and symptoms include someone who is quiet, withdrawn, sad, has poor posture, a slow gait, or agitation. The subjective signs and symptoms of depression may range from the simple blues to an intolerable feeling that there is no solution to life's problems. When the patient believes there is no solution, ideations of suicide or an actual suicide attempt may be made. This is when prehospital care providers frequently encounter the depressed patient.

Suicide

The idea of suicide is one that the patient usually entertains over a period of time. Signs and symptoms that a person is contemplating suicide include a lack of interest in activities or events that have been previously important, giving away prized possessions, getting personal and business affairs in order, or a sudden lift in mood. A history of these behaviors can be elicited from friends or family.

The role of the prehospital health-care provider is to treat any life-threatening injuries and to report all suspicions to the emergency department personnel. Details concerning the suicide attempt that should be discussed with health-care providers at the receiving facility include any history of suicide attempts, the presence of a farewell note, or any comments made by the patient that may indicate anger at the foiled attempt or plans for future attempts. Ultimately a judgment must be made concerning the lethality of the suicide attempt so that appropriate definitive care can be arranged. Did the attempt involve a plan that was well thought out? Was the attempt foiled by shear accident? Did the patient take precautions to avoid discovery? (Kitt & Kaiser, 1990). If prehospital care personnel have the ability to judge the scene or elicit such information from the patient, family, or friends, it is vital that all details be documented and passed on in a verbal report.

Manic States

Manic states are characterized by overactivity, behavioral excess, and hostility. The classic example of a manic state is the patient with a panic attack. The patient complains of insomnia, anorexia, and profuse sweating. On examination the rescuer may find tachycardia, tachypnea, diaphoresis, fear, apprehension, agitation, tremors, restlessness, or giddiness. The patient often describes these symptoms as having a sudden onset. With severe anxiety, the patient may have an intense cardiac and respiratory response with constriction of the chest muscles. This may result in a choking feeling, and the patient will inform the rescuer of being unable to breathe. A vicious cycle may be created if patients believe they are having a myocardial infarction; they become more anxious, which exacerbates all the signs and symptoms. Frequently, patients are misdiagnosed as having amphetamine or cocaine poisoning, mitral valve prolapse, hyperthyroidism, hypocalcemia, hypoglycemia, or pulmonary emboli.

Organically Induced Disorders

Organically induced disorders are psychiatric emergencies caused by an underlying medical condition. Examples include acquired immunodeficiency syndrome (AIDS) encephalopathy, cocaine psychosis, and neuroleptic malignant syndrome.

AIDS encephalopathy is the progressive inability to perform normal tasks and may be caused by central nervous system infections or tumors. Signs and symptoms include forgetfulness, difficulty concentrating, mental slowing, impaired judgment, personality changes, mood changes, psychotic behavior, leg weakness, hand tremor, and impaired coordination.

Cocaine psychosis is the result of long-term abuse of cocaine. Actual chemical changes in the brain can cause paranoia, despondency, euphoria, delusions, hallucinations, and delirium.

Neuroleptic malignant syndrome is a potentially lethal complication of antipsychotic drug therapy. Signs and symptoms include fever, malaise, muscle rigidity, altered level of consciousness, and autonomic nervous system dysfunction. The syndrome is frequently confused with meningitis and focal brain lesions.

Thought Disorders

Thought disorders are characterized by hallucinations and paranoid behavior. Two examples are the disorders of schizophrenia and paranoia, both common disorders. Patients with schizophrenia can function well in society until their "reality-check system" is broken down. A "reality-check system" enables people to function under acceptable terms in society. For example, if you have ever "put your foot in your mouth," the reaction of those around you is a social sanction that you are acutely aware of and serves to teach you that what you have said is not acceptable. When this system breaks down in the patient with schizophrenia, dramatic responses result. For example, the patient may engage in loud, bizarre, or offensive behavior such as public nudity or masturbation. The patient may also have delusions that are grandiose or persecutory in nature or hallucinations that are derogatory to the patient. Bizarre or infantile speech may be present. The patient may also demonstrate social withdrawal or preoccupation with inner thoughts that are often sexual or religious in nature. A flat affect (emotionless) with quick mood shifts that do not correlate with circumstances may also be exhibited. The patient is at risk for suicide, self-mutilation, assaultive behavior, and damage to property. Frequently, schizophrenia is mistaken for organic brain syndrome, steroid toxicity, or alcohol withdrawal.

Paranoia is a condition characterized by well-organized delusions or grandiose ideas. The patient appear composed, articulate, well dressed, and educated. The chief complaint may be logical, such as numbness in the arms and legs. After further probing, however, the patient may attribute the numbness to radar beams being shot into the body by neighbors.

Assessment

Assessment of the patient with a psychiatric emergency begins with the primary survey as for any patient in the prehospital arena. Rapid assessment of airway, breathing, and circulation and stabilization of life-threatening injuries are the top priorities of care.

History

To obtain an adequate history, it is advised to interview the psychiatric patient first rather than other people at the scene or referring facility, otherwise the client may believe that the transporting team is joining the enemy. If the patient is unable or unwilling to speak, the history is elicited from the referring facility personnel, family, friends, or bystanders. What is the chief complaint and history of its progression? What the patient believes about the cause of pain is important. If the patient has a disorder in thought processes, pain may be attributed to a punishment from God, radar beams from neighbors, or poisoning attempts made by family members. This may be the initial clue that the patient has a psychiatric disorder.

The medical history may help to reveal a cause of the change in mental status. Cancer, renal disease, and endocrine and vascular disorders are a few examples. What are the patient's allergies? Has the patient recently started taking any new medications that may be related to an allergy? For example, the patient allergic to penicillin may have started self-medication to treat a sore throat with a friend's ampicillin.

What current prescribed medications does the patient use? Pay close attention to any drug that may cause a change in mental status as a side effect, such as steroids, cardiac drugs, anticoagulants, or chemotherapy. Does the patient use any psychotropic drugs? Check the medication bottles for the date and number of pills issued. If the pills were issued 2 days ago and a significant number (more than expected) have been taken, a potential overdose should be considered.

Ask the patient about any use of illegal drugs. Many health-care providers expect patients to lie about this issue. However, if asked with a nonjudgmental attitude and if the patient is told that all information will be used for medical purposes only, the patient may be quite honest.

Inquire about any significant recent changes in the patient's life. Have there been any losses such as the death of a loved one, the loss of a job or a house? A loss of self-control, during which the patient behaved in an unacceptable manner, can produce extreme feelings of guilt or low self-esteem. For example, if a speeding car struck a pedestrian child, the driver may have a severe anxiety attack at the scene.

Physical Assessment

A small but important portion of the physical assessment is completed in the primary survey. The secondary survey, a head-to-toe assessment, is then performed, as for the intoxicated patient, looking for subtle signs and symptoms of potential complications and general information concerning the patient. Be aware that behavior frequently speaks louder than words. The patient may claim being fine and voice a desire to be left alone; however, simple observation may reveal pallor, diaphoresis, a stern facial expression, and restlessness, which should tell the prehospital care personnel that all is not well.

An in-depth mental status examination may be necessary to evaluate the patient's ability to understand and cooperate throughout the transport. Key elements of the mental status examination include the following:

Appearance and behavior: posture, manner of dress, facial expressions, personal hygiene, mood, motor activity, and specific mannerisms.

Speech: slurred, excessive, or loud or the patient refuses to speak.

Thought content: preoccupied with personal illness, suicide, or homicide; are thoughts oriented and organized, or does the patient exhibit flight of ideas?

Cognitive function: orientation, ability to concentrate, recent and remote memory, judgment, and abstract reasoning.

The remainder of the secondary survey is as previously described for the intoxicated patient. Available diagnostic data should be reviewed to rule out medical reasons for a patient's behavior.

Nursing Diagnoses and Interventions

Nursing diagnoses and general interventions related to the transport of the patient with a psychiatric emergency are given in the Boxes 10-21 and 10-22. Evaluative criteria are also included.

General interventions for the care of the patient with a psychiatric emergency include stabilization of airway, breathing, and circulation with continued monitoring and intervention as necessary, recognition of the patient with the potential for out-of-control behavior, and the provision of safety precautions. Of these interventions, the recognition of the patient with the potential for out-of-control or violent behavior is the most difficult. Unless a relationship has been established with a patient over a period of time, it is virtually impossible to predict accurately the effects of stress. Some of the more common indications of potential violence are identified in Box 10-23. Experience also plays a valuable role in the recognition of potential violence and should never be dismissed. "Gut reactions" should always be followed.

Safety precautions include the use of physical and chemical restraints, as well as deciding the most appropriate method of transport. Once again, both of these precautions should be guided by a protocol to legally protect the transport team.

Restraints, both physical and chemical, should be used to protect the patient and the members of the transport team. Restraints should never be used in an punitive fashion. Explain to the patient why physical restraints are necessary. If possible, allow the patient to have some control and be involved in decision mak-

---

Box 10-21
ANXIETY: NURSING DIAGNOSIS, INTERVENTIONS, AND EVALUATIVE CRITERIA

Diagnosis	Interventions	Evaluative Criteria
Anxiety due to situational stress, anxiety disorder, or underlying medical condition.	Listen supportively. Allow the patient to verbalize anxiety. Treat the underlying medical cause. Assess the patient's ability to cooperate throughout transport. Administer antianxiety medications per protocol. Apply physical/chemical restraints for the patient's and transport team's safety.	The patient's anxiety will decrease throughout transport as evidenced by verbalization of the patient (i.e., patient states feeling of being less anxious), by a decrease in the speech and restlessness of the patient, and by a decrease in heart and respiratory rates.

Box 10-22
IMPAIRED THOUGHT PROCESS: NURSING DIAGNOSIS, INTERVENTIONS, AND EVALUATIVE CRITERIA

Diagnosis	Interventions	Evaluative Criteria
Impaired thought process due to underlying medical/psychiatric disorder.	Assess orientation and reorient as necessary. Give simple directions. Administer sedatives per protocol. Apply physical/chemical restraints for the patient's and transport team's safety.	The patient will remain oriented as evidenced by the ability to answer simple questions appropriately and follow simple directions. The patient's alteration in thought process will not result in injury to the patient or any member of the transport team.

Box 10-23
INDICATIONS OF POTENTIAL VIOLENCE

The patient has a history of violence and injuries sustained in domestic or other (bar) fight.

The patient is under arrest in restraints/handcuffs.

Observation of behavior reveals:
1. Pacing, restlessness
2. Raising of voice/shouting/screaming
3. Use of abusive or profane language
4. Boasting of prior violence
5. Stating loss of control
6. Threatening violence
7. Paranoid or delusional statements
8. Psychotic thinking
9. Body language:
   a. Fist and/or jaw clenching/folded arms
   b. Tightly gripping objects
   c. Violent gestures
   d. Intense facial expressions of anger, hostility, or fear (glaring)
10. Physical clues:
    a. Soiled, disheveled, or bizarre appearance
    b. Openly carrying a weapon
    c. Reddened face

---

ing concerning the restraining process. For example, protocol at the University of Cincinnati Center for Emergency Care requires the placement of opposite limbs in leather restraints for any patient who has overdosed. If possible, patients are asked which limbs are to be restrained. With the appropriate explanation, most patient cooperate in this process.

Once simple restraints are applied, clear limits should be set on the patient's behavior. The patient should be advised in a concise and clear fashion which behaviors are and are not acceptable. If unacceptable behaviors (e.g., striking out with a nonrestrained limb) are demon-

strated, the patient should be made aware of the consequences. When setting limits be sure that they are reasonable, clear, and enforceable. Follow-through is essential, since everyone tests limits.

If the patient is completely out of control and full physical restraints are necessary, they should be applied as a team effort. If acting as a first responder, request and wait for the appropriate help to arrive. Establish a plan of action with all team members and approach the patient as a team. Classes on physical crisis management are offered by many psychiatric emergency services. The University of Cincinnati offers a workshop specifically for nonpsychiatric personnel on the management of aggressive patients. Such classes are highly recommended for all prehospital care providers.

Chemical restraints range from simple sedatives to paralyzing agents. Use of these and all medications should be guided by protocols. Paralytic agents should be used for medical purposes only (e.g., control or protection of the airway). If airway management is not indicated, then the most appropriate means of transport should be considered. For example, an aeromedical transport team may refuse to transport a patient who is out of control if in the team's judgment the patient's behavior poses a threat to their safety. An alternate means of assisting the patient to receive definitive care should be arranged.

CASE STUDY

The mobile care transport team was dispatched to a small community hospital to transport a patient with a history of attempted suicide by carbon monoxide inhalation to the level I trauma center for hyperbaric therapy. Upon their arrival at the referring facility, the mobile care team received the following report.

The patient, Mr. Green, was a 26-year-old man. The squad at the scene reports that Mr. Green was found in an enclosed garage with the car motor running. He was discovered by his sister after she was notified by Mr. Green's employer that he did not show up for work. Upon further investigation, the squad at the scene reported finding an empty bottle of diazepam (Valium) 10 mg tablets and bourbon along with a suicide note on the kitchen table. It was not known when these substances were ingested. Mr. Green's sister relates that 10 years ago their parents had been killed in an auto accident. Mr. Green had bouts of depression and previous suicide attempts. Two weeks ago, Mr. Green's wife of 3 years died of cancer. The Valium had been ordered for Mr. Green's anxiety. The original prescription was written for 20 tablets and was dated for 2 months ago. It was unknown how many pills Mr. Green may have ingested.

Initial vital signs at the scene were BP, 80; palp, 136; RR, 10—with Kussmaul respirations noted. Mr. Green was unconscious. Oxygen was started at 100% F&O$_2$, and respirations were assisted with a bag-valve-mask device. Upon Mr. Green's arrival at the referring facility, two large-bore intravenous lines were started and running at a wide open rate. Carboxyhemoglobin and alcohol levels were drawn. Mr. Green's respirations continued to be assisted.

Upon arrival of the transport team, Mr. Green was unconscious with a Glasgow coma scale score of 3; his pupils were equal at 4 mm and very sluggish to react. His vitals signs were BP, 90; palp, 120; RR, 24/BVM; and Temp, 99.8(R). The diagnostic data showed a carboxyhemoglobin level of 50%, an alcohol level of 0.2% (2 mg/ml), and a finger-stick blood sugar of 80. Mr. Green was stabilized based on the ABC priority of care.

Mr. Green was immediately intubated for several reasons. The standard of care for carbon monoxide is high-flow oxygen. However, and more important, Mr. Green needed his airway to be protected because of the high risk of emesis. The most efficient and safest way to deliver oxygen would be through an endotracheal tube.

Mr. Green's breath sounds were clear and equal bilaterally. Once intubated, oxygen saturation remained at 98%. Although his blood pressure was low, Mr. Green's peripheral pulses were strong and regular. The cardiac monitor showed sinus rhythm without ectopic beats. A Foley catheter was inserted to assist in monitoring perfusion throughout transport.

Mr. Green's decrease in neurological status could have been attributed to several factors. The combination of benzodiazepines, alcohol, and carbon monoxide was sufficient alone to produce the suppression. Even though the squad at the scene did a good investigation, there was still the possibility that Mr. Green may have ingested more unknown pills. According to their protocol, the team administered naloxone and glucose with no response.

Mr. Green was undressed so that he could be observed for any further signs of self-inflicted trauma. None were observed.

A brief secondary survey was completed and was essentially unremarkable. Soft restraints were applied in case Mr. Green's mental status improved and he became combative. Mr. Green was "packaged" and transport initiated.

Once en route, medical control was contacted. Orders were given to administer flumazenil (Mazicon) intravenously because of the severe CNS depression. The transport team administered 0.2 mg. of flumazenil, IVP, over 30 seconds. Mr. Green had no response. A second dose of 0.3 mg. IVP was given with still no response. Most patients with a pure benzodiazepine overdose will have an increase in their level of consciousness (eye opening, an increase in respiratory rate, or reaction to pain). If mental status does increase, it may be temporary, since the duration of the benzodiazepines may be greater than the duration of the flumazemil depending on the amount of substance ingested. Mr. Green did not respond to the flumazenil. Did this mean that he had a massive overdose or perhaps he had not taken any at all? No one knew at this time. Mr. Green's transport was completed uneventfully.

Upon arrival at the receiving facility, Mr. Green was placed on a ventilator and received emergent hyperbaric therapy. His benzodiazepine level was zero. Mr. Green did recover and was admitted to the psychiatric care unit for extensive treatment, since his suicide attempt was rated high on the lethality scale.

REFERENCES

Bjorn, P.R. (1991). An approach to the potentially violent patient. *Journal of Emergency Nursing, 17*(5), 336-339.

Broering-Ramey, B. (1993). Acute ethylene glycol poisoning. *Journal of Emergency Nursing, 19*(2), 86-88.

Burgess, A.W. (1990). *Psychiatric nursing in the hospital*

and the community. East Norwalk, CT: Appleton & Lange.

California EMS Authority (1990). Hazardous materials exposure: Arsine gas. *Journal of Emergency Nursing, 16*(4), 300-302.

Clark, S. (1988). The violated victim: Prehospital Psychological care for the crime victim. *Journal of Emergency Medicine Service, 13*(3), 48-51.

Daniels, P., & LePard, A. (1991). Organophosphates: the pervasive poison. *Journal of Emergency Services, 16*(11), 76-79.

Duffy, N. (1993). A 33-year-old woman with a propranolol and chlorpromazine overdose with applied nursing diagnosis. *Journal of Emergency Nursing, 19*(1), 13-18.

Foley, J. (1993). Recognition and treatment of neuroleptic malignant syndrome. *Journal of Emergency Nursing, 19*(2), 139-141.

Frederick, L. (1992). Defending your life: How to manage violent patients and scenes. *Journal of Emergency Medical Services, 17*(6), 64-67.

George, J.E., & Quathrone, M. (1989). The intoxicated E.D. trauma patient: A case report. *Journal of Emergency Nursing, 15*(5), 444-445.

Gough, A., & Markus, K. (1989). Hazardous materials protection in E.D. practice: Laws and logistics. *Journal of Emergency Nursing, 15*(6), 447-480.

Hadley, S. (1992). Working with battered women in the emergency department: A model program. *Journal of Emergency Nursing, 18*(1), 18-23.

House, M.A. (1990). Cocaine. *American Journal of Nursing, 90*(4), 41-45.

Jezierski, M. (1992). Guidelines for intervention by E.D. nurses in cases of domestic abuse. *Journal of Emergency Nursing, 18*(1), 28a-30a.

Kennedy, M.G. (1991). Dealing with violent patients in flight. *Journal of Emergency Nursing, 17*(5), 295-298.

Kinkle, S.L. (1993). Violence in the ED: How to stop it before it starts. *American Journal of Nursing, 93*(7), 22-24.

Kirk, M., & Bowers, L. (1991). Cluing in on the acutely poisoned patient. *Journal of Emergency Medical Services, 16*(5), 64-82.

Kitt, S., & Kaiser, J. (1990). *Emergency nursing: A physiological and clinical perspective.* Philadelphia: W.B. Saunders.

Kurlowicz, L.H. (1990). Violence in the emergency department. *American Journal of Nursing, 90*(9), 38-40.

Lee, G. (Ed.). (1991). *Flight nursing: Principles and practice.* St. Louis: Mosby.

McDonald, A.J., & Abrahams, S.T. (1990). Social emergencies in the elderly. *Emergency Medical Clinics of North America, 8*(2), 443-458.

Merker, J.S. (1986). Psychiatric emergency evaluation. *Nursing Clinics of North America, 21*(3), 387-397.

Neff, J., & Kidd, P. (1993). *Trauma nursing: The art and science.* St. Louis: Mosby.

Nuckols, C.C., & Greeson, J. (1989). Cocaine addiction: Assessment and intervention. *Nursing Clinics of North America, 24*(1), 33-43.

Ramoska, E.A., et al. (1993). A 1-year evaluation of calcium channel blocker overdoses: Toxicity and treatment. *Annals of Emergency Medicine, 22*(2), 196-200.

Rea, R., et al. (1987). *Emergency nursing core curriculum.* Philadelphia: W.B. Saunders.

Reynolds, E.A., et al. (1989). Delivering and documenting care in child abuse cases. *Journal of Emergency Medical Services, 14*(10), 71-76.

Rodgers, G.C., & Matyunas, N.J. (1986). Gastrointestinal decontamination for acute poisoning. *Pediatric Clinics of North America, 33*(2), 261-285.

Ruckman, L.M. (1992). Rape: How to begin the healing. *American Journal of Nursing, 92*(9), 48-51.

Saunders, C.E., & Ho, M.T. (1992). *Current emergency diagnosis and treatment.* East Norwalk, CT: Appleton & Lange.

Splawn, G. (1991). Restraining potentially violent patients. *Journal of Emergency Nursing, 17*(5), 316-317.

Thomas, C. (Ed.). (1977). *Taber's cyclopedic medical dictionary.* Philadelphia: F.A. David.

Whitehead, C. (1991). After the violation: Treating rape victims. *Journal of Emergency Medical Services, 16*(4), 48-54.

ADDITIONAL RESOURCES

The Chemical Transportation Emergency Center (CHEMTREC)
800-424-9300

National Organization for Victim Assistance (NOVA)
717 D. Street, NW, Suite 200
Washington, D.C. 20004
(202) 393-6682

National Center on Child Abuse and Neglect
330 C. Street, SW
Washington, D.C. 20201
(202) 245-0586 or Clearinghouse (703) 821-8955

Clearinghouse on Family Violence
P.O. Box 1182
Washington, D.C. 20013
(703) 821-2086

Drug manufacturers can provide in-depth information on their products including information on antidotes in case of overdose.

Local drug and poison control centers.

"Violence in the Emergency Room" videotape produced by American Journal of Nursing Company. 1-800-CALL-AJN.

CHAPTER 11

Transport of Patients with Infectious Diseases

OBJECTIVES

1. List three laws established by the Occupational Safety and Health Administration that apply to prehospital nursing
2. Give two reasons why caring for patients with infectious diseases in the prehospital arena is different from caring for them in the hospital
3. Identify a potential patient care situation in which proper body substance isolation can prevent contamination or cross contamination

COMPETENCIES

1. Follow OSHA's regulations when bagging, decontaminating, and disposing equipment
2. Stock the prehospital vehicle with the proper protective barriers for prehospital nursing
3. Act as a leader and educator for other prehospital personnel in preventing the spread of infectious diseases

Implementing and using practices of infection control result in a safer environment for health-care workers and patients. Following universal precautions for health-care providers can be difficult in the most controlled environments. Prehospital care nurses are confronted and challenged by additional concerns that must be addressed before practicing in the prehospital arena effectively. To treat patients in a prehospital care environment, nurses need not only to maintain clinical skills but also to understand and use infection control practices. The prehospital nurse's role changes in the treatment of patients in the field, and likewise, the utilization of universal precautions and the prevention of the spread of communicable diseases will differ. This chapter explores issues that pertain to prehospital nurses and recommends ways nurses can be proactive under the most unusual circumstances. It is critical for prehospital nurses to be both anticipatory and flexible in treating patients successfully and in maintaining infection control.

The Occupational Safety and Health Administration (OSHA) has defined certain terms relating to infection control (Box 11-1). OSHA's definitions are used throughout this chapter.

Box 11-1
DEFINITIONS RELATING TO INFECTION CONTROL

- *Blood:* human blood, human blood components, and products made from human blood.
- *Bloodborne pathogens:* pathogenic microorganisms that are present in human blood and can cause disease in humans. These pathogens include, but are not limited to, human immunodeficiency virus (HIV).
- *Contaminated:* the presence or the reasonable anticipated presence of blood or other potentially infectious materials on an item or a surface.
- *Decontamination:* the use of physical or chemical means to remove, inactivate, or destroy bloodborne pathogens on a surface or item to the point where they are no longer capable of transmitting infectious particles and the surface or item is rendered safe for handling, use, or disposal.
- *Exposure incident:* a specific eye, mouth, other mucous membrane, nonintact skin, or parenteral contact with blood or other potentially infectious materials that results from the performance of an employee's duties.

- *Regulated wastes:* liquid or semiliquid blood or other potentially infectious materials, contaminated items that would release blood or other potential infectious materials in a liquid or a semiliquid state if compressed, items that are caked with dried blood or other potentially infectious materials and are capable of releasing these materials during handling, contaminated sharps, and pathological and microbiological wastes containing blood or other potentially infectious materials.
- *Source individual:* any individual, living or dead, whose blood or other potentially infectious material may be a source of occupational exposure to the employee.
- *Sterilize:* the use of a physical or chemical procedure to destroy all microbial life including highly resistant bacterial endospores.
- *Work practice controls:* controls that reduce the likelihood of exposure by altering the manner in which a task is performed (e.g., prohibiting recapping of needles).

Note. From *Occupational Exposure to Bloodborne Pathogens: Final Rule* (29 CFR Part 1910.1030) by Occupational Safety and Health Administration, 1991, Washington, D.C.: U.S. Department of Labor, OSHA.

BARRIERS TO INFECTION CONTROL PRACTICES

Prehospital nurses face challenges that are different from those in the hospital. These differences must be expected, anticipated, and addressed at all times. It has been well documented that prehospital care providers are exposed to a greater amount of blood and body fluids, including unknown contact. Safety is a recurring issue that prehospital nurses must face and is the first priority in the prehospital setting, even above patient care. Nurses who venture into an unsafe scene and put the team and patient at risk are no different from nurses who do not use universal precautions and put themselves, other team members, and patients at risk. Astute prehospital care nurses must be familiar with infection control practices in various clinical settings and be proactive in the administration of these practices. In some instances this is even more of a burden because these nurses are exposed to the most peculiar and unexpected situations.

There are definite differences between prehospital nursing and nursing within an institution. For instance, in the hospital the nurse knows when the patient is returning from surgery and is able to prepare for the patient's return. Protective barriers such as gloves, towels, and plastic pads are readily available in the patient's room. Gloves are usually mounted on the wall. Practicing in the prehospital arena is different because of the uncertainty of receiving a potentially infectious patient. The prehospital nurse's resources are limited to what was brought along to the scene. For example, the nurse sees a patient that clearly needs treatment, but the intervention will cause exposure to bloody secretions. If gloves, mask, and goggles were not brought to the scene, then a dilemma arises. Does the nurse delay intervention to return to a vehicle to obtain these protective barriers, or does the nurse treat the patient unprotected? The prudent nurse would anticipate the necessity for protective barriers and have them available at all times. Even in the emergency department, the patient arrives in a setting where protective barriers and equipment are available. In the prehospital care setting nurses have to make sure that not only medical equipment is available to treat the patient but also that the protective barrier equipment is also readily available.

Another challenge prehospital nurses face is performing technical skills while wearing gloves. Starting an intravenous line in the field can be difficult. Nurses may feel that reaching into a car, the lack of light, an uncooperative patient, or the lack of personnel to assist are enough barriers to starting an IV line without the additional problem of not being able to feel the vein. To become proficient while using protective barriers, prehospital care nurses must learn to perform skills differently.

Another situation that puts prehospital care nurses at greater risk than hospital nurses is the fact that certain functions must be performed while in a moving vehicle. While starting an IV line in a moving squad vehicle, nurses face the additional challenge of instability. So not only do nurses have to be able to start an IV line while wearing protective gloves, but there is the additional challenge of sticking a moving target.

High-risk situations occur when members of the prehospital care team leave needles, sharps, or contaminated objects carelessly exposed. Prudent nurses place contaminated needles and equipment in a location where they will not cause injury or cross contamination. Two solutions would be to place sharps in small containers and to insert contaminated needles in small Styrofoam blocks.

The definition of infection control includes any efforts designed to prevent infection from occurring in both patients and health-care providers (OSHA, 1991). Infection control is a comprehensive, proactive approach to managing the risks associated with all infectious and communicable diseases (United States Fire Administration, 1992).

UNIVERSAL PRECAUTIONS VS. BODY SUBSTANCE ISOLATION

Prehospital care providers are routinely exposed to infectious, debilitating, and even life-threatening diseases. The nature of the job, including emergent rescues, multiple patients, weather conditions, working conditions, which could include giving care in the back of a moving vehicle, and crisis situations put prehospital nurses at a greater risk.

Now more than ever in the history of medicine, infection control is important because of the AIDS epidemic (U.S. Department of Labor, 1992). In 1992 the Centers for Disease Control and Prevention (CDC) estimated that 1 million people were infected with the AIDS virus. It has also been estimated that 90% of those individuals who are infected are unaware of their infectious status (United States Fire Administration, 1992). Health-care workers should be prudent and treat all body fluids as potentially infectious. It is difficult in the prehospital environment to determine which body fluids are infectious. For example, without adequate lighting it becomes difficult to determine if vomitus contains blood. The CDC guidelines recognize this difficulty and recommend treating all body fluids as potentially hazardous. The CDC has stated, "the unpredictable and emergent nature of exposures encountered by emergency and public-safety workers may make differentiation between hazardous body fluids and those which are not hazardous very difficult and often impossible" (United States Fire Administration, 1992, p. 11).

With the spread of communicable diseases the accessibility of protective barriers becomes as important as the nurse's medical equipment. Patients have a right to feel confident that health-care providers are doing everything possible to prevent the transmission of infectious diseases. Nurses would have a false sense of security if they treated only those patients they viewed as being at risk for infection rather than each patient.

Universal precautions are based on the concept that blood and certain body fluids of all patients should be considered potentially infectious for human immunodeficiency virus (HIV), hepatitis B virus (HBV), and other bloodborne pathogens (United States Fire Administration, 1992). The concept of body substance isolation (BSI) goes beyond the realm of universal precautions and assumes all body substances to be infectious. Sometimes in the prehospital setting it is uncertain from where the body fluid has originated or whether it is a combination of several types of fluids. BSI may be a more practical approach toward maintaining infection control in the prehospital setting because of the uncertainty of exposure in uncontrollable and often times unavoidable emergency situations. BSI can be accomplished by using simple protective barriers such as gloves, masks, protective eye wear, and gowns. The trend in the prehospital setting favors an increase in the num-

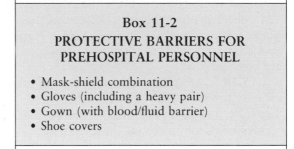

Box 11-2
PROTECTIVE BARRIERS FOR PREHOSPITAL PERSONNEL

- Mask-shield combination
- Gloves (including a heavy pair)
- Gown (with blood/fluid barrier)
- Shoe covers

ber of recommendations for using these protective devices. Box 11-2 lists protective barriers that could become part of a universal precaution protocol for prehospital personnel. Protective barriers are stored in plastic bags, one bag for each team member, thus ensuring proper size and preferred type of glove. The empty plastic bag, when properly labeled, is an ideal place to hold hazardous wastes until it can be disposed of properly. According to OSHA, red bags or red containers may be substituted for biohazard labels.

RISK OF EXPOSURE

The CDC reports that emergency medical workers are at an increased risk of being infected with HBV. The degree of risk correlates with the extent and the amount of exposure. The results of a study to estimate the frequency of occurrence of HBV in emergency medical technicians (EMTs) and paramedics showed employment in these occupations increased the risk of infection from three to five times that of the general population. All prehospital workers must assume an increase in overall risk (United States Fire Administration, 1992). So if nurses leave the hospital setting, which also is a high-risk area for infection, to begin prehospital work, the risk of exposure to infectious agents will increase.

Unfortunately, most of the data collected

about the transmission of HBV and AIDS have been collected on medical professionals from within institutions. We can only infer from these data and apply those to the prehospital care provider.

The CDC lists an increased incidence in the reported cases of HBV in the United States. They also estimate that 12,000 health-care workers whose jobs expose them to blood become infected each year. Studies indicate that 10% to 30% of health-care or dental workers show serologic evidence of past or present HBV infection (U.S. Department of Health and Human Services, 1989).

The potential for HBV transmission in the workplace is greater than for HIV transmission. The probability of high-risk individuals having HBV surface antigens for the general population is 5% to 15%. Individuals who have no vaccination or prophylaxis for HBV and who receive a needle-stick exposure from an infected HBV individual have a 6% to 30% chance of becoming infected, whereas the risk of infection with HIV after a needle-stick exposure from a known HIV-infected person is 0.05%. This rate is probably significantly lower because of the lower concentrations of virus in the blood of an HIV-infected person.

Tuberculosis (TB) is listed by the CDC as the leading infectious cause of death in the world. Every year since 1953, which is when reporting began, the number of cases has dropped off by 6%. In 1986 there was the first reported increase. Box 11-3 lists factors contributing to this increase. CDC estimates that there are 39,000 more cases than would have been expected had the downward trend continued (Simone, 1993).

Between 1985 and 1990 CDC reported that the areas with the largest numbers of AIDS cases also had the most TB cases. CDC now lists coinfection with HIV as being the strongest known risk factor associated with the progression of TB infection to TB disease (Simone, 1993).

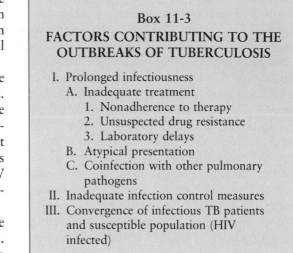

Box 11-3
FACTORS CONTRIBUTING TO THE OUTBREAKS OF TUBERCULOSIS

I. Prolonged infectiousness
  A. Inadequate treatment
    1. Nonadherence to therapy
    2. Unsuspected drug resistance
    3. Laboratory delays
  B. Atypical presentation
  C. Coinfection with other pulmonary pathogens
II. Inadequate infection control measures
III. Convergence of infectious TB patients and susceptible population (HIV infected)

Note. From "A Guide to Formulating a Comprehensive Program" by P. Simone, 1993, *Firehouse,* January, 64-66.

Health-care workers are concerned about the epidemic proportions of AIDS. Of all the AIDS cases reported to the CDC in 1987, 5.8% reported working in a health-related field. The CDC investigated these cases and concluded that of all those reported 95% were found to have high-risk factors for exposure to HIV (CDC, 1987).

Much attention has focused on the issue of confidentiality of reporting the status of AIDS patients to health-care workers. The CDC estimates that 90% of the people who are infected with HIV are unaware of their infectious status (United States Fire Administration, 1992).

Protective barriers become important when the infectious state of an individual is not known. All health-care providers must realize this fact and use precautions at all times, not just when a person is suspected of having the disease. One study conducted by Skahan (1993) at Johns Hopkins University asked its subjects if they thought they had risk factors for contracting HIV. The subjects were then divided into two groups, those who thought they could be infectious due to risk factors and those who did not think they had any risk factors. These subjects were then tested for HIV, and it was found that half of the subjects that were infected did not think they had any risk factors for AIDS. This study coincides with the CDC's estimation of peoples' awareness of their infectious status.

Given the incidence and risk of contracting HBV versus HIV, medical personnel have an increased risk of contracting HBV. Also, the risk of contracting AIDS after exposure to HIV is significantly lower than the risk of contracting hepatitis after HBV exposure. Because of the extreme anxiety about the transmission of AIDS, many forget that they are more susceptible to HBV than other infectious diseases. A pregnant prehospital worker is at an even greater risk for contracting all infectious diseases because of pregnancy-induced immunosuppressence (Denenberg, 1992).

The prehospital nurse must be cognizant of the characteristics and imminent dangers of other communicable diseases. These include, but are not limited to, TB, meningitis, rubella, measles, mumps, and chicken pox (United States Fire Administration, 1992).

VACCINES

The emergency worker, or anyone employed in other high-risk areas, should be made aware of the importance of vaccinations. The available vaccines for hepatitis B stimulate active immunity, providing over 90% protection. Even if the HBV vaccine is given within 1 week after HBV exposure it is still 70% to 88% effective. A combination of HB immunoglobulin and HBV vaccine if administered within a week following exposure is over 90% effective in preventing hepatitis B (U.S. Department of Health and Human Services, 1989; Weber, Hoffmann, & Rutala, 1991).

The National Flight Nurses Association's

(NFNA) position statement on hepatitis B vaccination recommends that all flight nurses obtain the vaccination and encourage others to do the same.

OSHA requires employers to offer this vaccination to high-risk employees at no charge. In addition, OSHA requires employers to obtain a signed declination paper from any employee who refuses the vaccination.

Currently, the brand name Heptavax vaccination has been replaced with a recombinant DNA yeast preparation. This preparation was introduced because of health-care workers' concern about the Heptavax vaccine, which is developed from pooled plasma, thus potentially increasing the risk of contracting infectious diseases from the vaccination itself. It was purported not to be a problem, but health-care providers were not convinced. The two compounds that replaced Heptavax were Recombavax and Engerex. Individuals allergic to yeast may want to investigate with their personal physician whether they should obtain the vaccine. An employee health physician may be another source of information because they will have current recommendations for prevention and treatment of infectious diseases.

It is important to follow-up on titers of the hepatitis B vaccine to determine if the immune system has developed antibodies to the virus. The vaccination itself is ineffective unless the antibody titers are sufficient to ward off the disease. Many health-care workers are unaware of their titer status. The HBV vaccination is ineffective if the titer is unknown. The titer should be drawn 1 to 6 months after the vaccination. In most cases a qualitative positive result is sufficient to document protection (SmithKline Beecham Pharmaceuticals, 1992).

Lamphear and colleagues' study (1993) looked at the incidence of HBV in health-care workers in relation to vaccine-induced immunity. The subjects were health-care workers who reported needle-stick and significant blood

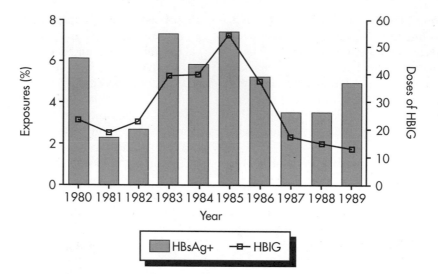

Fig. 11-1   Annual incidence of hepatitis B surface antigen among patients to whose blood and/or other body fluids health-care workers at the University of Cincinnati Hospital were exposed from 1980 through 1989 is shown in relation to the number of doses of hepatitis B immune globulin (HBIG) administered. (From "Decline of Clinical Hepatitis B in Workers at a General Hospital: Relation to Increasing Vaccine-Induced Immunity" by B.P. Lamphear, C.C. Linnemann, C.G. Cannon, & M.M. DeRonde, 1993, *Clinical Infectious Diseases,* *16,* 10-14.)

exposures to the employee health department. This study found a decrease in the number of times immunoglobulin was administered during the study period because employees had been receiving HBV vaccination (Figure 11-1). Figure 11-2 indicates the incidence of HBV for health-care workers and the rate of exposure to patients with HBV. A downward trend was noticed as the HBV vaccine was introduced in 1983 and workers acquired protective immunity (Lamphear, Linnemann, Cannon, & DeRonde, 1993).

GUIDELINES

The OSHA standard 1910.1030, titled *Bloodborne Pathogen Standard,* became effective March 6, 1992. Currently, it is standard to have a written policy outlining the details of possible exposure and guidelines for interventions to limit exposure to infectious diseases. Prehospital care nurses must take existing standards and policies and adapt them to the environment of prehospital nursing. This is especially important for prehospital care providers because they have an increased overall risk of blood and body fluid exposure.

Universal definitions and terms must be defined before there is a complete understanding of the guidelines. OSHA has standardized these definitions (see Box 11-1). These definitions should be used to maintain consistency throughout the health-care profession. Education is enhanced when everyone is operating from the same base of knowledge. A full list can be found in the Federal Register, *Occupational Exposure to Bloodborne Pathogens 29 CFR Part 1910.1030.*

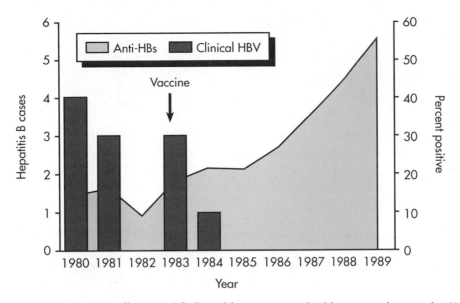

Fig. 11-2   Occupationally acquired clinical hepatitis B in health-care workers at the University of Cincinnati Hospital from 1980 through 1989 is shown in relation to the percentage of workers exposed to blood and/or other body fluids who had protective immunity (anti-HBs). Hepatitis B vaccine was made available beginning in 1983 as is indicated by the arrow. (From "Decline of Clinical Hepatitis B in Workers at a General Hospital: Relation to Increasing Vaccine-Induced Immunity" by B.P. Lamphear, C.C. Linnemann, C.G. Cannon, & M.M. DeRonde, 1993, *Clinical Infectious Diseases, 16,* 10-14.)

The CDC and the National Institute for Occupational Safety and Health (NIOSH) appear to be the forerunners in the development of standards for infection control, but OSHA is responsible for establishing the laws. Unfortunately, people do not heed guidelines until these become law. For the purposes of this chapter, OSHA guidelines are considered the Gold Standard because organizations are required by law to conform to OSHA rules and regulations. Nurses developing an infection control policy may want to consider reviewing information made available by CDC, NIOSH, and OSHA to guarantee the inclusiveness of their policies.

OSHA has developed regulations that prescribe safeguards to protect workers against the health hazards from exposure to blood and body fluids that contain pathogens, thereby reducing health-care workers' risks. The purpose of the regulations is to decrease the risk to this exposure. The controls that OSHA lists are aimed at reducing the employee's exposure in the workplace by either removing the hazard or isolating the worker. Each type of workplace must follow the guidelines that pertain to their specific environment. Federal OSHA authority applies to all private employers with one or more employees, as well as civilian employees in federal agencies. States can administer their own plans, but they must be at least as effective as federal requirements. There may be some discrepancy as to the judgment of "at least as effective," since this phrase is subjective.

OSHA requires all persons with the potential for exposure to infectious diseases to be adequately notified of their potential risk, and they

Box 11-4
KEY ELEMENTS OF TRAINING TO PREVENT EXPOSURE TO INFECTIOUS DISEASES

1. Identification of the tasks and procedures that each different job classification could encounter
2. Schedule of how and when the provisions of the standard will be implemented
3. Procedures for evaluating the circumstances of any exposure incident
4. Written exposure plan must be accessible to all employees and must be updated annually

Note. From *Occupational Exposure to Bloodborne Pathogens: Precautions for Emergency Responders,* by U.S. Department of Labor, Occupational Safety and Health Administration, 1992, Washington, D.C.: The Author.

must be properly trained in the prevention of that exposure. OSHA establishes minimum guidelines for training programs. Under the standard the plan should cover certain key elements (Box 11-4). All employees must have orientation and continuing education in infectious diseases including epidemiology, transmission, and prevention. The education must emphasize the use of protective barriers for all patients. Provisions of supplies necessary for universal precautions should be discussed, and monitoring of adherence to recommended protective measures must be documented.

Some of the specific practices included in the plan that affect prehospital care providers differently are discussed in the following sections. All areas of exposure are not covered, since it is assumed that prehospital care nurses are familiar with infection control practices.

Disposable airway equipment should be available in the prehospital care setting. In the hospital a reusable Ambu bag could be taken

to central service and sterilized, whereas in the prehospital setting there often is not time to disinfect equipment properly between patient uses. Every patient has the right to be treated with disinfected equipment. A simple solution for the prehospital nurse is to carry two disposable Ambu bags.

Containers for needles and sharps are not as immediately available in the prehospital care setting as they are in every corner of every room in the hospital. It is the responsibility of prehospital nurses to supply disposable containers as part of their equipment. Laying needles at their feet in the squad or in the field is an unacceptable practice, since this could easily result in a needle stick. Small needle containers can be purchased and placed in the back of squads or in equipment bags. Stix-a-bric, a Styrofoam box for uncapped needles, is convenient because it is small enough to be thrown as a whole into larger contaminated needle containers. New products, such as Saf-T-Caths, can decrease needle sticks because the needle is not exposed.

OSHA prohibits eating, drinking, smoking, applying cosmetics or lip balm, and handling contact lenses in patient care areas. Because of inclement weather conditions and extended periods of time involved, nurses may find it extremely difficult to abide by these rules. For example, after a transport, nurses must set priorities for personal needs, as well as prepare the vehicle for the next transport.

Hand washing is a procedure that must be altered in the prehospital setting, since running water is usually unavailable. Several products available for washing hands do not require rinsing. The product of choice is the alcohol-based foam spray, which is more pleasing and does not leave a sticky residue. Antiseptic towelettes are also available. These products have labels that list organisms against which they are effective.

OSHA standards also require that appropriate personal protective equipment be used to reduce the risk of exposure in the work area. Personal protective equipment includes gloves, face shields, masks, eye protection, gowns, and aprons. Prehospital and hospital workers find that protective equipment hinders their ability to work; however, protective equipment is the reality of today's health-care workers. They will have to adopt and adapt to different practice standards and skills to integrate the use of these items. Some skills will have to be relearned while wearing these protective items. As discussed previously, starting an intravenous line while wearing gloves is not an unobtainable skill, just different.

Disposal of protective items can be a problem in the prehospital setting, since space is limited for storing contaminated items during patient transport. Clearly marked areas for trash cans and disposable bags can be useful. Placing items in these areas during transport can prevent unnecessary cross contamination. This becomes especially important when other people are involved in treatment or in the decontamination process. All contaminated items must be bagged and properly labeled for later disposal. Prehospital care providers may dispose of contaminated materials in the hospital receiving the patient. Hospitals require prehospital workers to follow their policy when disposing of contaminated materials.

Decontaminating the helicopter or transport vehicle is of utmost importance after patient transport. Disinfecting must comply with OSHA guidelines. Infection control departments can help guide departments in the choice of disinfectants. The stretcher or litter from a helicopter must be properly disinfected after each use. Getting the helicopter or squad back into service is a priority, but infection control measures must not be overlooked in the process. Back-to-back flights challenge nurses to restock the necessary medical supplies quickly and also to decontaminate the vehicle. Decontamination supplies should be kept readily available to meet this need.

Labeling of contaminated equipment is required by OSHA. Bags and containers for contaminated items must be available. One alternative is to place all used equipment in plastic Zip-lock bags to be labeled later. After the transport the plastic bag makes it easier to determine how it should be labeled. Table 11-1 lists objects that require labeling.

At University Air Care in Cincinnati, Ohio, various practices for cleaning contaminated laryngoscope blades and handles were noted. Guidelines were implemented to provide a standard cleaning method, but some deviation still persisted. Flight nurses, flight physicians, and emergency department personnel were informally interviewed. Two questions were asked: Did they feel the cleaning method was followed routinely by the employees?; Would they want to put the "cleaned" metal laryngoscope blade into their own mouths? The answers to both questions were consistently "no." This led to an investigation for an improved method of disinfecting laryngoscope blades and handles. The prehospital setting was taken into consideration during this investigation. The solution believed to be the best involved autoclaving the contaminated blade and handle. However, often times prehospital care nurses must perform back-to-back patient transports, which makes it difficult for nurses to deliver equipment to central service for proper sterilization. One suggestion involved purchasing large quantities of blades and handles; when one handle and blade was used, it could be replaced with a sterilized one. It was quickly determined that this was not a viable option because of budget constraints.

After researching several avenues, disposable laryngoscope blades and handles seemed to be a viable alternative. Several products were researched and one met the hospital's standards, the Welch Allen disposable fiberoptic laryngoscopes. The handles are reusable and can be gas-sterilized. The blades are single use, sterile, and have a flexible flange that minimizes tooth injury during intubation. The blades and han-

Table 11-1   Labeling Requirements

Item	No Label Needed if Universal Precautions Are Used and Specific Use of Container is Known to All Employees	Biohazard Label	Red Container
Regulated waste container (e.g., contaminated sharps containers)		X or	X
Reusable contaminated sharps container (e.g., surgical instruments soaking in a tray)		X or	X
Refrigerator/freezer holding blood or other potentially infectious material		X	
Containers used for storage, transport, or shipping of blood		X or	X
Blood/blood products for clinical use	No labels required		
Individual specimen containers of blood or other potentially infectious materials remaining in facility	X or	X or	X
Contaminated equipment needing service (e.g., dialysis equipment, suction apparatus)		X plus a label specifying where the contamination exists	
Specimens and regulated waste shipped from the primary facility to another facility for service or disposal		X or	X
Contaminated laundry*	* or	X or	X
Contaminated laundry sent to another facility that does not use universal precautions		X or	X

Note. From *Occupational Exposure in Bloodborne Pathogens: Precautions for Emergency Responders* by U.S. Department of Labor, Occupational Health and Safety Administration, 1992, Washington, D.C.: The Author.
*Alternative labeling or color coding is sufficient if it permits all employees to recognize the containers as requiring compliance with Universal Precautions.

dles can be purchased individually or in box quantities.

PROTOCOL

Each employer is required by law to adopt an infection control policy that must meet minimum OSHA standards. The OSHA standards are meant to be flexible enough so that employers can individualize their programs to meet the needs of their patient populations and work environments. Each employee should provide input to the development of this plan. Compliance will increase if the employees feel they participated in the change process.

The development begins with a basic protocol. Changes are made to meet the individual needs of the department. After the protocol is established it is continually reviewed and updated. The prehospital arena is an ever-changing and unpredictable environment. One procedure that may work now may not be practical several months from now.

A prehospital care nurse is responsible to act as a liaison with other prehospital care providers on exposure issues. The prehospital nurse should be aware of institutional policies. Often, institutional infection control policies do not include procedures for prehospital care nurses and other prehospital care providers. Box 11-5 contains a sample of prehospital care guidelines for potential HIV exposure. Figure 11-3 is a sample of a request form for information by emergency workers, and Figure 11-4 is a response form to give information back to the prehospital care provider.

This specific policy listed in Figures 11-3 and 11-4 and in Box 11-5 provided workers with a consistent and convenient form for documentation and follow-up of an exposure. This form serves as the actual documentation of the exposure, making future access easy. It also provided some unexpected results. The knowledge of the prehospital worker increased, since the form lists the types of significant exposures. The more educated health-care workers are concerning infection control issues, the more they use and have faith in universal precautions. Anxiety levels decrease, resulting in fewer non-exposure requests. Patient confidentiality increased, since only valid exposures were pursued. Fewer patients and families were bothered with the requests for permission for blood testing. Costly, unnecessary laboratory testing decreased. The ultimate goal, protection for the worker, was maintained.

OSHA states the source individual's blood shall be tested as soon as feasible and after consent is obtained. The source patient or family may refuse to give consent to have blood drawn. "If consent is not obtained, the employer shall establish that legally required consent cannot be obtained" (OSHA, 1991). Individual states have laws pertaining to a situation where the source patient refuses consent and the hospital has a stored specimen of blood. In Ohio, an administrative decision can be made to overrule the source patient's refusal if a stored specimen of serum is available. At University of Cincinnati Hospital (1993) the Director of Medical Center Health Services is one person who can make this decision. The criterion for the decision is based on whether the exposure was significant.

EQUIPMENT

OSHA requires personal protective equipment to be used to reduce the risk of exposure in the workplace. The goal of personal protective equipment is to maintain BSI techniques. BSI eliminates direct contact with any body substance of the patient. OSHA's law requires that employers make available, at no cost to employees, appropriate personal protective equipment in the appropriate sizes to provide protection from blood or other potentially infectious materials (OSHA, 1991). "An employee may temporarily and briefly decline wearing personal protective equipment under

Text continued on p. 279.

REQUEST NO._____

UNIVERSITY OF CINCINNATI HOSPITAL

REQUEST FOR INFORMATION BY EMERGENCY SERVICES WORKER

PLEASE PRINT - Use Blue or Black Ink - PRESS HARD

This form is for use by emergency care workers to request information on the presence of a contagious or infectious disease (if known) of a person, alive or dead, who has been treated, handled, or transported to University Hospital by an emergency services worker.

Before you can be provided with this information, you must believe that you have suffered significant exposure through contact with the person about whom you are requesting the information. A significant exposure means:

A percutaneous (break in the skin or needle stick) or mucous membrane exposure (eyes, nose, mouth) to the blood, semen, vaginal secretions, or spinal, synovial (joint, bone, tendon), pleural (lung), peritoneal (abdomen), pericardial (heart), or amniotic fluid of another person.

Deposit top (white) copy in designated Emergency Department QA box. Submit yellow copy to your agency or employer. Retain pink copy.

1.   Regarding the exposure, what was

      Name of patient:_____

      Date:_____   Time:_____

      Place:_____

      Manner of exposure:
      _____ Dirty needle stick   _____ Broken skin exposure
      _____ Splash-eye, nose, mouth   _____ Unprotected mouth to mouth
      _____ Other, describe:_____
      _____

2.   Your name:_____

3.   Your address:_____

      City/State/Zip:_____

4.   Your telephone number: Home:_____ Work:_____

5.   Have you completed more than two (2) injections in Hepatitis B series? Yes_____   No_____

6.   Employer or volunteer agency for whom you were administering health care when exposure occurred:

      Employer or agency:_____

      Address:_____

      City/State/Zip:_____Phone:_____

7.   Name of your chief at above listed place of employment or volunteer agency:_____

This is to attest that the above statements are true and correct to the best of my knowledge and belief.

Your signature:_____ Date:_____

ACKNOWLEDGEMENT

Name of person receiving request:_____

Received: Date:_____   Time:_____

White-Emergency Department QA Box   Yellow-Agency/Employer   Pink-Requestor's Copy

6/26/92

Fig. 11-3   Sample of a request form by emergency workers for information. (From University of Cincinnati Hospital.)

UNIVERSITY OF CINCINNATI HOSPITAL

REQUEST NO._____

RESPONSE TO EMERGENCY SERVICES WORKER REQUEST FOR INFORMATION

PLEASE PRINT - Use Blue or Black Ink - PRESS HARD

THIS INFORMATION HAS BEEN DISCLOSED TO YOU FROM CONFIDENTIAL RECORDS PROTECTED FROM DISCLOSURE BY STATE LAW. YOU SHALL MAKE NO FURTHER DISCLOSURE OF THIS INFORMATION WITHOUT THE SPECIFIC, WRITTEN, AND INFORMED RELEASE OF THE INDIVIDUAL TO WHOM IT PERTAINS, OR AS OTHERWISE PERMITTED BY STATE LAW. A GENERAL AUTHORIZATION FOR THE RELEASE OF MEDICAL OR OTHER INFORMATION IS NOT SUFFICIENT FOR THE PURPOSE OF THE RELEASE OF HIV TEST RESULTS OR DIAGNOSIS.

1. Date of oral report:_____ Name of ESW:_____

    Person giving report:_____

    Comments:_____

2. Date of written report:_____

    Report sent to worker_____chief_____chief's name_____

    Person sending report:_____

3. Your request for information has been received. It has been determined that:

    a. _____ There is no known presence of a contagious or infectious disease at this time based upon the following:

        _____ No tests were performed.

        _____ The following tests were performed with negative results:

        _____ _____
        _____ _____
        _____ _____

    b. _____ There is the presence of a contagious or infectious disease. Testing on person in question was positive for:

        _____ _____
        _____ _____
        _____ _____

    c. _____ The person in question has refused HIV testing.

    d. _____ Patient discharged home.

    e. _____ Patient discharged to health care facility/coroner's office/funeral home.
        Address:_____

THIS RESPONSE PROVIDES ALL INFORMATION AVAILABLE AS OF THE DATE OF THIS WRITTEN RESPONSE.

4. Report included:
    _____ Name of disease   _____ Suggested precautions for preventing transmission.
    _____ Signs and symptoms of disease   _____ Recommended prophylaxis (if any)
    _____ Date of exposure   _____ Suggested follow-up
    _____ Incubation period of disease   _____ Appropriate counseling
    _____ Mode of transmission

5. It is expected that the worker will consult a physician in cases of true disease exposure. It is understood by provider of report and recipients that decisions related to prophylaxis, treatment, and counseling will be at the discretion of that physician.

White-Requestor's Copy   Yellow-Agency/Employer   Pink-University Hospital Infection Control Committee/Prehospital Training

6/25/92

Fig. 11-4 Sample of a response form for emergency workers' request for information. (From University of Cincinnati Hospital.)

Box 11-5
PREHOSPITAL CARE GUIDELINES FOR POTENTIAL HIV EXPOSURE

I. Purpose
To provide guidelines for potential HIV exposures involving emergency services workers.

II. Introduction
An emergency services worker who believes he has suffered a significant exposure through contact with a patient may submit to the health care facility a request to be notified of the results of any test performed on the patient to determine the presence of a contagious or infectious disease. The request shall include:
 1. The name, address, and telephone number of the emergency services worker submitting the request
 2. The name of the emergency services worker's employer or the entity where he is a volunteer, and his supervisor
 3. The date, time, location, and manner of the exposure
An emergency services worker is defined to include a peace officer, an employee of an emergency medical service, a firefighter, a volunteer firefighter, emergency operator, or rescue operator, or an employee of a private organization that renders rescue services, emergency medical care, or emergency medical transportation to accident victims and persons suffering serious illness or injury.

III. Definition of Exposure
The key step for determining which course of action to take regarding any exposure is, if possible, to accurately define the exposure. The following are specific guidelines concerning exposure of emergency services workers to potentially HIV infected patients or body fluids.
A. *Significant exposure:* Percutaneous or mucous membrane exposure of an individual to any of the following body fluids:
 1. Blood
 2. Semen
 3. Synovial fluid
 4. Spinal fluid
 5. Amniotic fluid
 6. Peritoneal fluid
 7. Pleural fluid
 8. Pericardial fluid
 9. Vaginal secretions
 10. Any fluid with suspected blood
B. *Nonsignificant exposures:*
Nonsignificant exposures are defined as follows: mucous membrane penetrating wound, or skin exposure to feces, nasal secretions, sputum, sweat, tears, urine, saliva, and vomitus, unless they contain visible blood.
C. *Indeterminate exposures:* All other exposures not listed above, including exposures in which it is difficult to determine or questionable whether any of the above exposures actually occurred.

IV. Exposure Management
A. *Significant exposure—actions taken*
If the emergency services worker chooses to register and be seen in the CEC, the following actions will be taken;
 1. The basic procedures as outlined in the needlestick, other percutaneous, and mucous membrane exposures are to be followed (Hospital Policy, II-3II).
 2. An HIV test is routinely drawn if the source individual consents to the HIV test and counseling is done by the physician as described by the University Hospital AIDS Guidelines.

Note. From University of Cincinnati Hospital.

Box 11-5
PREHOSPITAL CARE GUIDELINES FOR POTENTIAL HIV EXPOSURE—cont'd

3. Emergency services workers will be referred for follow-up to a private physician, medical director, or health agency responsible for the monitoring, evaluation, and review of the emergency services worker's occupational health.
4. The emergency services worker will receive counseling information regarding the exposure and potential risk to others during the observation period.
   a. Information will be obtained to determine if the emergency services worker is a member of a high-risk group.
   b. The emergency services worker will be advised to report any and all illnesses that occur within the initial 6-month period following exposure, specifically the occurrence of sore throat, skin rashes, fever, malaise, joint pain, muscle aches, enlargement of lymph nodes, and any acute infections.
   c. Instructions on an appropriate method to prevent sexual transmission of HIV during the observation period will be given.
   d. Women of childbearing age will be advised on family planning.
   e. Information will be provided regarding follow-up counseling if necessary, i.e., resources other than presently available.
5. If a source individual refuses or is unable to consent to HIV testing, the following guidelines are recommended.
   a. If blood has been taken for other medical indications and a significant exposure has taken place according to the definitions above, The Quality Assurance Coordinator/Prehospital Care will notify the Infection Control Committee, which will determine the need for HIV testing of the patient serum sample. The steps outlined in Section IV, of this document, will be followed in the emergency department.
   b. If the patient is comatose or deceased, a sample of blood will be taken in the emergency department and the Quality Assurance Coordinator/ Prehospital Care will notify the Infection Control Committee, which will determine the need for HIV testing of the patient serum sample. The steps outlined in Section IV, of this document, will be followed in the emergency department.
   c. If the patient is determined to be competent and refuses consent to HIV testing or any blood removal, the exposed emergency services worker will be treated according to Section IV, in this document. The faculty physician will document on the "Request to be Notified of the Presence of an Infectious Disease Form" that the patient refused consent to HIV testing or any blood removal and place the form in the Quality Assurance Coordinator's box.
6. *Nonsignificant exposure:* No specific testing or prophylaxis will be

Continued

Box 11-5
PREHOSPITAL CARE GUIDELINES FOR POTENTIAL HIV EXPOSURE—cont'd

administered, but the emergency services worker will be referred according to Section IV, item 3, of this document.

7. *Indeterminate exposure:* The same guidelines will be followed as outlined for significant exposure. Because indeterminate exposures still carry HIV exposure risk, the guidelines outlined in this document for significant exposures should be followed.

V. The Quality Assurance Coordinator/ Prehospital Care will give an oral notification of the presence of a contagious or infectious disease to the emergency services worker and designated supervisor within 2 working days of determining the presence of a contagious or infectious disease. A written notification, approved by the Infection Control Committee at University Hospital, will follow the oral notification within 3 work days. Both oral and written notification shall include:

1. The name of the disease
2. Its signs and symptoms
3. The date of the exposure
4. The incubation period
5. The mode of transmission of the disease
6. The precautions necessary for preventing transmission to others
7. The appropriate prophylaxis, treatment, and counseling for the disease

The notification will not include the name of the patient.

If the requested information is not available because the patient is no longer being treated at the University of Cincinnati Hospital, the emergency services worker will be notified of any institution to which the patient has been transferred and assisted in obtaining the requested information from that facility. If the patient has died, the emergency services worker will be given the name and address of the coroner or funeral director who received the patient.

VI. Guidelines Regarding the Use of AZT Prophylaxis

The use of AZT following blood and body fluid exposure is controversial. The data at present *do not* support the use of AZT following a occupational exposure in most instances. There may be more significant exposures, such as the transfusion or deep intramuscular needlestick of *known* HIV infected blood that might justify the use of AZT. In general, the use of AZT prophylaxis following a superficial scratch, needlestick, or laceration is not being recommended.

The decision to institute AZT prophylaxis must be individualized. An emergency services worker should consult with his private physician, medical director, or the agency that oversees his general health regarding this issue.

rare and extraordinary circumstances and when in the employee's professional judgment it prevents the delivery of health care or public safety services or poses a greater hazard to workers" (U.S. Department of Labor/OSHA, 1992).

As stated in the initial recommendations from OSHA, reasonable decisions should be made concerning these devices. In the extreme cases of exsanguination, all of these barriers should be used.

Nurses who work infrequently in the prehospital arena, such as transporting a patient to another facility, must add infection control to their awareness of essential equipment. The word *essential* is important, since infection control devices are just as important as a transport cardiac monitor or ventilator. They must be cognizant of infection control devices that may not be available in the transport vehicle so that personal protective barriers can be brought from the institution. These nurses may need to request their institutions to purchase special items that can be taken on these transports.

If universal precautions are not required for infection control, hand washing practices and general infection control measures must be followed. Universal precautions are meant to supplement rather than replace general guidelines for routine infection control.

According to OSHA guidelines, the employer has the obligation to purchase any equipment that is necessary for infection control purposes. Personal protective equipment consists of gloves, face shields, masks, eye protection, gowns, and aprons. This also includes miscellaneous pieces of equipment for individual use, for example, powderless gloves for workers with problems in skin breakdown. Extra small or extra large sizes may need to be ordered. Employers are responsible for making equipment available to the employee, but the employee is responsible for making sure the equipment fits correctly. In some instances, ill-fitting equipment may be the same as not having any equipment at all.

Disposable gloves should be standard equipment made easily accessible to the prehospital nurse. Gloves should be worn before approaching any patient care area. Extra pairs should always be available. Gloves should be changed between all patient contact, when possible, and should be replaced if their ability to function as a protective barrier is compromised.

No single glove type is appropriate for every situation. There have been no reported differences in barrier effectiveness between intact latex and vinyl. Thicker gloves may be more appropriate for the extrication process because of the exposure to metal and glass. The 1992 OSHA guidelines state the selection criteria should include dexterity, durability, fit, and the tasks that will be undertaken while the gloves are worn (U.S. Department of Health and Human Services, 1989). Box 11-6 contains CDC general guidelines for glove usage. "Wicking" becomes a problem when the gloves are exposed to disinfectants used for cleaning equipment. Wicking has occurred if hands are wet or soapy after glove removal. To prevent cross contamination through wicking, general-purpose utility gloves should be worn for disinfecting purposes.

Masks, safety goggles, and face shields should be easily accessible. These devices are worn when blood and other body fluid will likely be present. Table 11-2 lists recommended usages of protective equipment. The mask must be able to filter out .05 micron to be effective as a protective barrier. If large quantities of blood are expected to splash, an impervious gown should be worn. An extra change of clothing should be left at work.

Equipment must be researched and evaluated before placing the specifics into the final draft of the policy. Minimum state and institutional guidelines must be met, as well as OSHA guidelines.

The infection control or medical supply department can be helpful when evaluating equipment. Samples may need to be obtained and

---

Box 11-6
CDC GUIDELINES FOR GLOVE USAGE

1. Use sterile gloves for procedures involving contact with normally sterile areas of the body.
2. Use examination gloves for procedures involving contact with mucous membranes, unless otherwise indicated, and for other patient care or diagnostic procedures that do not require the use of sterile gloves.
3. Change gloves between patient contacts.
4. Do not wash or disinfect surgical or examination gloves for reuse. Washing with surfactants may cause "wicking," i.e., the enhanced penetration of liquids through undetected holes in the glove. Disinfecting agents may cause deterioration.
5. Use general-purpose utility gloves (e.g., rubber household gloves) for housekeeping chores involving potential blood contact and for instrument cleaning and decontamination procedures. Utility gloves may be decontaminated and reused but should be discarded if they are peeling, cracked, or discolored, or if they have punctures, tears, or other evidence of deterioration.

Note. From *Guidelines for Prevention of Transmission of Human Immunodeficiency Virus and Hepatitis B Virus to Health-Care and Public-Safety Workers* (DHHS [NIOSH] Publication No. 89-107) by U.S. Department of Health and Human Services, Public Health Service, National Institute for Occupational Safety and Health, 1989, Washington, D.C.: The Author.

tried before making a final decision. Purchasing small orders will prevent wasting money out of a budget for equipment that is not practical. If the equipment does not fit exactly, is not the right solution for the problem, or cannot be stored in an easily accessible place, the equipment becomes useless. Prehospital nurses have an advantage because they have contact with other prehospital departments and hospitals where they can get ideas about equipment that is either useful or nonfunctional.

Here is an example of how an infection control problem was solved at University Air Care, Cincinnati, Ohio. When exsanguinating patients are transported, blood runs down the patient platform in the helicopter and poses an infection control risk. When the helicopter is unloaded with the engines running, blood sprays out the back door. This blood is a risk for the unloading crew and for the crew that receives the patient. This problem was discussed with the medical crew and the medical supply director. The medical supply director suggested using a large piece of plastic the hospital stocks for lining a Hubbard tank. The price of this plastic is minimal compared with other wraps that are specifically prepared for containing blood. The Hubbard tank liner is placed in the middle of a linen roll with sheets and bath blankets. The pilots prepare the litter with this roll, and the patient is wrapped before the safety belts are placed. The belts provide support to contain the plastic within the sheet. The plastic sheet has proven to be a means to contain blood. This product is still being evaluated.

CLEANING OF EQUIPMENT

Disinfecting equipment is the last step in the infection control process, but in no way is it the least important. Reusable equipment that has been properly disinfected can be safely handled and used on the next patient without risk of transmitting disease. It is important to understand which type of cleaning each object re-

Table 11-2   Examples of Recommended Personal Protective Equipment for Worker Protection Against HIV and HBV Transmission* in Prehospital† Settings

Task or Activity	Disposable Gloves	Gown	Mask‡	Protective Eyewear
Bleeding control with spurting blood	Yes	Yes	Yes	Yes
Bleeding control with minimal bleeding	Yes	No	No	No
Emergency childbirth	Yes	Yes	Yes, if splashing is likely	Yes, if splashing is likely
Blood drawing	At certain times	No	No	No
Starting an intravenous (IV) line	Yes	No	No	No
Endotracheal intubation, esophageal obturator use	Yes	No	No, unless splashing is likely	No, unless splashing is likely
Oral/nasal suctioning, manually cleaning airway	Yes§	No	No, unless splashing is likely	No, unless splashing is likely
Handling and cleaning instruments with microbial contamination	Yes	No, unless soiling is likely	No	No
Measuring blood pressure	No	No	No	No
Measuring temperature	No	No	No	No
Giving an injection	No	No	No	No

Note. From *Guidelines for Prevention of Transmission of Human Immunodeficiency Virus and Hepatitis B Virus to Health-Care and Public-Safety Workers* (DHHS [NIOSH] Publication No. 89-107) by U.S. Department of Health and Human Services, Public Health Service, National Institute for Occupational Safety and Health, 1989, Washington, D.C.: The Author.

*The examples provided in this table are based on application of universal precautions. Universal precautions are intended to supplement rather than replace recommendations for routine infection control, such as hand washing and using gloves to prevent gross microbial contamination of hands (e.g., contact with urine or feces).

†Defined as a setting where delivery of emergency health care takes place away from a hospital or other health-care facility.

‡Refers to protective masks to prevent exposure of mucous membranes to blood or other potentially contaminated body fluids.

§While not clearly necessary to prevent HIV or HBV transmission unless blood is present, gloves are recommended to prevent transmission of other agents (e.g., herpes simplex).

Box 11-7
REPROCESSING METHODS FOR EQUIPMENT USED IN THE PREHOSPITAL HEALTH-CARE SETTING

Sterilization
Destroys

All forms of microbial life including high numbers of bacterial spores.

Methods

Steam under pressure (autoclave), gas (ethylene oxide), dry heat, or immersion in EPA-approved chemical "sterilant" for prolonged period of time, e.g., 6-10 hours or according to manufacturers' instructions. Note: liquid chemical "sterilants" should be used only on those instruments that are impossible to sterilize or disinfect with heat.

Use

For those instruments or devices that penetrate skin or contact normally sterile areas of the body, e.g., scalpels, needles, etc. Disposable invasive equipment eliminates the need to reprocess these types of items. When indicated, however, arrangements should be made with a health-care facility for reprocessing of reusable invasive instruments.

High-Level Disinfection
Destroys

All forms of microbial life *except* high numbers of bacterial spores.

Methods

Hot water pasteurization (80-100° C, 30 minutes) or exposure to an EPA-registered "sterilant" chemical as above, except for a short exposure time (10-45 minutes or as directed by the manufacturer).

Use

For reusable instruments or devices that come into contact with mucous membranes (e.g., laryngoscope blades, endotracheal tubes, etc.).

Intermediate-Level Disinfection
Destroys

Mycobacterium tuberculosis, vegetative bacteria, most viruses, and most fungi, but does not kill bacterial spores.

Methods

EPA-registered "hospital disinfectant" chemical germicides that have a label claim for tuberculocidal activity; commercially available hard-surface germicides or solutions containing at least 500 ppm free available chlorine (a 1:100 dilution of common household bleach—approximately ¼ cup bleach per gallon of tap water).

Use

For those surfaces that come into contact only with intact skin, e.g., stethoscopes, blood pressure cuffs, splints, etc., and have been visibly contaminated with blood or bloody body fluids. Surfaces *must* be precleaned of visible material before the germicidal chemical is applied for disinfection.

Low-Level Disinfection
Destroys

Most bacteria, some viruses, some fungi, but not *Mycobacterium tuberculosis* or bacterial spores.

Note. From *Guidelines for Prevention of Transmission of Human Immunodeficiency Virus and Hepatitis B Virus to Health-Care and Public-Safety Workers.* (DHHS (NIOSH) Publication No. 89-107) by U.S. Department of Health and Human Services, Public Health Service, National Institute for Occupational Safety and Health, 1989, Washington, D.C.: The Author.

Box 11-7
**REPROCESSING METHODS FOR EQUIPMENT USED IN THE PREHOSPITAL
HEALTH-CARE SETTING—cont'd**

Methods

EPA-registered "hospital disinfectants" (no
label claim for tuberculocidal activity).

Use

These agents are excellent cleaners and can be
used for routine housekeeping or removal of
soiling in the absence of visible blood contamination.

Environmental Disinfection

Environmental surfaces that have become
soiled should be cleaned and disinfected using any cleaner or disinfectant agent that is
intended for environmental use. Such surfaces include floors, woodwork, ambulance
seats, countertops, etc.

Important: To ensure the effectiveness of any
sterilization or disinfection process, equipment and instruments must first be thoroughly cleaned of all visible soil.

---

quires. Box 11-7 lists reprocessing methods for
equipment used in the prehospital health-care
setting.

Plastic leakproof bags should be available for
packaging contaminated materials and contaminated personal protective gear. Contaminated
materials must be completely separated from
any other stored items. Prehospital care providers dispose of contaminated materials at the receiving care facility. Specific regulations of the
receiving institutions should be known so that
contaminated material can be packaged and
disposed of according to their regulations. A
summary of OSHA's guidelines for labeling
contaminated materials can be found in Table
11-1.

Used needles and sharps should be placed in
a puncture-resistant plastic container. Needles
should never be recapped or manipulated in any
way after use. The prehospital nurse has a limited supply of medications; therefore it may be
necessary to recap syringes because the patient
may need to be remedicated. When a needle
does need to be recapped, OSHA recommends

a single-handed technique or replacing the cap
with a hemostat.

Although the risk of actual disease from contaminated linen is negligible (U.S. Department
of Health and Human Services, 1989), contaminated linen should be handled as little as possible. It should be placed in a plastic leakproof
bag for disposal. Boots and leather goods may
be brush-scrubbed with soap and hot water to
remove contamination.

Contaminated spills cannot be left at a scene.
Prehospital care nurses should be cognizant of
this fact and try to contain spills. A 1:100
household bleach solution or an approved ger-
micide solution should be used to clean spills
in the prehospital setting (U.S. Department of
Health and Human Services, 1989).

All reusable items, such as trash receptacles,
buckets, mops, and the actual transport vehicle
should be disinfected on a regularly scheduled
basis by the prehospital care provider. All of
these items should be recorded and documented
on a cleaning schedule. Walls and floors typically do not pose a serious threat to the health-

---

Box 11-8

EDUCATIONAL REQUIREMENTS OF AN INFECTION CONTROL PROGRAM

1. An accessible copy and explanation of the regulatory text
2. A general explanation of the epidemiology and symptoms of bloodborne diseases
3. An explanation of:
   a. The modes of transmission of blood-borne pathogens
   b. The written exposure control plan and how to obtain a copy
   c. The basis for selecting personal protective equipment including information on the types, proper use, location, removal, handling, decontamination, and disposal of personal protective equipment
   d. The use and limitations of safe work practices, engineering controls, and personal protective equipment
   e. The procedures to follow if exposure occurs, including methods of reporting and the medical follow-up that will be made available
   f. Information on warning signs, labels, and color coding
4. Information of hepatitis B vaccination such as safety, benefits, efficacy, and availability
5. Information on the postexposure evaluation and follow-up required in the event of an exposure and information on emergencies that relate to blood or other potentially infectious materials, follow-up procedures, and medical counseling

---

Note. From *Occupational Exposure to Bloodborne Pathogens: Precautions for Emergency Responders* (OSHA 3130) by U.S. Department of Labor, Occupational Safety and Health Administration, 1992, Washington, D.C.: The Author.

care provider in transmitting infectious diseases unless there has been direct contact with infectious fluids. Nurses must decide how these areas should be cleaned. If there has been a large amount of blood spilled on the floor from an exsanguinating patient, then more care needs to be taken during decontamination.

EDUCATION

Training is a necessary and important part of the infection control program. The 1992 OSHA guidelines list the parts of the training program that are necessary (Box 11-8). To comply with OSHA standards, all of these parts must be included. OSHA also requires that the instructor be knowledgeable in the specificities of the particular job requirements. For instance, a staff development educator without prehospital experience would not be an appropriate person to educate prehospital nurses. Most institutions have a designated day for instructing their nurses on infection control. Prehospital nurses, even though part of the institution, should prepare their own infection control in-services.

During the in-service training, the staff should be trained in the use of the specific equipment. Hands-on experience with certain equipment has proven to be beneficial. "The application step in the adult learning process cannot be over emphasized" (Rubin, 1993, p. 65).

As a group, the medical team should decide where to place the infection control equipment in their transport vehicle for easy access. As stated before, the infection control equipment becomes as important as medical equipment.

The employer is responsible for record keeping, including training records. Regular in-service should be scheduled and updates given as necessary.

The Indiana State Emergency Management Agency conducted a random survey of Indiana prehospital care providers to measure their attitudes, perceptions, and knowledge of infectious diseases and protective barriers (Linden & Beaver, 1992). They were asked about their education and in-service training in infection control. The survey reported that 71% reported receiving training in infection control in the past year. However, many emergency medical personnel lacked a reasonable degree of knowledge of infectious diseases (scores of 80% or better). Only 18% of the first responders achieved the "reasonable degree" of knowledge.

Often times EMS personnel openly express their concerns about the risk of exposure to HIV. In the study from Indiana, it was documented that the respondents demonstrated significant deficiencies in knowledge about AIDS and held suboptimal attitudes toward AIDS-related issues. (Linden & Beaver, 1992) In 1991 Linden and Beaver performed a study of EMTs and found that they made relatively little use of protective barriers and had exaggerated concerns about the risk of infection even when protective barriers were used.

The results of this study, as well as some health-care providers' inappropriate reactions to exposures, indicate that education should be an ongoing process. The National Flight Nurses Association's (NFNA) position statement is that prehospital care nurses must act as educators and assist with this dissemination of correct information concerning infectious diseases. The first step in this process is for nurses to be knowledgeable so that the correct information can be disseminated. Nurses should be leaders in this area, and this includes being aware of personal attitudes and setting a good example.

QUALITY ASSURANCE

OSHA guidelines from 1991 stated that management is responsible for observing and documenting usage of appropriate protective barriers during patient care and cleaning equipment. In the prehospital setting it is impossible for the manager to observe nursing actions directly.

The manager should be a good role model and provide employees with education; it is up to individual nurses to comply. Based on NFNA and American Nurses Association (ANA) standards nurses should be leaders.

As stated earlier in the chapter, an employee has the right to use personal judgment to decline the use of universal precautions. The employee must document this declination. A manager must follow through and determine if changes should be made to prevent recurrences. An infection control policy should be continually reviewed and updated on a regularly scheduled basis to reflect changes in the prehospital environment.

Prehospital care providers perform their duties under extremely variable conditions. Thus control measures that are simple and uniform across all situations have the greatest likelihood of gaining worker compliance.

Each program has to determine ways to monitor compliance. This can be accomplished by implementing a quality assurance program. The threshold for compliance to quality assurance should be expected to be 100%. Policies should be formulated to give the exact nature of decontaminating equipment. A written record with dates and signatures can be maintained to monitor compliance with cleaning schedules of reusable objects such as buckets, mops, sponges, and the inside of the transport vehicle.

SUMMARY

The number of people with infectious diseases is increasing. The nature of the job puts prehospital nurses at a greater risk for contracting infectious diseases, particularly since the prehospital environment exposes the nurse to inherently unpredictable risks of exposures. General infection control measures should be adapted to these work situations. Implementing and using infection control practices result in a

Table 11-3   Nursing Diagnoses, Interventions, and Evaluative Criteria for Preventing Infection and Establishing Safety

Diagnosis	Interventions	Evaluative Criteria
High risk for infection related to an overall increase risk of infection for prehospital care providers as evidenced by uncontrollable emergent situations, higher percentage of patients with bloody secretions, lack of light, and close working conditions.	Anticipate need for infection control practices. Utilize universal precautions. Utilize body substance isolation when it is difficult to determine the source of the body fluid. Follow OSHA guidelines in proper packaging, labeling, disinfecting, and disposing of contaminated material. Use thicker gloves when decontaminating. Obtain hepatitis B vaccination. Prevent injury.	The nurse will practice primary prevention and be infection free.
High risk for injury related to the work environment.	Think safety. Make safety a number one priority. Recognize high-risk areas for potential injury. Do not recap needles unless using a one-handed technique or with an instrument such as a hemostat. Use sharps containers. Use thicker gloves when working around extrication.	The nurse will be injury free.

safer environment for all. Nurses are role models and educators for other prehospital workers.

OSHA's definition of infection control includes any efforts designed to prevent infection from occurring in both patients and health-care providers. Infection control is a comprehensive, proactive approach to managing the risks associated with infectious diseases. The main goal of infection control practices is primary prevention. It is more productive for nurses to be knowledgeable about the transmission of infectious diseases and to use appropriate interventions than to worry about what to do if they get the disease. Nurses should think safety, work smart, and start the vaccination series.

Table 11-3 summarizes key points for preventing infection and establishing safety in the prehospital care environment.

REFERENCES

Denenberg, R. (1992). Women, immunity, and sex hormones. *Treatment Issues*, Summer/Fall, 6-10.

Lamphear, B.P., Linnemann, C.C., Cannon, C.G., & DeRonde, M.M. (1993). Decline of clinical hepatitis B in workers at a general hospital: Relation to increasing vaccine-induced immunity. *Clinical Infectious Diseases, 16*, 10-14.

Linden, K.W., & Beaver, K.L. (1992). AIDS-related issues and EMS personnel: Results of the Indiana emergency workers survey. Unpublished raw data, Purdue University.

Nelson, D.E. (1990). Self-perception of risk of acquiring AIDS. Unpublished raw data.

Nelson, D.E., Sigell, L.T., Rucker, R.D., & Driggens-Smith, S. (1990). Reaching everyone! AIDS and Cincinnati's health. *Abstract Presented at the Second Annual NADR National Meeting, Bethesda, Maryland.*

Occupational Safety and Health Administration. (1991). *Occupational exposure to bloodborne pathogens: Final rule* (29 CFR Part 1910.1030). Washington, D.C.: U.S. Department of Labor, OSHA.

Rubin, D.L. (1993). A guide to formulating a comprehensive program. *Firehouse,* January, 64-66.

Simone, P. (1993). Symposium on AIDS. *Tb and AIDS.* Symposium conducted by the University of Cincinnati Hospital Nursing Department, Cincinnati.

Skahan, K. (1993). Symposium on AIDS. *Women and children with AIDS.* Symposium conducted by the University of Cincinnati Hospital Nursing Department, Cincinnati.

SmithKline Beecham Pharmaceuticals. (1992). *Hepatitis B: What public safety workers need to know.* USA: The Author.

University of Cincinnati Hospital. (1993). *Bloodborne pathogen exposure control plan.* Cincinnati, OH: Medical Center Health Services.

U.S. Department of Health and Human Services. (1987). *Recommendations for prevention of HIV transmission in health-care settings* (Vol. 36/No. 2S), *Morbidity and Mortality Weekly Report.* Atlanta: Centers for Disease Control and Prevention.

U.S. Department of Health and Human Services, Public Health Service, National Institute for Occupational Safety and Health. (1989). *Guidelines for prevention of transmission of human immunodeficiency virus and hepatitis B virus to health-care and public-safety workers* (DHHS [NIOSH] Publication No. 89-107). Atlanta: Centers for Disease Control and Prevention.

U.S. Department of Labor, Occupational Safety and Health Administration. (1992). *Occupational exposure to bloodborne pathogens: Precautions for emergency responders* (OSHA 3130). Washington, D.C.: The Author.

United States Fire Administration. (1992). *Guide to developing and managing an emergency service infection control program* (FA-112). Emmitsburg, MD: The Author.

Weber, D.J., Hoffmann, K.K., & Rutala, W.A. (1991). Management of the healthcare worker infected with human immunodeficiency virus: Lessons from nosocomial transmission of hepatitis B virus. *Infection Control and Hospital Epidemiology, 12,* 625-630.

CHAPTER **1 2**

Pediatric Transfer and Transport

OBJECTIVES

1. Identify indications for the transport of the ill or injured child
2. Describe the physiological and psychological considerations related to the transport of the ill or injured child
3. Describe the components of a pediatric transport team
4. Describe the nursing care of the ill or injured child before and during transport

COMPETENCIES

1. Identify the physiological and psychological differences between the adult and pediatric patient
2. Identify the equipment needed for the transport of the ill or injured child
3. Perform an assessment of the ill or injured child
4. Prepare the child for transport
5. Perform specific interventions related to the child's illness or injury during transport

Children require transfer and transport when they have potentially serious or life-threatening health conditions. *Transfer* is the process whereby health-care professionals recognize the child's serious health condition and realize that definitive care at a tertiary care center is needed. *Transport* is the act of moving the child from the referring hospital to the tertiary care center by air or ground transportation. Throughout the transport the child is cared for by experienced health-care professionals, and each segment of care is provided at a higher level than the one preceding it (Pon & Notterman, 1993).

The critically ill or injured child is transported by either a specialized pediatric transport team or by selected nurses or physicians from the referring hospital. In either circumstance, the nurse who accompanies the child must be able to safely and effectively care for the child during the transport. There are two types of transfer: one-way and two-way (Pon & Notterman, 1993). *One-way* transfer involves transfer of the child from the referring facility to the tertiary care center. Disadvantages of this system include lack of adequate equipment to care for pediatric patients, as well as lack of personnel who are adept at caring for critically ill or injured children. *Two-way* transfer is when the tertiary care center dispatches a specialized transport team to the referring center and transfers the child to the tertiary care center. Specialized equipment and team expertise in the care of children are the hallmark of this system. Unfortunately, inclement weather or response time may cause delays in transport.

Nurses who provide care for children may find themselves involved either as part of a designated transport team for two-way transfers or as part of a hospital or prehospital system that conducts one-way transfers. Nurses in either situation must be comfortable in the care of critically ill or injured children. The purposes of this chapter are to provide a basic overview of the treatment rendered to children requiring transport and to outline a step-by-step method for preparing the child and team for transport.

INDICATIONS FOR PEDIATRIC TRANSPORT

Kissoon, Frewen, Kronick, and Mohammed (1988) reported that 85% of the children cared for by their pediatric transport team over a 4-year period were 6 years of age and younger. The most frequent health condition involved the central nervous system (53%), and the least frequent condition was multiple trauma (2.7%) (Kissoon, Frewen, Kronick, & Mohammed, 1988). Common reasons for pediatric transport include the following:

- Upper airway emergencies (croup, epiglottitis, and foreign body obstruction)
- Respiratory distress and respiratory failure
- Shock states (hypovolemic, septic, and cardiogenic)
- Postcardiopulmonary resuscitation
- Increased intracranial pressure (ICP) from head injuries or brain tumors
- Uncontrolled seizure activity
- Infectious disease emergencies (e.g., meningitis)

- Metabolic conditions including diabetic ketoacidosis (DKA)
- Poisonings

PHYSIOLOGICAL AND PSYCHOSOCIAL CONSIDERATIONS

The child's physiological and psychosocial differences must be considered when determining the child's need for transfer and when preparing the child for transport. Airway, breathing, and circulation management are the priorities of care, but some additional factors must be considered when transferring and transporting children. The following considerations help the transport nurse to care for the child safely and effectively.

Airway and Ventilation

Because the infant's and younger child's airway is narrow in diameter, it is easily obstructed. Therefore every attempt is made to protect the child's airway, which becomes even more tenuous if the child has an infection or is injured. For the child with suspected epiglottitis or upper airway obstruction, the child should be positioned comfortably; the child should not be placed in a supine position because the airway may become compromised. Every effort is made to keep the child calm, since agitation can cause complete airway obstruction. In the transport of a child with a potential for airway compromise, the parent(s) should be present during the transport, if at all possible. For ground transport, a parent can be secured on the stretcher and allowed to hold the child on the lap. The child is then secured as best as possible. The presence of a parent during air transport is determined by the size of the helicopter, season of the year, and the transport system's rules about transporting family members. Family presence during transport may help to calm the child, thereby preserving airway integrity. No invasive procedures are attempted, including cardiac monitoring. Astute observation of the child's work of breathing is paramount. If the transport time is long or if the child is in impending respiratory failure, the airway must be secured before transport. In the case of epiglottitis, the airway is secured in the operating room by an experienced pediatric critical care physician or anesthesiologist. Throughout the child's intubation, sedation and paralyzation are recommended. The child cannot be transported without such medications because of the risk of self-extubation during transport. Once the child is intubated, 100% oxygen must be delivered through a bag-valve-mask device or a ventilator. A nasogastric tube must also be inserted to prevent gastric distention and subsequent diaphragmatic pressure.

If the decision is made to transport the child without a secure airway, the equipment to maintain airway patency must be prepared and available during transport. Should the child become unable to maintain a patent airway, several maneuvers can be attempted. The jaw-thrust (used in the trauma patient) or head-tilt/chin-lift maneuver (used in the nontrauma patient) can be used to open the airway. An oropharyngeal airway can be inserted in the unconscious child who does not have a gag reflex; insertion is determined by measuring from the corner of the mouth to the angle of the jaw. The airway is inserted with a tongue blade directly into the mouth; it is not turned 90 degrees as in the adult, since tissue damage may occur. A nasal airway (trumpet) can be inserted into the child with a gag reflex. This airway is inserted by measuring from the naris to the tragus of the ear and can be lubricated before insertion. Suction must be available and in working order should vomiting occur. An appropriately sized bag-valve-mask device and oxygen are available should the child require positive pressure ventilation.

Because children have fewer alveoli and therefore less respiratory reserve that adults, attention to the work of breathing is essential.

The child in respiratory distress is maintained in a position of comfort throughout the transport; therefore safety and securing measures may have to be adapted. For example, the stretcher straps can be criss-crossed over the child's chest to secure the child. Also, harness devices are available to better secure the child. If the child displays signs of impending respiratory failure, transport is not attempted until the child is stabilized. Signs of impending respiratory failure include the following:

- An increased work of breathing
- Retractions
- Head bobbing
- Nasal flaring
- Grunting
- Decreased activity level
- Decreased interest in the environment
- Pale skin
- Delayed capillary refill
- Poor air exchange
- Increased inspiratory-expiratory ratio
- Pulse oximetry readings below 90% on oxygen
- Tachycardia

In early respiratory distress the child is tachypneic; bradypnea is a signal of impending respiratory failure. Oxygen is *never* withheld from a child and is delivered through a variety of methods. Nasal cannula prongs are cut and lubricated before placement in the nares to prevent mucosal irritation. The cannula is taped to the child's face to secure its placement. A properly fitting oxygen mask does not cover the child's eyes and face. If the mask is too large or the child becomes agitated with its application, the mask is held near the child's face, and the child is able to breathe the oxygen. Another method of oxygen administration is the "blow-by" method, in which blue corrugated tubing is connected to the oxygen tubing; the blue tubing is held by the child's face, and the child breathes the oxygen. (Figure 12-1). Pulse oximetry can be used to measure the child's oxygen saturation levels.

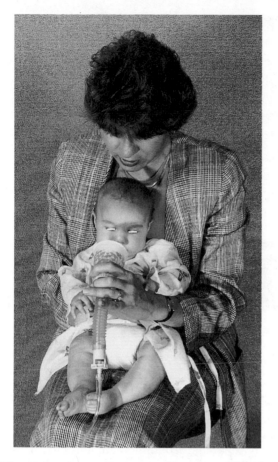

Fig. 12-1   A paper cup may distract a child who needs oxygen.

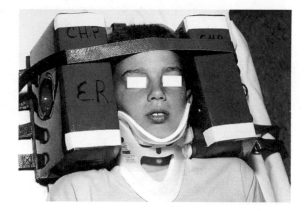

Fig. 12-2   A method of immobilizing a child's cervical spine.

Special attention to the airway is essential in the injured child. In addition to using the jaw-thrust technique, the cervical spine must be stabilized. The cervical spine must remain midline to prevent hyperextension of the neck, which could lead to a spinal cord injury. Spinal immobilization includes the application of a cervical collar, the use of a cervical immobilization device, and a long back board or commercially available pediatric immobilization device. The cervical collar fits correctly if the chin rests in the chin holder, the collar does not cover the ears, and the bottom of the collar rests above the upper sternum (Bernardo & Waggoner, 1992). A collar that is too large may push the jaw backward and cause an airway obstruction; a collar that is too small will not provide adequate alignment and may compromise the airway (Bernardo & Waggoner, 1992). When a cervical immobilization device is used, the chin strap is not applied, since the strap may push the jaw backward, thus compromising the airway and increasing the risk of aspiration should vomiting occur (Lang, 1993) (Figure 12-2). Various methods can be used to strap the child onto the long back board; one method is depicted in Figure 12-3. An infant can be secured in a car seat if the car seat is intact; one method for securing an infant in a car seat is depicted in Figure 12-4.

Circulation

Children have greater cardiac reserves than adults and can maintain their circulatory perfusion for a prolonged period of time. In early shock the child is tachycardic, tachypneic, and has a slightly elevated blood pressure. If these are unrecognized or untreated, profound shock occurs. Signs of impending shock are decreased capillary refill, cool, clammy skin, mottled skin color, tachycardia, tachypnea, and altered level

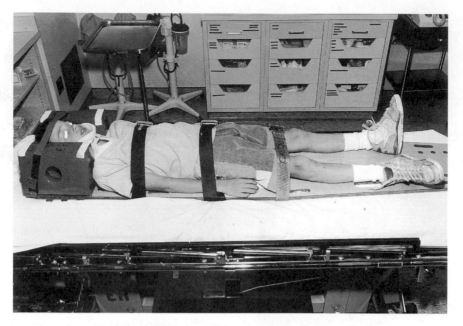

Fig. 12-3   Immobilization of a pediatric patient on a backboard.

of consciousness (does not recognize family members or show interest in the environment). A decreased blood pressure is a *late* sign of shock, as well as bradycardia and apnea. If the child exhibits signs of shock, transport is delayed until stabilization is attempted. Stabilization includes airway and breathing management, followed by the initiation of two large-bore intravenous catheters (22 gauge and larger). Because intravenous attempts may be difficult, an intraosseous device is inserted after three attempts or 90 seconds. Central line insertion or venous cutdown is reserved for practitioners skilled in this technique. An arterial line may be initiated if the transport is prolonged, a practitioner is experienced in the technique, and the equipment to perform the procedure and monitor the arterial blood pressure are available.

Depending on the type of shock, intravenous fluids are administered at different rates. For hypovolemic shock, lactated Ringer's solution or normal saline solution is administered. Three fluid boluses are administered at 20 ml/kg each. It is helpful to have a stopcock connected to the intravenous tubing to facilitate delivery of the medications and boluses. The child is reassessed for improvement after each bolus; improvement is measured by an increase in blood pressure, decrease in heart rate, an increase in peripheral perfusion, and improved mentation. If the hypovolemic child does not respond to these three boluses, then a bolus of packed cells is administered at 10 ml/kg. If the blood is available, it should not be withheld from the child in hypovolemic shock; it should, however, be warmed before administration to prevent hypothermia. If available, 5% albumin or Plasmanate can be administered.

The child can be in hypovolemic shock from

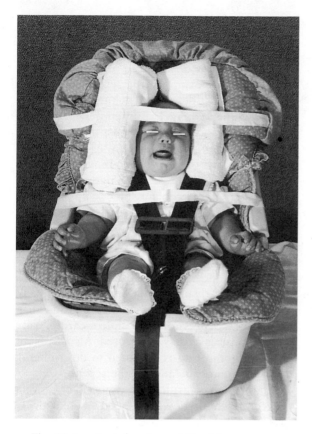

Fig. 12-4   An infant immobilized in a car seat.

gastroenteritis with prolonged vomiting and diarrhea. The child with severe dehydration has the following features:

- Decreased skin turgor
- Sunken eyes
- Dry mouth, lips, mucous membranes, and skin
- Tachycardia
- Tachypnea
- Decreased urine output
- Decreased attention to the environment
- Infants may not have tears and may have a sunken fontanel

Management of the child with dehydration includes fluid resuscitation with lactated Ringer's or normal saline at 20 ml/kg for the first hour. Subsequent hourly rates and types of fluids are based on the laboratory results (decreased CO_2, improved base excess, improved bicarbonate, and decreased blood urea nitrogen and creatinine levels). Glucose is added to subsequent intravenous fluids to prevent hypoglycemia.

The child in septic shock may have petechiae, along with the aforementioned signs of shock. Intravenous fluids of lactated Ringer's or normal saline are given, along with fluid boluses. Albumin or Plasmanate can also be given. After bolusing, maintenance fluids are administered. Glucose monitoring is necessary to prevent hypoglycemia. If there are no changes in the child's situation, vasopressor therapy with a continuous infusion of dopamine may be administered. Antibiotic administration is also initiated. Insertion of an arterial line may also be considered.

In cardiogenic shock intravenous fluids of lactated Ringer's or normal saline are given. However, fluid intake is restricted to avoid fluid overload. If vasopressor therapy is needed, dobutamine is the drug of choice.

Neurological Status

Changes in level of consciousness are difficult to measure in children. The best determinant is the child's ability to recognize the family and familiar objects. The child's attention to the environment is another indicator of level of consciousness. The child who appears unconcerned about or uninterested in the busy emergency department environment or does not mind separation from the parents is worrisome. After airway, breathing, and circulation management is ensured, further neurological evaluation is warranted.

The Glasgow coma scale helps to document trends in neurological functioning. The pediatric Glasgow coma scale is better for infants and young children because it is more descriptive in *best verbal response*. Best verbal response includes coos, babbles, smiles (5 points); irritable, crying (4 points); cries, screams to pain (3 points); moans, grunts (2 points); and no response (1 point). Sequential neurological testing with this scale helps to determine neurological changes during transport.

Increases in ICP are either chronic or acute. Chronic increased ICP is observed in children with hydrocephalus who may not have a ventriculoperiotoneal shunt. These children may have a large head and sunset eyes. Acute increased ICP is measured by changes in mental status, irritability or combativeness, lethargy, vomiting, and papilledema. Retinal hemorrhaging is a sign of shaken impact syndrome, warranting investigation into possible child maltreatment. Pupillary changes and bradycardia are *late* signs of increased ICP. In the child with increased ICP, endotracheal intubation is accomplished using rapid sequence intubation. Hyperventilation is initiated to decrease ICP. Mannitol is administered as indicated. Intravenous fluids are restricted, and the head of the bed is elevated 30 degrees. A quiet and calm environment is highly recommended to decrease ICP fluctuations.

Children with ventriculoperitoneal shunts may develop shunt infections or shunt malfunction. The child with a shunt infection is febrile, irritable, complains of a headache, and has an elevated white blood cell count. The child with a malfunctioning shunt exhibits signs of increased ICP, as noted previously. For the child with a shunt malfunction who has increased ICP, narcotic analgesics are not administered to relieve the headache, since this may cause respiratory depression.

If increased ICP is suspected in the child with meningitis, a lumbar puncture is not attempted because of the potential for brain stem herniation. Infectious disease precautions, such as masks, should be worn in the case of suspected meningitis. In the child with suspected meningitis, the referring hospital may defer the lumbar puncture until the pediatric transport team arrives or the child is admitted to the tertiary care center.

Seizure activity in infants and children is different from that observed in adults and varies with ages. For example, the seizure activity in the infant includes lip smacking, nystagmus, and yawning. Younger children may have petit mal seizures, in which the seizure activity is limited to twitching of the extremities. Grand mal seizures consist of tonic/clonic movements with a loss of consciousness. The length and type of seizure activity are documented. The airway is opened with the chin-lift method and suctioned as needed. Oxygen is administered, and an intravenous catheter is inserted. The child with a first-time seizure is managed with phenytoin (Dilantin) and phenobarbital, followed by lorazepam (Ativan) or diazepam (Valium), as needed. Since anticonvulsant therapy can cause respiratory depression, the child's cardiorespiratory status is closely monitored. Also, bedside glucose monitoring is obtained to determine if hypoglycemia is a cause of the seizure.

Changes in neurological status may be observed in children with diabetic ketoacidosis (DKA). DKA is treated differently in children as compared with adults, since rehydration, not glucose lowering, is the goal of care. Children with DKA are recognized by altered mental status, Kussmaul respirations, fruity breath, and signs of dehydration. The parents report a history of frequent urination and drinking. Airway, breathing, and circulation interventions are immediate priorities. Glucose testing can reveal a glucose as high as 1200. Rehydration is initiated through intravenous solutions of normal saline; insulin is not considered at this time because the goal is to lower the child's glucose level no faster than 100 mg/dl/hour, and this should be monitored closely. Lowering the glucose level faster than this rate will lead to an increase in ICP. Other considerations include adding sodium bicarbonate and potassium to the intravenous solutions based on laboratory analyses of blood and urine. Careful intake and output monitoring is documented. An indwelling bladder catheter is also inserted and secured.

THE PEDIATRIC TRANSPORT TEAM

Pediatric patients should be transported by health-care professionals who are educated and

---

Box 12-1

EDUCATION GOALS FOR PEDIATRIC TRANSPORT TEAM MEMBERS

1. Obtain and record a concise but complete patient history
2. Perform a complete physical examination and record the findings
3. Learn the pathophysiology of pediatric (and neonatal) respiratory, cardiac, neurological, infectious, metabolic, toxicological, traumatic, and other surgical disorders
4. Learn to identify respiratory failure and the indications for respiratory support
5. Learn to identify and differentiate between the causes of shock and the indications for circulatory support
6. Identify the problems affecting an acutely ill child
7. Establish a management plan and initiate appropriate intervention
8. Stabilize the child's condition before transport by preventing or correcting hypoxemia, hypercarbia, acidosis, and hypothermia, among other conditions
9. Communicate and interact effectively with patients and both the referring and receiving health-care team
10. Maintain critical care during the transport
11. Learn the impact of aeromedical transportation on the child's physiology

---

Note. From "Staff and Equipment for Pediatric Critical Care Transport" by S.E. Krug, 1992, *Current Opinion in Pediatrics, 4,* pp. 447-448.

skilled in the care of children (Day, McCloskey, Orr, Bolte, Notterman, & Hackel, 1991). Krug (1992) identified 11 educational goals for transport team members (Box 12-1). These healthcare professionals who make up the pediatric transport team include a qualified pediatric medical specialist and professionals qualified to care for critically ill children in the transport environment (American Academy of Pediatrics [AAP], 1988). The American Academy of Pediatrics (AAP) (1988) recommends that physicians (minimal third-year resident level of training), nurses, respiratory therapists, and emergency medical technicians and paramedics have expertise in pediatric care. The minimal requirements for a pediatric transport nurse, according to the AAP (1988) are a registered nurse licensed to practice within the state and a minimum of 1 year of pediatric critical care experience. The transport nurse must be experienced, organized, and have the ability to adapt to obstacles encountered in an ever-changing environment. Furthermore the AAP (1988) recommends that a critical number of patients must be transported so that transport team members maintain their skills. Formal and continuing education for all team members includes didactic and skill sessions related to the care of children, the usage of equipment, and the effects of the transport environment on the child and team (AAP, 1988). Such continuing education includes the emergency nursing pediatrics course (ENPC) (Emergency Nurses Association), pediatric advanced life support (PALS) (American Heart Association and American Academy of Pediatrics), and neonatal advanced life support (NALS) (American Academy of Pediatrics).

These recommendations are not uniform from hospital to hospital. For example, nurses who transport patients may routinely work in the pediatric intensive care unit or emergency department and may be called out for transport as needed; or nurses may be dedicated to pediatric transport only, with a separate budget and staff. The dedicated transport nurse system is far superior to the nondedicated transport nurse system for the following reasons (Day, et al., 1991):

1. Patient care may decline in the area from which the nurse is "reassigned" when dispatched for transport.
2. Planning and implementation of the transport go more smoothly with a dedicated team, since delays are prevented.
3. Equipment tracking and maintenance are improved.
4. Separate transport policies, procedures, and protocols, as well as quality improvement measures, can be developed and executed.
5. Follow-up communication with the referring hospitals and education outreach programs are enhanced.

The transport physicians may be experienced in critical care or emergency medicine; they can be attending physicians or fellows and be board-eligible or board-certified in their fields. Their technical skills and experience, however, are variable. Each pediatric transport should be supervised by a designated, experienced attending pediatric critical care or emergency physician (Day, et al., 1991).

The presence of a physician for every patient transport is addressed through research. McCloskey, King, and Byron (1989) surveyed pediatric transport physicians to determine if their presence was needed on transports. In at least 46% of the transports, the physicians believed that their expertise was not required. These researchers concluded that, based on their other findings of few required procedures and medications, a physician may not always be needed on pediatric transports.

In a later study, McCloskey, Faries, King, Orr, and Plouff (1992) sought to determine when a pediatric transport team was required to transport a child to a tertiary care center. A survey of transport physicians after the transport showed that in 43% of the cases the physicians believed their presence was needed. Af-ter reviewing the team's records they found that children less than 1 year of age who were endotracheally intubated and had unstable vital signs were predictive of the need for a pediatric transport team. For some hospitals, then, the transport team composition could be tailored to best meet the anticipated needs of the patient (Day, et al., 1991).

The pediatric transport team must be available 24 hours a day, 7 days a week. Optimally the team is on call from the hospital; however, some teams take call from their homes. Ideally the time from notification to departure of ground or air transport systems should be approximately 10 minutes. The recommended time from notification to departure by ground transport is about 30 minutes (Aoki & McCloskey, 1992; Day, et al. 1991); less than 45 minutes is recommended for air transport (AAP, 1986) for gathering of team members. "If the team consistently takes much longer than 40 minutes to leave, the tertiary level hospital must reevaluate the design of the transport system in an effort to decrease that time period" (Aoki & McCloskey, 1992, p. 338). Again, a quality improvement system to monitor and track response times should be in place.

Preexisting arrangements with helicopter, fixed-wing aircraft, and ambulance service must be in place. It is the responsibility of the transport team director to ensure the team's safety by investigating these flight and ambulance services for their maintenance, safety, equipment reliability, and pilot/driver/EMT or paramedic experience (Day, et al., 1991). A standard amount of time from their notification to their arrival at the hospital must be a mutual agreement. Agreements concerning the type of equipment each service provides and equipment and vehicle maintenance must also be secured.

NOTIFICATION FROM THE REFERRING FACILITY

The receiving hospital must have an organized system for directing incoming calls to the appropriate pediatric transport personnel. Some facilities have a dispatch system that co-ordinates the direction of the call to the appropriate pediatric transport person. The dispatcher receiving the call must be knowledgeable and experienced in triaging the call to the appropriate transport person and should be experienced with basic pediatric medical terminology. A minimum requirement for the dispatcher is EMT training. A quality improvement mechanism to measure the accuracy and effectiveness of the communications system should be in place (Day, et al., 1991).

When the call from the referring facility is received by the dispatcher, the dispatcher obtains a brief initial report. This information includes the name of the hospital, city and state, phone number, the caller, the name and age of the patient, the patient's diagnosis, and the patient's location in the referring hospital (e.g., emergency department, intensive care unit, or pediatric unit). Then the dispatcher notifies the entire pediatric transport team with one telephone call or radio notification. With the caller on the telephone, the pediatric transport physician is conferenced with the caller. This process should not exceed 5 minutes' time.

The pediatric transport physician obtains further information from the caller at the referring hospital. This information is documented in a transport log for future reference, since the log becomes part of the medical record. The physician obtains further patient assessment data, which include respiratory status, neurological status, and pertinent laboratory results and diagnostic findings. Recommendations for interventions are then made. In the meantime the dispatcher has already notified the ground or air transport service for the appropriate mode of transport.

PREPARATION FOR TRANSPORT

Each member of the transport team has responsibilities for preparation for transport. The transport nurse begins to prepare the equip-

ment for transport. This equipment is dedicated to the transport team only and should be in an accessible location, always prepared and double checked (Table 12-1). Standardized equipment is taken on all transports. The prepared equipment pack includes supplies and medications (Box 12-2). The nurse obtains the appropriate type of cardiac monitor (life pack 10 for a child, or a neonatal monitor for an infant) and a pulse oximeter. The nurse determines the number of intravenous pumps that may be needed, with the minimum number being two, and these should be small, battery-operated, syringe-type continuous infusion pumps. If air transport is indicated, the stretcher is already prepared with the oxygen tank, monitor, and equipment pack. Equipment preparation time should not exceed 5 minutes.

As time permits, the nurse prepares for the patient based on the information obtained by the transport physician. Preparation includes preparing intravenous fluids and resuscitation medications. Heat packs are also taken for infants less than 4 to 5 months of age and children with known hypothermia or postresuscitation.

The respiratory therapist is responsible for obtaining the portable ventilator (for example, Omni-vent or Uni-vent) as indicated, as well as the respiratory equipment pack. Infants in isolettes require an appropriate infant ventilator (e.g., Health-Dyne ventilator). A circuit consisting of a Laerdal resuscitation bag connected to the ventilator circuit adapted with changeable positive end-expiratory pressure (PEEP) valves and peak inspiratory pressure (PIP) control is useful if manual ventilation (such as a transport less than 15 minutes) is an option for some transport teams. This circuit, besides providing PEEP and PIP changes, also allows the transport team members to be able to sit securely in their seats without leaning over the patient. This equipment ideally is stored in one location and dedicated to the transport team.

The team meets in a predesignated central location, such as the helipad or emergency de-

Table 12-1 Quick Reference to Pediatric Emergency Equipment*

Equipment	Premature	Neonate	6 Mo.	1 Y	2 Y	3 Y	4 Y
Airway							
Oral airway† (size)	Infant	Infant/Small	Small	Small	Small	Small	Medium
Endotracheal tube‡ (mm) (* = cuffed)	2.5-3.0	3.0-3.5	3.5-4.0	4.0-4.5	4.0-4.5	4.0-4.5	5.0-5.5
Laryngoscope blade† (s, straight; c, curved)	0 s	1 s	1 s	1 s	1 s	1 s	2 s/c
Suction cathe-ter‡ (French)	5	6	6	8	8	8	10
Breathing							
Face mask† (size)	Premie NB	NB	NB	Pediatric	Pediatric	Pediatric	Pediatric
Bag-valve de-vice† (size)	Infant	Infant	Infant	Pediatric	Pediatric	Pediatric	Pediatric
Chest tube† (French)	10-14	12-18	14-20	14-24	14-24	14-24	20-32
Circulation							
Over-the-needle cathe-ter§ (gauge)	22-24	22-24	22-24	20-22	20-22	20-22	20-22
Intraosseous device (gauge)	18	15	15	15	15	15	15
Gastrointestinal/Genitourinary							
Nasogastric tube‖ (French)	5	5	8	8	10	10	10
Urinary cathe-ter† (French)	5 feeding tube	5-8 feeding tube	8	10	10	10	10-12

*This reference demonstrates suggested sizes only. Always consider each child's size and health condition when selecting appropriate equipment for procedures.
†Committee on Trauma, *Advanced Trauma Life Support Student Manual*. Chicago: American College of Surgeons, 1989, 231.
‡Endotracheal intubation. In Motoyama E. and Davis P. (Eds). *Smith's Anesthesia for Infants and Children*. St. Louis: Mosby, 1990, 275.
§Chameides L. (Ed). *Textbook of Pediatric Advanced Life Support*. Dallas: American Heart Association and American Academy of Pediatrics, 1988, 105.
‖Skale N. *Manual of Pediatric Nursing Procedures*. Philadelphia: JB Lippincott, 1992, 407.

5 Y	6 Y	7 Y	8 Y	9 Y	10 Y	11-18 Y
Medium	Medium	Medium	Medium/large	Medium/large	Medium/large	Large
5.0-5.5	5.5-6.0	5.5-6.0	6.0*-6.5*	6.0*-6.5*	6.0*-6.5*	7.0*-8.0*
2 s/c	2 s/c	2 s/c	2-3 s/c	2-3 s/c	2-3 s/c	3 s/c
10	10	10	10	10	10	12
Pediatric	Pediatric	Pediatric	Adult	Adult	Adult	Adult
Pediatric	Pediatric	Pediatric/adult	Adult	Adult	Adult	Adult
20-32	20-32	20-32	28-38	28-38	28-38	28-38
18-22	18-20	18-20	16-20	16-20	16-20	14-18
15	—	—	—	—	—	—
10	10	12	12	12	12	14-16
10-12	10-12	10-12	12	12	12	12-18

Box 12-2
CONTENTS OF THE PACIFIC EMERGENCY PACK: AN EXAMPLE OF A PEDIATRIC EMERGENCY TRANSPORT PACK

Compartment A
Pocket #1

500-ml bag of 10% dextrose in water
Stopcocks: Cobes (3) and Pharmaseal (1)

Pocket #2

250-ml bag of 5% dextrose/0.25 normal saline solution (NSS)
250-ml bag of 0.9 NSS

Pocket #3

Cobe arterial pressure line tubing: 4
Minidrip
Extension set: 2
T-connector: 2

Loops

60-ml Luer-Lok syringes: 4
30-ml syringes: 2
20-ml syringes: 2
18-gauge needles: 10
Syringes: 5 each of 5 ml and 10 ml

Zipper compartment

Pressure kit
250-ml bag of 0.9 NSS
1 ml heparin 1000 U/ml

Compartment B
Pocket #1

Pediatric and adult nonrebreather masks
Nasal cannulas (adult, pediatric, infant)

Pocket #2

Venturi mask and Venturi setup
Nebulizer kit
Albuterol (Proventil) prediluted (3)

Loops

Oral airways: 1 each of 70, 80, 90, and 100 mm

NSS bullets (5)
Flashlight

Zipper compartment

Nasopharygeal airways: 14, 16, 18, 20, 22, 24, 26
8 Feeding tube
#10 Replogle catheter
#10 Anderson sump
Catheter tip syringe
2 Surgilubes
1-inch tape

Compartment C
Plastic bag

Extension set
3-ml syringe
30-ml syringe
1-inch white adhesive tape
1 vial 0.9 NSS (10-ml vial)
1 heparin lock (10 USP units/ml)
T-connector
18-gauge fill needle
Alcohol wipes (10)
Ames Gulcometer kit
Glucofilm test strips (1 bottle)
1 paper towel

Compartment D

Yellow drug box
Cutdown set
Infant O_2 hood
Nellcor probes (neonatal, infant, pediatric, adult)

Universal precaution set

3 pairs nonsterile gloves
3 masks/goggles or shields
3 gowns

Box 12-2
CONTENTS OF THE PACIFIC EMERGENCY PACK: AN EXAMPLE
OF A PEDIATRIC EMERGENCY TRANSPORT PACK—cont'd

Monitor supplies (located in respiratory
drawstring bag)

Infant EKG electrodes (2)
Adult EKG electrodes (2)
Transducer
Rectal probe (corometric)
Skin probe covers

Compartment E
Plastic bag

Extension set
Infant disposable blood pressure cuff
Neonatal disposable blood pressure cuff
3-way stopcock
Doppler gel
Handheld manometer
Thermometer

Within pocket

Infant, child and adult blood pressure cuff
   with adaptable manometer for all three cuffs

Compartment F
Zipper compartment

Umbilical catheters: 2 each of sizes 3.5 and
   5.0
Umbilical tape
Cook catheter access tray
Cook catheters and wires: 5 Fr/5 CM DB; 5
   FR/8 CM DB; 3 FR/8 CM SGL
1 extra guidewire: C-DOC/diameter, 18;
   length, 50; curve, 0-3
Fuhrman pleural and pneumopericardial drain-
   age set
Trocar catheters: 10 French and 16 French
Large sterile Y adaptors (2)
Heimlick valve
2 packs 3 × 9 Vaseline gauze

Front of Main Compartment
Endotracheal tubes

Uncuffed: 2 each of sizes 2.0, 2.5, 3.0, 3.5
Cuffed ETT: 4.0 (2 each)
Small and medium stylet
Cuffed: 2 each of 5.0, 6.0, 7.0, 8.0
Large stylet
Magill forceps
Kolodny forceps

Intubation pack

½- and 1-inch roll adhesive tape
2 packets surgilube and benzoin
2 size-C batteries
2 small and 2 large laryngoscope bulbs
Bite block
14 French O_2 suction catheter
Laryngoscope handle
Miller blades: 1 each of 0, 1, 2, 3
Macintosh 3 and Wis-Hipple 1.5

Arrest/intubation medications

Epinephrine 1:10,000: Bristojet (0.1 mg/ml)
Calcium chloride 10%: (100 mg/ml) 10-ml
   vial
Lidocaine 2%: Bristojet (20 mg/ml)
Sodium bicarbonate 50-ml vial: (1 meq/ml)
Atropine (0.4 mg/ml vial) 3 each of 1-ml vials
Mannitol 25% vials: 2 each
Vecuronium and sterile water (2 each)
NSS 0.9-vials: 2 each of 10 ml
Ketamine: 20-ml vial (10 mg/ml)
Pentothal Bristojet: (250 mg/10 ml) 2 each
   (beside arrest pack)
Terbutaline: 10 ampules (1 mg/ml) in box
Pack of nonsterile 4 × 4s

Respiratory support

Laerdal resuscitation bags (adult and infant)
Extension tubing (for manometer)

Continued.

Box 12-2
CONTENTS OF THE PACIFIC EMERGENCY PACK: AN EXAMPLE
OF A PEDIATRIC EMERGENCY TRANSPORT PACK—cont'd

Swivel adaptor
Gas diverter
Manometer
Manometer adaptor
PEEP valves: 2.5, 5.0, 10

Rear of Compartment
Intravenous access pack

Outside pockets: 6 each of 1-ml syringes and
   8 each of 3-ml syringes and 15 alcohol
   wipes
Inside pack: Infant cloth restraints
2 filter needles
2 benzoin swabs
20 alcohol wipes
3 sterile 2 × 2s
2 skin prep wipes
4 Betadine wipes
Neonatal armboard
Infant armboard
1- and ½ -inch white adhesive tape
T-connectors (3)
Butterfly catheters: 2 each of 23 and 25 gauge

10-ml vials of 0.9 NSS: 4 each
Medi-Port access needle
Intraosseous needle, 15-gauge adjustable
Tourniquet
IV Quik catheters: 24 (5 each)
                   22 (3 each)
                   18, 16, 14 (1 each)
1 insulin syringe

Loops

4 1-ml syringes (in package)
4 3-ml syringes (in package)
5% Albumin (250 ml)
Resuscitation facemasks: 1 each of newborn,
   infant, toddler, child, and adult
Suction catheters: Yankauer suction catheter
                   14 French O_2 suction cathe-
                   ter
Suction catheters: 2 each of
   6, 8, 10, 14
2 sterile gloves
1 #8 DeLee suction trap

---

partment ambulance entrance. The equipment is loaded into the vehicle and secured. Finally the transport team secures itself in the vehicle.

NURSING RESPONSIBILITIES EN ROUTE TO THE HOSPITAL

En route to receiving the child, the team makes specific care plans. These plans include medications, antibiotics, or types of intravenous fluids. Each team member has assigned responsibilities that must be carried out on arrival. The team also finishes the medication calculations and anticipates and prepares equip-

ment that might be needed. For example, if airway compromise is anticipated, the team prepares the appropriately sized endotracheal intubation equipment, including endotracheal tubes one size smaller and one size larger than calculated, as well as any medications for rapid-sequence intubation (Table 12-2), as time permits. En route time varies from minutes to hours, depending on the mode of transport, distance, and weather conditions. Updated information may be relayed to the team, such as the results of any diagnostic tests or interventions suggested by the pediatric transport physician at the time of the initial call. This information

Table 12-2   Medications for Rapid-Sequence Intubation

Medication	Dose Range	Indications	Comments
Atropine	0.1 mg/kg 0.5 mg/kg maximum	Prevents bradycardia	Elect not to use if child is tachycardic
Lidocaine	1 mg/kg	Decreases intracranial pressure; decreases vagal stimulation	
Sedation			
Fentanyl	2 mcg/kg	Sedation	May cause hypotension
Midazolam (Versed)	0.035 mg/kg 0.2 mg/kg maximum	Sedation	May cause hypotension; give over 2 minutes
Thiopental (Pentothal)	3-5 mg/kg		May cause respiratory depression and hypotension
Paralysis			
Vecuronium	0.1 mg/kg to 0.2 mg/kg	Paralyzation	Apnea; must be able to manually ventilate patient; administer *after* sedation

may be relayed by cellular telephone or radio frequency.

NURSING RESPONSIBILITIES UPON ARRIVAL

When the transport team arrives at the referring hospital, they are, in effect, agents of their own hospital. The patient, then, is actually admitted to the receiving hospital and is cared for accordingly (Day, et al., 1991). This belief, then, negates the need for multistate licensure if the pediatric transport team accepts patients from outside of the state in which they are licensed to practice (Day, et al., 1991).

Upon arrival the pediatric transport nurse introduces the transport team to the referring hospital staff, patient, and family. The transport nurse conducts a cursory visual assessment of the child. If the child appears to be in stable condition, the transport nurse obtains a report from the referring nurse. If the child appears unstable (e.g., active seizures), the transport

nurse forgoes the report and focuses attention on the child's needs. Universal precautions are always maintained. If infectious diseases are suspected, such as meningococcemia, face masks are indicated.

The priorities of assessment and interventions are airway, breathing, and circulation. The airway is assessed for patency, with any snoring or stridor noted. The patency of any airway adjuncts, such as an endotracheal tube, is assessed. If the airway is not patent, maneuvers to open the airway are made. Positioning and suctioning are attempted; endotracheal intubation is indicated in the child who is in impending respiratory failure or who is unable to maintain the airway. The team prepares the medications for rapid-sequence intubation, places the patient on a cardiac monitor and pulse oximeter, and prepares the endotracheal tube tape. The child is preoxygenated with 100% oxygen before the intubation attempt. While the physician or designated transport team member is performing the intubation, the respiratory therapist is preparing the ventilator. Cricothyrotomy and tracheostomy are rarely performed by the pediatric transport team; however, if such a procedure is needed, the necessary equipment must be readily available in the transport team equipment pack.

Next, the child's breathing is assessed. The child's work of breathing is observed by symmetrical chest rise and fall, respiratory rate and effort, and skin color. Breath sounds are auscultated in the lung fields; retractions, wheezing, and adventitious sounds are noted, as well as the absence of breath sounds. Supplemental oxygen devices are assessed, including the type of oxygenation device, the percent of oxygen, and liter flow. The child's tolerance of the supplemental oxygen is noted. If the child is not receiving any oxygen but appears to need it, the oxygen is applied at this time in a manner tolerated by the child. Bag-valve-mask ventilation is initiated if the child is apneic or is in respiratory failure. The bag should be able to deliver a minimum of 450 ml of air. If present, the pop-off valve must be occluded to allow for sufficient ventilation. The mask must fit the child's face snugly and must not cover the eyes. An adult bag can be used effectively in the apneic child if a pediatric-size bag is not available, since the child is ventilated only until the chest rises. If the child is intubated, the ventilator is prepared by the respiratory therapist. Ventilator settings are determined by the chest rise and fall and lung compliance. Administration of 100% oxygen is standard in the vast majority of patients.

The child's circulatory status is assessed by capillary refill, skin color and temperature, peripheral pulses, and an apical heart rate and blood pressure. Signs and symptoms of shock are assessed. If the child appears to be in shock, at least one intravenous line is initiated. If an intravenous line is not secured within three attempts, an intraosseous device is initiated. However, equipment for central line placement must be available. When the IV is initiated,

---

Box 12-3
PEDIATRIC FLUID CALCULATIONS

Fluid Boluses

20 ml/kg of normal saline solution or lactated Ringer's solution administered two times. If no improvement in the child's condition is observed, consider administering blood at 10 ml/kg

Maintenance Fluid Calculations

100 ml/kg for the first 10 kg
50 ml/kg for the next 10 kg
20 ml/kg for the remaining kg

---

blood is sent for further tests relative to the patient's condition. Glucose testing is conducted to determine hypoglycemia (see Box 12-3 for intravenous fluid considerations). All pediatric IV lines must be infused with an infusion pump to ensure accuracy of delivery. If the patient is unstable, a stopcock is placed on the IV tubing. Also, needleless intravenous administration systems should be used for safety. When moving, such as in an ambulance or helicopter, it is easier to infuse a medication through the stopcock than to risk needle-stick injury. If IV lines are already in place, they are assessed for patency, which may include removing the current dressing, applying a new one, and immobilizing the extremity. A T-connecter is applied to the IV catheter to facilitate medication delivery. IV fluids are assessed for their appropriateness and rate, as well as the amount that has been infused.

Next, a brief neurological assessment is obtained; this includes pupillary reactivity and best motor, verbal, and eye opening responses. The child's level of consciousness is ascertained. This includes the child's ability to recognize the family, know name and age, ability to obey simple commands, and interest in the environment. Posturing and seizure activity are also noted. The pediatric Glasgow coma scale is helpful in measuring mental status. Finally, a rapid head-to-toe assessment is conducted, much the same as in the adult patient. During the assessment the nurse observes for signs of child maltreatment, including the following:

- Bruises about the face, neck, back, abdomen, and thighs
- Bruises in the shape of an object, such as a looped electrical cord or belt buckle
- Bruises in various stages of healing
- Bruises from rope marks or restraining devices found around the neck, wrists, or ankles
- Clearly demarcated, deep, circumferential burns to the hands or feet
- Burns to the perineum
- Burns in various stages of healing
- Cigarette burns
- Contact burns that appear in the shape of the burning object, such as an iron or radiator
- Blood or bruising in the genital region
- Radiographs showing multiple fractures in various stages of healing, as well as rib fractures

When asking the parent about any bruises, the nurse listens to the parent and then determines two things: first, if the child is developmentally capable of engaging in such an activity; and second, if the physical assessment findings are congruent with such an activity.

If it is determined that the child's condition is stable, the transport team obtains further information, such as which medications the child has received, the amount of IV fluids infused, and abnormal laboratory results or X-ray findings. Intake and output records are obtained. If antibiotics had been administered, it is important to know the dose of the antibiotic and the amount of diluent in which it was administered so that an accurate intake record can be maintained.

STABILIZATION FOR TRANSPORT

After the airway is secured, ventilation and circulation are established, and additional interventions are conducted before leaving the referring hospital. These interventions depend on the child's needs and health condition. If the patient is intubated, the endotracheal tube is retaped before transport if it is not well secured to prevent dislodgement. Intravenous sites are securely taped, and their patency is ensured. Indwelling Foley catheters and nasogastric tubes are also secured. Stabilization medications, such as anticonvulsants, must be administered before departure to ensure seizure control. Antibiotics may be delivered en route to the hospital, since they are not necessary for stabilization.

Temperature status is reverified before departure to make sure the child is not hypothermic. Family members are brought into the patient's room before departure if they have not already been present. The transport team discusses with them the child's condition and the impending transport; parental permission is obtained for transport and care at the receiving hospital. The transport nurse and therapist, as well as the referring hospital staff, move the patient onto the transport stretcher. All monitors and equipment are secured. The patient is secured onto the stretcher and is reassessed after the transfer from the emergency department stretcher to the transport stretcher. The family visits with the child and is provided with directions to the receiving facility, as well as telephone numbers if not accompanying the child during transport. The family may want to give the child something of theirs to hold, such as a scarf, so that the child knows that the family will return. The child's transitional or security object is brought along. The family is encouraged to drive safely.

The family may not always be permitted to accompany the child because of safety and space reasons, especially during air transport. However, during the ground transport of a stable child or of the child with potential airway

Table 12-3   Common Medications Used in Children

Medication	Dose	Comments
Arrest Medications		
Epinephrine	0.01 mg/kg (0.1 ml/kg)	Betaadrenergic high-dose epinephrine 1:10,000 is under study
Atropine	0.01 mg/kg	Stimulates heart rate in bradycardia
Sodium bicarbonate	1-2 meq/kg (1-2 ml/kg)	Used in documented acidosis; infants <1 mo, dilute 1:1 due to increased risk of intraventricular hemorrhage
Glucose		
50%	1-2 ml/kg	Used in older children; can cause reflex hypoglycemia; used in younger children and sometimes used in infants instead of 25% dextrose; obtain from an intravenous bag of 10% dextrose in water
25%	1-2 ml/kg	
10%	1-2 ml/kg	
Naloxone (Narcan)	0.25 ml/kg	Half-life is 60 minutes; observe for respiratory depression after this time
Anticonvulsants		
Phenytoin (Dilantin)	20 mg/kg	Use a cardiac monitor; give *slow* IV push; count apical heart rate; observe for bradycardia; can cause severe hypotension in the child with shock; incompatible with glucose solutions; use with caution if dopamine is infusing
Diazepam (Valium)	0.1 mg/kg	Can cause apnea; have resuscitation equipment available
Lorazepam (Ativan)	0.05 mg/kg dilute 1:1 with normal saline	Watch for respiratory depression, hypotension, and sedation
Phenobarbital	15-20 mg/kg	Watch for sedation, respiratory depression, and hypotension
Antibiotics		
Ampicillin		
Neonates		
< 7 days:	50-150 mg/kg/24 hours; divided every 8-12 hours	Can be given IV push over 5 minutes; does not need dilution
> 7 days:	75-200 mg/kg/24 hours; divided every 6-8 hours	
Children:	50-100 mg/kg/24 hours; divided every 6 hours	

Table 12-3   Common Medications Used in Children—cont'd

Medication	Dose	Comments
Cefotaxime (Claforan)	50-200 mg/kg/24 hours; divided every 4-6 hours	Dilute with 10 ml of normal saline solution; can be given IV push
Gentamicin		
Neonates		
< 1 week:	2.5 mg/kg/dose; divided every 12 hours	Infuse over 30 minutes
Infants/children:	6.0-7.5 mg/kg/24 hours; divided every 8 hours	
Nafcillin		
Children:	100-200 mg/kg/24 hours; divided every 6 hours	
Ceftriaxone (Rocephin)		
Infants/children:	50-75 mg/kg/24 hours; divided every 12-24 hours	
Meningitis:	100 mg/kg/24 hours; divided every 12 hours	Administer over 20 minutes; dilute
Cefuroxime (Zinacef)		
Neonates:	20-40 mg/kg/24 hours; divided every 12 hours	
Infants/children:	50-100 mg/kg/24 hours; divided every 6-8 hours	

compromise, one parent may be permitted to go with the team. The patient, family member, and team are secured into the vehicle. The bedside time should average 20 minutes but may be shorter or longer depending on the patient's needs.

TRANSPORT OF THE PEDIATRIC PATIENT

Before leaving the referring hospital, a transport team member calls to the receiving facility to update them on the child's condition. The transport team member recommends which unit the child should be admitted based on the child's condition and travel time. During transport to the receiving facility, the transport nurse's primary responsibility is maintaining the child's stabilization and safety. The main oxygen tanks are used to supply the oxygen adequately during the transport. The equipment is secured, and certain equipment may be plugged in to prevent power depletion. The ambient temperature is controlled to allow for optimal patient comfort. The nurse's position in the vehicle depends on the child's status. If the patient is intubated, the physician or designated team member responsible for airway control is positioned at the head of the stretcher. The therapist is usually seated at the foot of the stretcher with the ventilator, and the transport nurse is seated in between. The nurse monitors the child's vital signs at least every 15 minutes (every 5 minutes if the child is in critical condition) and observes for changes in the child's condition. Medications are administered as necessary, such as antibiotics, anticonvulsants, or paralyzation/sedation medications (Table 12-3). During prolonged transport, temperature and glucose monitoring may be indicated.

Psychosocial support is continued throughout the transport. The nurse explains procedures to the child using age-appropriate language. The nurse continues to reassure the child that the parents will meet them at the hospital. The nurse engages the stable child in conversations or quiet play. Security objects, such as a blanket, pacifier, or a parent's article of clothing, are brought with the child to provide comfort. The paralyzed and sedated child also is given explanations for everything that happens. Soft touch and a soothing, quiet voice help to calm the anxious child. To decrease the noise during air transport, older children may appreciate head phones. Also during air transport, the child is prepared for the sensations experienced during takeoff and landing. About 5 to 10 minutes from the receiving facility, the designated team member calls to give the estimated time of arrival and an update on the child's condition.

ARRIVAL AT THE RECEIVING FACILITY

Upon arrival at the receiving facility the transport team takes the patient to the predetermined unit and assists with the transfer of the patient from the stretcher to the bed. The transport nurse gives a report to the receiving nurse. Equipment such as IV pumps and ventilators are switched over. The transport nurse completes the required documentation and leaves it with the receiving nurse. Finally, the equipment is cleaned, restocked, and returned to its designated place.

FOLLOW-UP

After the child is admitted to the receiving hospital, the transport nurse contacts the refer-

ring hospital to inform them of the patient's status during transport and the patient's location in the hospital. Transport nurses follow-up on their patients and provide feedback to the referring hospital every few days.

Problems with the child's care provided by the referring hospital should be approached in a nonthreatening manner by either the transport nurse or the medical director. Depending on the type of problem, such as fluid overload or hypothermia, the transport team may elect to approach the subject with the staff nurse while at the referring institution. Other problems, such as empty oxygen tanks or medication errors, should be addressed to the referring hospital's department head within a few days after the transport. Usually, if given in a nonthreatening manner, constructive criticism is well received by the referring institution. The transport team may also elect to provide outreach classes or case reviews on the care of the pediatric patients to the staff.

CASE STUDY—TRANSPORTING A CHILD WITH A TRANSPORT TEAM

A 4-year-old boy is brought by his mother to a small hospital emergency department with a complaint that he has a fever and is not eating or drinking. The emergency department staff assesses the child, and it is determined that transfer to the nearby pediatric tertiary care center is warranted. The physician calls the center's pediatric transport team to transport the child.

At 10:24 AM the dispatcher at the pediatric tertiary care center receives a call from the emergency department physician at a nearby hospital. The physician tells the dispatcher that a 4-year-old child may need transfer to the tertiary care center. The dispatcher notifies the transport team members, all of whom carry radios. The transport physician, a pediatric intensive care fellow, is connected by telephone to the referring physician. The transport physician is told that this 4-year-old boy came to the emergency department with a complaint of a fever of 103°, decreased oral intake, and gastrointestinal disturbances. The referring physician also states that he was thinking about sending the child home, but the lateral neck radiographs showed possible epiglottitis; however, the radiographs were of poor quality. Based on this information, the transport physician informs the referring physician that the pediatric transport team would transport the patient. During this conversation, the dispatcher already has called for the ambulance, as the referring hospital is only 10 minutes from the tertiary care center.

The transport nurse obtains the necessary equipment from the designated transport equipment storage area and meets the transport physician in the emergency department. The ambulance and team depart for the referring hospital at 10:38 AM, 14 minutes after the initial call was received.

The transport physician and transport nurse plan for the patient's care en route. The team considers the possibility of epiglottitis remote, based on the physician's description and on the fact that many radiographs fail to diagnose epiglottitis.

At 10:45 AM, the transport team arrives at the referring hospital. They find the patient in a room with his mother and grandmother at his side. As the team enters the room, they note that the child is in a sitting position but is slouching down and forward. He appears listless and lethargic; his eyes are rolled back, and his mouth is open. The child's shirt had been removed, and suprasternal and intercostal retractions are noted; his respiratory rate is counted at 16 breaths per minute. Upon auscultation, bilateral breath sounds are present, and fair air exchange is noted.

The transport team immediately realizes that the radiographic diagnosis of epiglottitis was correct; this patient has epiglottitis and is on the brink of complete respiratory failure. Even though the child is unaware of his environment, the transport nurse calmly explains to him what she is doing as she places him on a pulse oximeter and cardiac monitor. She would *not* perform these interventions in the child who appeared anxious and was actively protecting his airway. The child does not have an intravenous catheter in place, and the team elects not to place one because this maneuver would cause pain and possibly upset the child. Since the team is only 10 minutes away from the tertiary care center, and the referring hospital has no in-house operating

room staff on the weekend, the team elects to return to their facility quickly.

As the transport nurse and referring physician carefully transfer the child onto the ambulance stretcher, the transport physician calls back to the dispatcher and gives the dispatcher a report. The dispatcher is directed to have the operating room team and ear, nose, and throat (ENT) surgeon ready. The transport team secures the child and departs at 10:56 AM (8 minutes after arrival).

The transport nurse quickly removes from the transport equipment the bag-valve-mask device, as well as supplies for performing a cricothyrotomy or endotracheal intubation. Blow-by oxygen is utilized for the child to prevent causing further anxiety. During the 10 minutes' drive to the tertiary care center, both the physician and nurse closely monitor the child. They realize they have an unstable child with impending respiratory failure but know that it would be safer to have the child treated in the operating room at the tertiary care center.

The child continues to be unstable during the transport, with pulse oximeter readings at 93% saturation. Five minutes away from the tertiary care center, the nurse notes that the child is having premature ventricular contractions. At 2 minutes away, the dispatcher is provided with updated information; the dispatcher is told to have an elevator waiting for the team to go directly to the operating room.

At 11:06 AM the transport team arrives at the tertiary care center and delivers the patient to the waiting operating room team. The ENT surgeon quickly intubates the child, and the child is transferred to the pediatric intensive care unit.

The transport nurse cleans and replaces the equipment and then telephones the referring hospital and updates the emergency department nurse who cared for the child. The referring nurse thanks the transport nurse for calling and tells the nurse that the emergency department physician wanted to send the patient home. The nursing staff believed the child was ill enough to require admission to the tertiary care center. The nursing staff at the referring hospital feel vindicated that they made the correct decision to act as the child's advocate and to facilitate the child's treatment process.

CASE STUDY—TRANSPORTING A CHILD WITHOUT A TRANSPORT TEAM

A 10-month-old female is brought by paramedics to the local emergency department. Her color is ashen, and she is unresponsive. She is quickly taken to a treatment room where her assessment continues. Her respirations are shallow at 32, with good air exchange noted. Her heart rate is 166, and her peripheral pulses are weak and thready. Capillary refill is greater than 3 seconds, and she is cool and clammy to the touch. Her blood pressure is 70/P, and her temperature is 103° rectally. Oxygen is administered, and an intravenous catheter is secured. After two normal saline solution boluses are administered, the infant is more responsive to the environment. Her perfusion improves, her blood pressure increases to 90/P, and her heart rate decreases to 144. With further testing, a diagnosis of septic shock is made, and antibiotics are administered.

The physician places a call to the tertiary care center with a pediatric transport team that is 2 hours away by ground transportation. The physician is told that because of inclement weather conditions, their helicopter is unable to fly. After further consultation, the physician decides that it would be better to send the child to the tertiary care center with staff members from their own facility. The decision is made that you are the staff nurse who will accompany the child because of your background in pediatric nursing. Also, you have been caring for this infant during her emergency department treatment. Because of the patient's potential for decompensation due to her shock state, a nurse anesthetist is selected to accompany you. What do you do to prepare for this transport?

As this case study demonstrates, there may be situations in which a critically ill or injured child is transported to a receiving facility by health-care professionals who are not members of an organized pediatric transport service. Such situations include weather conditions that prohibit the pediatric transport team from transporting the patient; the referring hospital's belief that the patient is stable enough to not require a specialized team; the unavailability of the specialized team; the decision of the referring and receiving hospitals to transport the patient with a nurse; or the referring facility's unwillingness to wait for the pediatric transport team's arrival. Under such circumstances the same principles that apply to pediatric transport teams are useful.

The decision to transfer and transport the child to a tertiary care center is made by the physician caring for the child, as well as the physician receiving the child. The receiving physician arranges the child's acceptance at the receiving hospital. The details of the transport are decided upon, such as the mode of transportation and who will accompany the patient.

Once these matters are decided, the health-care professionals who will accompany the patient are selected. The nurse accompanying the child must be experienced in the care of children, as well as emergency, critical care, or transport nursing. If a physician is to go on the transport, the physician also should have experience in the care of children and emergency or critical care medicine. Finally the respiratory therapist should have experience with pediatric airway and ventilatory management. Other personnel that can accompany the pediatric patient include nurse anesthetists, anesthesiologists, or critical care physicians.

Although there are no established guidelines on who can and cannot transport children, the referring hospital must have transfer and transport guidelines in place that clearly outline these criteria.

When determining who should accompany the child to the receiving facility, the involved legalities must be considered. Because members of the referring hospital are responsible for the child until arrival at the receiving hospital, they must provide the same quality of care to the child as they would to the adult patient in the same situation. This means that the personnel accompanying the child on the transport must have the equipment and medication, as well as the cognitive and technical skills, to care for the child properly. Under no circumstances should a child be transported without the attendance of health-care professionals who are educated and technically skilled in pediatric care.

Generally a nurse can transport the child if the patient is stable and decompensation is not anticipated. A physician and nurse can transport the unstable child or the child who has the potential to become unstable during the transport. Examples of such patients include those with upper airway emergencies (epiglottitis, croup), septic shock, respiratory distress/failure, major trauma with head injury, and shock. Children who are endotracheally intubated and receiving ventilatory assistance are accompanied by a nurse, physician, and respiratory therapist. The respiratory therapist also accompanies a nurse if the child has severe asthma that requires frequent aerosol treatments during a long transport.

Steps in Preparing the Child for Transport

Once the decision is made to transport the child without an organized transport team, the child's condition should be further stabilized according to the medical direction received from the receiving facility. The designated transport personnel are summoned, and they prepare the necessary equipment. Ideally, their equipment should be kept in a separate location for easy retrieval. The minimal equipment for the transport includes the following:

- Oxygen tank
- Airway management equipment
- Suction device
- Oxygen masks
- Bag-valve-mask device with reservoir
- Cardiac monitor
- Pulse oximeter
- Intravenous catheters
- Intravenous solutions, tubing, and Buretrol
- Intravenous infusion pump
- Medications

- Emesis basins
- Blankets
- Heat source

All equipment must be in good condition and working order. As the transport team prepares to leave, each member agrees to be responsible for a specific aspect of the child's care.

Before leaving the referring facility, the transport personnel double check the patency of the child's airway, oxygen device, intravenous sites, as well as the patency of any chest tubes, nasogastric tube, and Foley catheter. All interventions must be done before leaving the referring hospital; anticipated interventions must also be performed at this time, such as a second intravenous site. Documentation forms are also obtained, as well as a copy of the child's medical record and radiographs. Calculations of any fluid boluses or medications that may be needed on the transport should be made at this time. Standing orders for anticonvulsants, sedation and paralyzation, antibiotic therapy, and so forth must be in place if a physician is not going on the transport. The family should be allowed to enter the treatment room to see the child before transport and provided with directions to the receiving hospital. The child and team are secured in the ambulance or helicopter. Once in the vehicle, the child's airway, oxygen, IV sites, and other tubes for patency are reassessed.

Once en route, the child is closely monitored. Again, emotional support and comfort measures go a long way in making the child feel safe. Reading a story or holding the child's hand may also help the child relax.

When the team is within 15 minutes of the receiving facility, they contact the receiving physician to provide an update on the child's condition and the estimated time of arrival. Upon arrival the transport nurse gives a report to the receiving nurse. A copy of the patient's transport record is retained by the referring nurse, and it becomes part of the child's medical record.

Table 12-4   Nursing Diagnoses, Interventions, and Evaluative Criteria for Transport of the Pediatric Patient

Diagnoses	Interventions	Evaluative Criteria
Ineffective airway clearance.	Open the child's airway using the jaw-thrust or chin-lift maneuver.	The child will have a patent airway.
	Inspect the airway for the presence of blood, vomitus, teeth, or foreign bodies.	
	Listen for stridor, coughing, or crowing.	
	Observe for drooling, for breath odor.	
	Suction the airway with a Yankauer catheter.	
	Insert an appropriately sized oral or nasopharyngeal airway.	
	Prepare for endotracheal intubation.	
	Secure the endotracheal tube.	
	Prepare for needle cricothyrotomy.	
Ineffective breathing pattern.	Assess the child's breathing pattern.	The child will have:
Impaired gas exchange.	Observe for retractions, nasal flaring, and head bobbing.	Adequate ventilatory effort.
	Assess the child's responsiveness to the environment.	Equal and bilateral breath sounds.
	Auscultate breath sounds in all lung fields.	A functioning chest-drainage collection system.
	Listen for adventitious sounds, such as rales, rhonchi, wheezing, or absence of breath sounds.	Pulse oximetry readings above 93%.
	Observe for chest symmetry.	Ventilatory functioning at the recommended parameters.
	Observe for signs of trauma (contusions, abrasions, penetrations, paradoxical movements).	Appropriate mentation for age.
	Administer oxygen through a nasal cannula, face mask, or blow-by method.	
	Assist with ventilations in the child with absent or slow respirations by using a bag-valve-mask device with a reservoir connected to 100% oxygen.	
	Place the child on a pulse oximeter and cardiorespiratory monitor.	
	Prepare to place the child on a mechanical ventilator once endotracheal intubation is completed.	
	Prepare for needle thoracostomy and chest tube placement.	
	Obtain a chest radiograph.	
	Assist with obtaining arterial blood sampling for analysis.	
Decreased cardiac output.	Control active bleeding.	The child will have:
Fluid volume deficit.	Assess central and peripheral pulses.	Active bleeding under control.
	Assess skin color, temperature, and capillary refill.	Patent intravenous access.
	Assess the child's responsiveness to the environment.	Fluid replacement.

Nursing Diagnosis	Interventions	Expected Outcomes
	Place child on a cardiorespiratory monitor. Obtain blood pressure readings. Secure intravenous access with the largest-bore catheter possible. Administer crystalloid fluids. Secure an intraosseous device if three intravenous access attempts are unsuccessful or 90 minutes has elapsed. Prepare for central line insertion or venous cutdown. Prepare to administer fluid boluses. Prepare to administer blood products. Provide for active warming measures.	Ongoing cardiorespiratory and pressure monitoring.
Pain. *Fear.* *Anxiety.*	Explain all events to the child using nonthreatening language. Allow the child to ask questions. Encourage the parent to touch the child and talk with the child before transport. Allow the child to have a security object during transport. When possible, give the child time to prepare for painful procedures. Recognize pain in infants, children, and adolescents. Provide pharmacological and nonpharmacological interventions for pain relief. Evaluate the effectiveness of pain-relief measures.	The child will have: A basic understanding of what will happen on the transport. Minimized or complete pain relief. Feelings of comfort and safety.
Altered family processes. *Parental role conflict.* *Altered parenting.*	Explain the transport process to the family. Obtain the family's consent for transport. Allow the family to ask questions. Be honest in communicating with the family. Allow the family to see the child before transport. Encourage the family to touch and to talk to the child. Allow siblings to be with the child before transport. Allow the family to give the child one of their belongings to carry on the transport. If one family member is to accompany the child, explain the family member's role during the transport. Ask the family what helps the child feel safe or comfortable; ask the family what words the child uses for pain, hurt, urination, and so forth. Give the family directions to the receiving facility.	The family will have: An understanding of what will happen with their child during the transport. Knowledge of the transport process. An understanding of what their roles will be during the transport process.

Prepare for the transport by obtaining the necessary equipment as the emergency staff stabilizes the patient and obtains the family's consent for transport. The nurse anesthetist brings the necessary equipment for intubation, as well as medications for rapid-sequence intubation. The nurse anesthetist also calculates the dosages for these medications.

The prehospital team arrives with the ambulance. They tell you that they have AC capabilities and a full H cylinder of oxygen. You can use their cardiac monitor, too. You obtain a battery-operated syringe-type IV pump from the pediatrics unit; this pump also runs on AC power. Finally, you gather equipment and supplies that you anticipate may be needed, such as intravenous catheters, fluids including 5% albumin, cardiac arrest medications, pulse oximeter, thermometer, bedside glucose measuring device, and syringes. A stopcock is already in place on the intravenous tubing to facilitate fluid boluses.

The physician writes down orders and parameters for when to deliver fluid boluses, administer vasopressors, and deliver anticonvulsant medications. The infant is secured onto the stretcher, and the oxygen and intravenous catheters are double checked for patency. You gather the emergency department record, radiographs, and nurses' notes. The family has written directions to the tertiary care center, and the prehospital team has verified the directions. The total time for preparation is 35 minutes.

En route to the tertiary care center, you monitor the infant and record vital signs every 15 minutes. One hour into the transport, the infant's blood pressure decreases to 68/P, her heart rate increases, and her perfusion once again becomes poor. You give a 20 ml/kg fluid bolus of normal saline, as written in the order sheet. Since there is no improvement in the child's condition, you follow your next order to administer a 20 ml/kg bolus of 5% albumin. This time the infant's blood pressure increases to 74/P with no change in heart rate or perfusion. Following the written orders, you begin a dopamine infusion at 10 mcg/kg/minute. Ten minutes after starting the dopamine, the infant's perfusion has improved, and her blood pressure is now 94/P. The infant is now responding by opening her eyes and moving around.

You continue to closely monitor the infant's airway patency, respiratory status, and perfusion status. You also measure the infant's temperature and glucose level. On arrival at the tertiary care center, you relinquish care to the emergency department staff, who have been expecting the patient. You give report to the infant's nurse and deliver the medical records. You copy your transport record and leave the original with the emergency department staff. The parents arrive and are escorted into the treatment room to see their baby. The emergency department staff thank you for a job well done.

Table 12-4 contains a summary of the nursing care of the pediatric patient during transport.

REFERENCES

American Academy of Pediatrics (1988). Guidelines for air and ground transportation of pediatric patients. *Pediatrics, 78*(5), 943-950.

Aoki, B.Y., & McCloskey, K. (1992). *Evaluation, stabilization, and transport of the critically ill child.* St. Louis: Mosby.

Bernardo, L.M., & Waggoner, T. (1992). Pediatric trauma. In S.B. Sheehy (Ed.), *Emergency nursing: Principles and practice,* (pp. 683-690). St. Louis: Mosby.

Day, S., McCloskey, K., Orr, R., Bolte, R., Notterman, D., & Hackel, A. (1991). Pediatric interhospital critical care transport: Consensus of a national leadership conference. *Pediatrics, 88*(4), 696-704.

Kissoon, N., Frewen, T.C., Kronick, J., & Mohammed, A. (1988). The child requiring transport: Lessons and implications for the pediatric emergency physician. *Pediatric Emergency Care, 4*(1), 1-4.

Krug, S.E. (1992). Staff and equipment for pediatric critical care transport. *Current Opinion in Pediatrics, 4,* 445-450.

Lang, S. (1993). Procedures involving the neurological system. In L.M. Bernardo & M. Bove (Eds.), *Pediatric emergency nursing procedures* (pp. 143-161). Boston: Jones & Bartlett Publishers. Inc.

McCloskey, K.A., Faries, G., King, W.D., Orr, R.A., & Plouff, R.T. (1992). Variables predicting the need for a pediatric critical care transport team. *Pediatric Emergency Care, 8*(1), 1-3.

McCloskey, K.A., King, W.D., & Byron, L. (1989). Pediatric critical care transport: Is a physician always needed on the team? *Annals of Emergency Medicine, 18*(3), 247-249.

Pon, S., & Notterman, D.A. (1993). The organization of a pediatric critical care transport program. *Pediatric Clinics of North America, 40*(2), 241-261.

CHAPTER 13

Transport Considerations for Specific Patient Populations

OBJECTIVES

1. Identify the physiological and anatomical changes that occur with aging and discuss how transport may affect these changes
2. Identify the physiological and anatomical changes that occur with pregnancy and discuss how transport may affect these changes
3. Describe some of the sources of communication problems related to patients who require transport

COMPETENCIES

1. Perform a primary and secondary assessment of the elderly patient
2. Develop a plan of care for the pregnant patient
3. Employ alternative communication techniques for the patient with a communication problem

Certain patient populations pose additional care challenges before and during transport. The patient's age, size, ability to communicate, and need for additional equipment will require the nurse to anticipate and adjust care before and during transport.

Three patient populations are addressed in this chapter: the elderly patient, the pregnant patient, and the patient with a communication problem.

CARE AND TRANSPORT OF THE ELDERLY PATIENT

The population of the United States is aging, and by the year 2020 it is estimated that nearly 50 million people will be over the age of 65 (Champion, Copes, Buyer, Flanagan, Bain, & Sacco, 1989). With the advent of new treatments, illnesses that used to cause early death, such as cancer and cardiovascular disease, are survivable for multiple years.

The elderly population now make up a significant proportion of those who sustain injuries from falls, motor vehicle crashes, and penetrating trauma (Champion, et al., 1989). About 30,000 deaths occur each year in the elderly as the result of injuries from falls and motor vehicle crashes (Dandan, 1992). Falls are the leading cause of injury and mortality in the elderly and generally result from environmental obstacles and changes related to age.

Motor vehicle crashes are the most common cause of death in those between the ages of 65 to 74 (Burns & Bayley, 1992). Elderly patients are also at risk of being severely injured from thermal burns, which are associated with high mortality.

Because of the physiological changes that occur with aging, the elderly patient is susceptible to complications from shock or head injury. Subdural hematomas are three times more common in the elderly who has a head injury than in the general population (Dandan, 1992).

It is important to keep in mind when caring for the elderly patient who is acutely ill or injured that the illness or injury may be incurred in addition to other chronic illnesses. Chronic illnesses such as diabetes, arthritis, or hypertension further complicate patient treatments and responses.

ASSESSMENT OF THE ELDERLY PATIENT

In the assessment of the elderly patient, physiological changes and their effect on aging need to be considered. These include the following (Burns & Bayley, 1992; Dandan, 1992; Kauder & Schwab, 1991; Newman, 1993):

1. Changes in lung tissue cause stiffening and potential ventilating problems.
2. Decreased alveoli may lead to an increased risk of hypoxia.
3. Diminished gag reflex increases the risk for aspiration and the development of pneumonia.
4. Degenerative changes in the heart cause less effective contractions, decreased cardiac reserve, and decreased ability to respond to such stressors as blood or fluid loss.
5. Increased peripheral vascular resistance causes an increase in systolic and diastolic blood pressures that may lead to a misinterpretation of shock parameters related to blood pressure.

6. Prescribed medications such as beta blockers used to treat hypotension affect the patient's pulse, allowing the possible misinterpretation of shock parameters.
7. Neurological changes include a decrease in the number of neurons, diminished emotional response, confusion, memory loss, and decreased motor and sensory responses.
8. Decreased visual acuity and peripheral vision may increase the risk of injury, particularly the risk of being struck by a vehicle.
9. Skin changes include body fat in an increase in proportion to muscle mass; decreased sensitivity to heat and cold places the elderly patient at risk of injury or the development of hypothermia because of decreased muscle mass, slower metabolic rate, and decreased ability for vasoconstriction.
10. Calcium loss from bone leads to the development of osteoporosis and potential for fractures.
11. Altered response to pharmacological agents such as morphine or benzodiazepines.

History

When obtaining a history from an elderly patient, the nurse must be sure to allow sufficient time for the patient to comprehend the question as well as to respond. The interview should begin with questions related to the current problem. In addition to the usual components of history, additional pieces of information that should be obtained from the elderly patient include the following:

I. Chronic illnesses
   A. Diabetes
   B. Cardiovascular disease
   C. Arthritis
   D. Stroke
II. Medications
   A. Over-the-counter drugs

B. Prescribed medications
1. Beta blockers
2. Calcium channel blockers
3. Angiotensin-converting enzyme inhibitors
4. Diuretics
5. Nonsteroidal antiinflammatory agents
6. Anticholinergics
7. Anticholesterolemics
8. Sedatives
III. Alcohol ingestion
IV. Immunization history

Physical Assessment

The components of the physical assessment of the elderly do not differ from those in the assessment of any other patient; however, what may be considered abnormal in other patient populations may be normal in the elderly. A summary of some of those findings follows.

Inspection

- Decreased chest excursion and depth of respirations
- Peripheral edema
- Distended neck veins
- Slowed motor reactions
- Limitation of joint movement
- Joint or spine deformities
- Diminished balance
- Skin changes
  - Increased dryness
  - Decreased adipose tissue
  - Protruding bones
  - Loss of body hair
  - Skin purpura
  - Pressure sores

Palpation

- Altered response to pain
- Changes in skin temperature
- Changes in pulse quality
- Cardiac dysrhythmia
  - Premature ventricular contractions (PVCs)
  - Atrial fibrillation

Auscultation

- Decreased breath sounds in the bases
- End-expiratory crackles
- Early systolic murmur
- Presence of an S_4

The Potential for Abuse

Unfortunately the potential for elderly abuse has increased significantly over the past few decades (Janing, 1992; Newman, 1993). When obtaining a history and performing a physical assessment of the elderly patient, the nurse needs to keep in mind the possibility of abuse. Historical data that may indicate abuse include the following:

1. The elderly patient not being allowed to speak for themselves
2. History of alcohol or substance abuse
3. Lack of family support
4. Injuries not consistent with the patient's physical capabilities
5. Inappropriate prescribed medication use

Physical signs of abuse may include:
1. Cuts and bruises
2. Dehydration
3. Poor hygiene
4. Malnutrition
5. Strong odor from incontinence
6. Infected burns

GENERAL INTERVENTIONS FOR THE ELDERLY PATIENT
Before Transport

The interventions for the care of the elderly patient who is ill or injured are essentially no different when preparing them for transport than for any other patient with an illness or injury. However, because the elderly patient may have other complicating illnesses, may not respond to physiological and psychological stresses, and may be at risk for developing specific problems such as hypothermia, nursing and collaborative interventions need to be focused on anticipating and preventing problems

(Thompson, McFarland, Hirsch, Tucker & Bowers, 1993).

The nurse needs to be cognizant of the fact that the elderly patient may have some other concerns in addition to the specific illness or injury. These include fear of what is going to happen, particularly when they need to be taken away from a familiar environment; potential loss of independence related to the illness or injury; fear of procedures that may need to be performed; the prospect of death; and finally, facing the possibility of long-term care and assistance because of the illness or injury (Henry & Stapleton, 1992; Judd, 1991).

Specific interventions include the following:

1. Obtain a history related to the illness or injury
2. Obtain a history of previous illnesses
3. Obtain information about the patient's current medications including prescribed and over-the-counter drugs
4. Perform a primary and secondary assessment focusing on the patient's chief complaint and keeping in mind the psychological and physiological effects of aging
5. Place oxygen on the patient
6. Obtain intravenous access (carefully monitor the effects of fluid resuscitation)
7. Place patient on a cardiac monitor
8. Place patient on a pulse oximeter and end-tidal CO_2 monitor as indicated by the patient's disease process
9. Perform a baseline neurological assessment including assessment of the patient's mental status, speech pattern, articulation, judgment, and motor and sensory response
10. Provide methods to protect the patient from becoming hypothermic (application of blankets, use of warm fluids, warm humidified oxygen)
11. Assess the patient's level of pain and provide pain management, carefully moni-

toring for relief and reactions such as respiratory depression or hypotension
12. Involve the patient's family as appropriate
13. Explain all procedures to the patient
14. Address patients by their last name unless given their permission to use their first name
15. Provide interventions for the patient based on the specific problem (e.g., myocardial infarction)

Care of the Elderly Patient during Transport

1. Continuous monitoring of the patient's airway, breathing, and circulation
2. Provide interventions as indicated
3. Ensure that the patient is appropriately restrained in the transport vehicle
4. Talk to the patient during the transport process providing information as needed and when any changes occur

CARE AND TRANSPORT OF THE PREGNANT PATIENT

The care and transport of the patient who is pregnant offer a unique challenge. The majority of pregnant patients who are being transferred are ill and at risk of premature delivery (Nelson, 1988). The nurse and transport team are caring not only for the mother but also for the fetus.

The rate of maternal death is 20 to 30 for every 100,000 live births (Miller & Wilson, 1992). Many potential complications may occur during pregnancy, including hemorrhage, eclampsia, preeclampsia, infection, vascular accidents, embolism, premature labor and premature rupture of membranes, and injury from a traumatic event. Trauma is the most common cause of death in women of childbearing age. Approximately 6% to 7% of women who are traumatically injured are pregnant (Drost, Rosemurgy, Sherman, Scott, & Williams, 1992).

Care of the patient during transport includes assessment and interventions related to the unique patient complaint. Technological advances have made available noninvasive blood pressure and cardiac monitoring, as well as fetal monitoring (Poulton & Gutierrez, 1992). Poulton and Gutierrez (1992) found that portable external fetal monitors could be easily applied and were not adversely affected during the transport process while providing an additional method of fetal monitoring. The authors suggest that changes in fetal status may require simple but important interventions during transport such as changing the position of the mother and applying supplemental oxygen (Poulton & Gutierrez, 1992).

Specific indications for the transport of the pregnant patient may include the following:

- Preeclampsia
- Eclampsia
- Pregnancy-induced hypertension
- Hemolysis, elevated liver enzymes, and low platelet (HELLP) syndrome
- Premature labor
- Premature rupture of membranes
- Vaginal bleeding
  - Placenta abruptio
  - Placenta previa
- Multiple pregnancies
- Perimortem cesarean section
- Traumatic injury

When making the decision to transport a pregnant patient in active labor, several things need to be considered: the skills of the transport team, the distance of the transport, the level of care available at the referring facility, the age of the fetus, and the amount of cervical dilatation (Elliott, Spii, & Balazs, 1992). In their study of 54 patients in active labor (cervical dilatation of 7 cm or greater), Elliott, Spii,

and Balazs found that the nurse's judgment provided the best means for evaluating whether a patient in active labor should be transported.

Physiological and Anatomical Changes That Occur with Pregnancy

The pregnant patient undergoes both physiological and anatomical changes that affect both the mother and infant. These include the following (Cardona, 1988; Henninger, 1992; Manley, 1993; Rhodes, 1990; Sherman & Rosemurgy, 1990; Skinner, 1991):

1. Cardiovascular
   a. Increase in intravascular volume up to 50%
   b. Increase in heart rate (15 to 20 beats per minute)
   c. Increase in cardiac output from 5 to 7 liters per minute
   d. Changes in blood pressure that may result in a fall of 5 to 15 mm Hg during the second and third trimesters
   e. 90% of pregnant women have a flow-related murmur
   f. Left axis deviation on a twelve-lead EKG
   g. Increase risk of PVCs
   h. "Anemia of pregnancy"; hematocrit may vary 3% to 6% below normal
2. Pulmonary
   a. During late pregnancy, diaphragm will elevate from the gravid uterus and decrease the residual capacity
   b. Oxygen consumption increases between 15% to 20%
   c. Decreased Pco_2, which leads to respiratory alkalosis
3. Anatomical changes
   a. Fetus protected by the pelvis during early pregnancy; it loses this protection as it grows
   b. Increased vascularization of the pelvis
   c. Pressure on inferior vena cava from the

gravid uterus may decrease blood return as much as 30%

d. Compression on distal aorta and vena cava may alter cardiac output

ASSESSMENT OF THE PREGNANT PATIENT
History

1. Age of the patient
2. Chief complaint
3. Mechanism of injury
4. Medical history
   a. Hypertension
   b. Diabetes
   c. Alcohol or substance abuse
5. Medications
6. Allergies
7. Obstetrical history
   a. Gestational age of the fetus (estimated date of conception)
   b. Gravida and para
   c. Previous deliveries (vaginal, cesarean section)

d. Previous delivery complications
e. History of preterm labor
f. Length of previous labors
g. History of multiple pregnancies

Physical Assessment
Inspection

1. General appearance of the patient
   a. Skin color
   b. Signs of coagulopathy (bruising, bleeding from intravenous sites)
2. Height of the patient's fundus (Figure 13-1); see Box 13-1 for methods of measuring
3. Visual inspection of the vagina and perineum
   a. Bulging
   b. Crowning

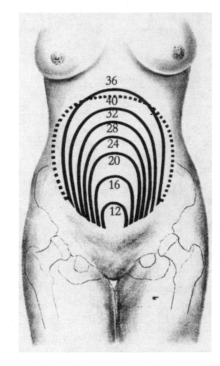

Fig. 13-1   Size of the uterus in relation to the length of pregnancy. (From *Mosby's Guide to Physical Examination* by H.M. Seidel, et al., 1992, St. Louis, Mosby.)

Box 13-1
METHODS TO MEASURE THE HEIGHT OF THE FUNDUS

McDonald's Method

Measure with tape from symphysis pubic to fundus. 1 cm = 1 week of gestation.

Rapid Estimate Method

0 to 12 weeks: uterus confined in the pelvis
20 to 24 weeks: uterus at the level of the umbilicus
36 weeks: uterus at the level of the diaphragm

Note. From "Obstetric" by B. Henninger. In *Trauma Nursing* (p. 462) by E. Bayley & S. Turcke (Eds.), 1992, Boston: Jones & Bartlett.

    c. Bloody fluid
    d. Greenish fluid
    e. Placenta
    f. Arms, legs
4. Seizure activity
5. Patient's response to labor
    a. Facial gestures
    b. Bearing down

Palpation

1. Blood pressure, peripheral and central pulses
2. Skin temperature
    a. Diaphoresis
3. Uterine tenderness and rigidity
4. Assessment of contractions:
    a. Presence
    b. Strength
    c. Frequency
    d. Pattern
5. Determine fetal position
6. Vaginal examination when indicated and prescribed by protocol

Auscultation

1. Blood pressure
2. Pulse quality
3. Maternal breath sounds
4. Fetal heart tones
5. Fetal monitoring when available

GENERAL INTERVENTIONS FOR THE PREGNANT PATIENT
Before Transport

1. Perform a baseline assessment
2. Obtain history of the patient's chief complaint, current symptoms, and treatment
3. Apply supplemental oxygen
4. Obtain fetal heart tones
5. Place patient on an external fetal monitor when available and obtain baseline reading
6. Start large-bore intravenous line
7. Check concentration, dosage, and rate of any medications that are being administered (Box 13-2) (Skidmore-Roth, 1993).

8. Place drugs on intravenous infusion pumps or monitors as indicated
9. Perform a vaginal examination when indicated or prescribed (assess for cervical contractions and dilatation, bleeding, leakage of fluid, and any presenting parts)
10. Determine the potential for delivery during transport
11. Identify a possible place for definitive care during transport if the team needs to stop
12. Prepare equipment for potential delivery during transport
    a. Emergency delivery kit
    b. Neonatal resuscitation kit
    c. Method to keep the child warm (transport isolette, "bubble bags," cap)

Box 13-2
DRUGS USED IN THE CARE OF THE PREGNANT PATIENT

Preeclampsia and Eclampsia

Magnesium sulfate
Hydralazine
Benzodiazepines

Premature Labor

Terbutaline
Ritodrine
Magnesium sulfate

Diabetic

Insulin
50% dextrose solution

Nausea and Vomiting

Droperidol

Additional Drugs

Calcium gluconate (for magnesium sulfate toxicity)
Oxytocin (uterine contraction after delivery)
Methylergonovine maleate (uterine contraction after delivery)

Box 13-3
UTAH VALLEY REGIONAL MEDICAL CENTER
MATERNAL TRANSPORT TEAM
STANDING ORDERS

Preeclampsia

1. Prepare magnesium sulfate 40 g in 1000 ml lactated Ringer's or normal saline solution. Give 4-g bolus over 30 minutes then run at 2 to 3 g/hr.
2. Maintain intravenous infusion as needed.
3. If intravenous magnesium sulfate is not feasible, administer magnesium sulfate deep intramuscularly, Z track, 5 g in each hip. May use 1 ml of 2% lidocaine in each syringe.
4. Position Foley catheter to down drain.
5. Check vital signs every 15 to 30 minutes.
6. Check for toxemia every 15 to 30 minutes.
7. Obtain laboratory values (hematocrit, platelets, magnesium level, prothrombin and partial thromboplastin times, fibrinogen), if available.
8. Assess fetal well-being.
9. Give nothing by mouth.
10. Monitor intake and output.
11. Assess cardiac, lung, and kidney status.
12. Give hydralazine (Apresoline), 5 to 10 mg IV push for diastolic blood pressure greater than 110. Hold for heart rate greater than 110, repeat in 10 to 15 minutes three times if necessary. Diastolic blood pressure not to be less than 94 to 100 mm Hg.

Eclampsia

1. Refer to standing orders for preeclampsia.
2. If patient has a seizure, infuse 4 g of magnesium sulfate over 4 minutes intravenously, then 3 g/hr.
3. If seizures do not stop, give Valium 1 to 10 mg IV. Push 1 mg/min until seizures stop.
4. If second series of seizures occurs within 20 minutes, an additional 2 to 4 g bolus of magnesium sulfate may be given IV push over 2 to 4 minutes (1 g/min).
5. Have 10 ml ampule of calcium gluconate on hand. Give 5 to 10 meq IV over 3 to 5 minutes if unable to elicit deep tendon reflexes or is unresponsive.
6. Check blood pressure frequently.
7. After seizure:
   a. Turn the patient to left side
   b. Establish airway
   c. Provide nasopharyngeal suction as needed
   d. Administer O_2 7-10 liter/min.
8. Assess fetal well-being.
9. Assess cardiac and lung status.

Magnesium Sulfate Toxicity

1. Assess reflexes/clonus, respiratory rate, change in level of consciousness, and magnesium sulfate level if possible.
2. Administer 10% solution calcium gluconate 1 g IV push, repeat in 5 minutes if respiratory rate is not normal.

Nonresponsiveness

1. Begin advanced cardiac life support interventions.

Severe Pulmonary Edema

1. Intubate/ventilate.

Preterm Labor

1. Perform vaginal examination to determine appropriateness to transport.
2. If the patient's labor is controlled by IV ritodrine or terbutaline, transport patient without changing the medication.
3. Administer terbutaline 0.25 mg subcutaneously every 15 to 30 minutes as needed during transport.

> ## Box 13-3
> ## UTAH VALLEY REGIONAL MEDICAL CENTER
> ## MATERNAL TRANSPORT TEAM
> ## STANDING ORDERS—cont'd
>
> Hold for maternal pulse greater than 140 beats/minute.
> Assess lung and cardiac status before administering drug.
> 4. Administer magnesium sulfate intravenously, 40 g/1000 ml lactated Ringer's solution; first give 4-g bolus over 30 minutes, then infuse at 3 g/hr per pump.
> 5. Nothing by mouth, with ice chips and sips if needed.
> 6. Obtain laboratory values if possible: complete blood cell count, K+, glucose, uric acid.
> 7. Pulmonary edema—intubate/ventilate.
>
> ### Premature Rupture of Membranes
>
> 1. No vaginal examination if patient is not laboring.
> 2. If laboring, see Preterm Labor orders.
> 3. Administer terbutaline 0.25 mg subcutaneously as needed every 30 to 60 minutes for contractions during transport.
> 4. Obtain laboratory values: hematocrit, white blood cell count, if available.
> 5. Assess cardiac and lung status.
>
> ### Vaginal Bleeding
>
> 1. No vaginal examination unless order by perinatologist.
>
> 2. Keep pad count on bleeding.
> 3. Have IV infusing with normal saline.
> 4. Obtain laboratory values: hematocrit, platelets, white blood cell count, prothrombin and partial thromboplastin times, if available.
> 5. Assess fetal well-being before transport.
> 6. If blood has been typed and cross matched, bring units with transport.
>
> ### Diabetic
>
> 1. Obtain laboratory values: blood sugar, complete blood cell count, and sequential multiple analysis 6 and 12.
> 2. For ketoacidosis: take insulin with patient on transport.
>   a. Dip urine for ketones
>   b. 1000 ml normal saline run at 250 ml/hr
>   c. Obtain blood gases if possible
> 3. Call for insulin dosage orders.
>
> ### General Verbal Orders
>
> 1. For nausea in flight, administer droperidol (Inapsine) ¼ ml intravenous push once for flight.
> 2. Assess fetal monitor strip; elicit a fetal heart rate acceleration before transport.
> 3. Perform a complete but brief history and physical before transport.

During Transport

1. Place patient in a left lateral recumbent position to displace the uterus from the inferior vena cava
2. If the patient's cervical spine is immobilized, place pillows or sheets under the backboard to displace the uterus
3. Place safety straps low on the patient's pelvic girdle
4. Monitor vital signs
5. Monitor fetal heart tones or fetal monitoring device
6. Intervene as indicated

Box 13-4
**UTAH VALLEY REGIONAL
MEDICAL CENTER
MATERNAL LIFE FLIGHT
PROTOCOL FOR TRANSPORT OF
DIABETIC PATIENT**

Purpose

To establish protocol for the transport of the diabetic patient by the maternal transport team.

Protocol
Before transport

1. Check temperature, pulse, respirations, blood pressure, and fetal heart tone.
2. Assess for contractions. If contracting, assess contractions for quality, duration, and frequency.
3. If contracting, perform vaginal examination.
4. Obtain information—time of last insulin dose and type of insulin. *Obtain insulin bottle for transport.*
5. Establish intravenous infusion with 16-gauge catheter of normal saline.
6. Check for signs of insulin shock and diabetic coma.
7. Have glucose level determined before transport.
8. Record information.
9. Call perinatologist.

During transport

1. Check pulse and respirations every 30 minutes.
2. Continuous fetal monitoring.
3. Check for signs and symptoms of insulin shock and diabetic coma.
4. Record information.

---

7. Monitor the effect of tocolytic agents on the patient
8. Monitor and intervene for any seizure activity
9. Provide medication for anxiety, nausea, and vomiting as needed by the patient
10. Decrease stimulation as much as possible by:
    a. Explaining what is going to happen during transport before it happens
    b. Providing hearing protection
    c. Considering letting a family member accompany the patient
11. Perform assessment and interventions for specific emergencies (Boxes 13-3 to 13-10)
12. Be prepared for emergency delivery (Figures 13-2 to 13-4)
13. Be prepared for neonatal resuscitation (Figure 13-5)

CARE AND TRANSPORT OF THE PATIENT WITH A COMMUNICATION PROBLEM

Communication has been described as a process through which messages are sent by one individual and received by another. It is a dynamic process susceptible to changes in both the persons engaging in the process and the environment in which the process takes place. The stresses of illness and injury can impair this process.

Examples of patients who may have a communication problem include the unconscious patient, patients with an altered mentation (head injury, stroke, drug intoxication, or psychogenic), pediatric and elderly patients, patients with sensory deficits (visually or hearing impaired), and those with cultural differences.

Indications of a potential communication problem may be seen when the patient is disoriented or does not respond to the nurse, when the patient's behaviors manifest fear or anxiety, or the patient ignores or withdraws from the nurse (Riley & Cleary, 1987).

Box 13-5
UTAH VALLEY REGIONAL MEDICAL CENTER
EMERGENCIES DURING TRANSPORT

Purpose

To establish a protocol for the maternal transport team for emergency situations during transport.

Protocol

Seizures

Symptoms: Severe headaches, visual disturbances, scotomas, diplopia, blurred vision, vomiting and/or epigastric pain

1. Insert tongue blade.
2. Protect patient and physically support to keep on stretcher.
3. Administer diazepam (Valium) 10 mg IV push.
     If diabetic: draw blood sugar—assume insulin reaction (give 25 ml, D_{50} IV push).

Establish respiratory support according to transport protocol and administer O_2 as needed.

Postseizure

1. Clear airway, suction if necessary, and administer O_2.
2. Continue respiratory support as needed.
3. Reassure patient and offer emotional support.
4. Check vital signs every 5 minutes until stable with continuous fetal monitoring.

Hemorrhage

If bleeding begins:
1. Turn up IV (use lactated Ringer's or Plasmanate).
2. Pilot to set down at nearest hospital. Convey patient to hospital for evaluation and possible delivery.
3. Monitor blood pressure and pulse.
4. Monitor fetal heart tone.

5. Elevate feet if possible.
6. Establish radio contact with perinatologist for further orders.
7. Establish and maintain respiratory support according to transport protocol.

Ruptured uterus

If patient has increased or sudden extreme abdominal pain, sudden cessation of contractions in laboring, previously scarred uterus, or symptoms of shock, or small parts of fetus can be palpated through abdominal wall:

1. Check pulse, respirations, and blood pressure every 5 minutes and monitor fetal heart tone if possible on fetal monitor.
2. Increase IV fluids to maintain blood pressure.
3. Establish IV infusion—use lactated Ringer's or Plasmanate.
4. Establish and maintain respiratory support according to transport protocol.
5. Get to nearest hospital.
6. Maintain radio contact with perinatologist.

Impending delivery

1. Place patient in lithotomy position.
2. Control expulsion of fetus.
3. Hold head of baby down and clear airway with bulb suction.
4. Stimulate fetal back to stimulate respirations. If no response, begin infant CPR as outlined in protocol.
5. Clamp and cut cord and direct distal blood flow to baby.
6. Collect cord blood.
7. Don't pull on cord attached to placenta.
8. Massage uterus to assist placental expulsion.
9. Add oxytocin (Pitocin) 20 units intravenously.

Continued.

Box 13-5
UTAH VALLEY REGIONAL MEDICAL CENTER
EMERGENCIES DURING TRANSPORT—cont'd

10. (Return to Utah Valley Regional Medical Center.)
11. Maintain contact by radio with perinatologist.

Prolapsed cord

Predisposing factors: Prematurity, breech presentations, transverse lie, multiple pregnancy, premature rupture of membranes without engagement, and polyhydramnios

1. Insert gloved hand in vagina and elevate presenting part of cord.
2. Follow fetal pulse.
3. Put mother in knee-chest position.
4. Mask O_2 at 8 L to patient.
5. With stable fetal heart tone, continue to Utah Valley Regional Medical Center.

6. If unable to maintain stable fetal heart tone, with elevation of presenting part, land at nearest hospital for delivery.

Fetal distress

1. If fetal bradycardia is detected:
   a. Use continuous fetal monitoring of fetal heart tone.
   b. Perform vaginal examination for possible cord prolapse.
   c. Turn patient to left side.
   d. Give oxygen at 8 L to mother.
   e. Put patient in knee-chest position if appropriate.
2. If bradycardia persists and is severe (90) and prolonged, direct pilot to land at nearest hospital unless less than 10 minutes from Utah Valley Regional Medical Center.

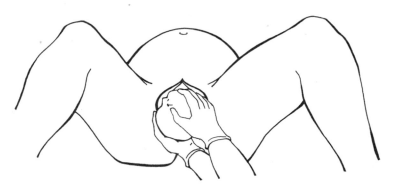

Fig. 13-2   Delivery of the head. Place in a dependent position. (From *Emergency Nursing: Principles and Practice* by S.B. Sheehy, 1992, St. Louis, Mosby.)

Box 13-6
UTAH VALLEY REGIONAL MEDICAL CENTER TRANSPORT OF PATIENT WITH PREGNANCY-INDUCED HYPERTENSION

Purpose
To establish protocol for transport care of the patient with pregnancy-induced hypertension.

Protocol
Before transport

1. Check blood pressure, temperature, pulse, and respirations, and fetal heart tone.
2. Assess presence or absence of contractions, noting frequency, duration, and quality.
3. Perform vaginal examination for dilatation, station, and presentation.
4. Establish intravenous infusion with 16-gauge catheter.
5. Use Foley catheter with urometer.
6. Assess status of magnesium sulfate therapy:
    a. Check blood pressure as compared with prenatal, admitting, and previous blood pressure.
    b. Reflexes.
    c. Output for past hour.
    d. Respirations above 12 per minute.
    e. Amount of magnesium sulfate given, if any.
    f. Urine protein level.
    g. Administer magnesium sulfate either intravenously or intramuscularly per order of perinatologist if not already started.

7. Collect intake and output record for past 24 hours.
8. Record all information on maternal transport form.
9. Obtain consent forms for transfer.
10. Obtain copies of patient records.

During transport

1. Maintain total hourly input at 150 ml/hour. If urine output is less than 30 ml/hour, increase to total input of 200 ml/hour by intravenous fluids.
2. If administering magnesium sulfate intravenously, maintain 20 g magnesium sulfate in 1000 ml. Infuse 5% dextrose in 0.2 normal saline; run at 100 ml/hour (2 g/hour rate).
3. Check vital signs, blood pressure, pulse, and respiration every 15 minutes and continuous fetal monitoring.
4. Discontinue magnesium sulfate if:
    a. Respirations are less than 12 per minute.
    b. Reflexes are totally absent.
    c. Patient is unresponsive.
    d. Sudden flushing, sweating, hypotension, or flaccid.
5. May give 10 ml of 10% calcium gluconate intravenously slowly for magnesium intoxication.
6. Have airway and tongue blade.
7. Nothing by mouth.
8. Follow strict intake and output.

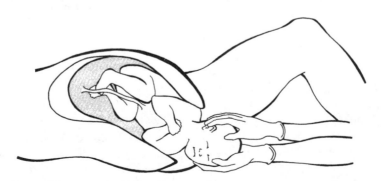

Fig. 13-3   The infant's head needs to be carefully supported during delivery. (From *Emergency Nursing: Principles and Practice* by S.B. Sheehy, 1992, St. Louis, Mosby.)

Box 13-9
UTAH VALLEY REGIONAL MEDICAL CENTER MATERNAL LIFE FLIGHT PROTOCOL FOR TRANSPORT OF PATIENT WITH PREMATURE RUPTURE OF MEMBRANES

Purpose

To establish protocol for the maternal transport team for the transport of the patient with premature rupture of membranes.

Protocol

Before transport

1. Confirm diagnosis of premature rupture of membranes, noting color of fluid and amount.
2. Perform sterile vaginal examination for prolapse of cord (unless otherwise ordered by perinatologist).
3. Assess for contractions.
4. Check temperature, pulse, respiration, and fetal heart tone.
5. Compare admission temperature with subsequent temperature.
6. Establish intravenous line if indicated.
7. Record information.
8. Give terbutaline (Brethine) 0.25 mg subcutaneously as needed every 30 to 60 minutes for contractions before departure and during transport.
9. Check laboratory values of hematocrit and white blood cell count, if available.
10. Call perinatologist.

During transport

1. Check vital signs every 30 minutes.
2. Continuous fetal monitoring.
3. Record information.

Box 13-10
UTAH VALLEY REGIONAL MEDICAL CENTER MATERNAL LIFE FLIGHT PROTOCOL FOR TRANSPORT OF PATIENT WITH MULTIPLE PREGNANCY

Purpose

To establish protocol for maternal transport nurse to transport patient with multiple pregnancy.

Protocol

Before transport

1. Perform vaginal examination for dilatation, station, and presentation of presenting part.
2. Check blood pressure, temperature, pulse, respiration, and fetal heart tone.
3. Assess for contractions. If patient is having contractions, assess contractions for quality, duration, and frequency.
4. Establish intravenous line.
5. Record information.
6. Call perinatologist and inform of patient condition; if delivery is imminent, obtain orders for administration of any medications.

During transport

1. Check vital signs every 30 minutes.
2. Continuous fetal monitoring.
3. Observe for contractions.
4. Record information.

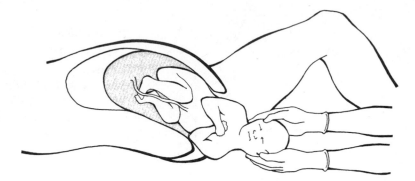

Fig. 13-4   Delivery of the shoulders. Once the shoulders are delivered the rest of the infant generally will rapidly follow. (From *Emergency Nursing: Principles and Practice* by S.B. Sheehy, 1992, St Louis, Mosby.)

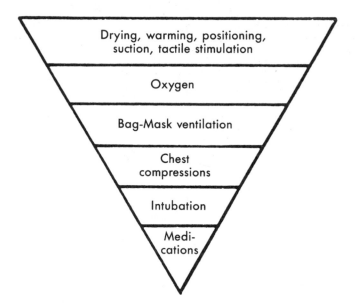

Fig. 13-5   Neonatal resuscitation. (From *Textbook of Advanced Pediatric Life Support* by the American Heart Association, 1988, Dallas, The Author.)

CARE OF THE PATIENT WITH A COMMUNICATION PROBLEM
Before Transport
1. Assess the patient's ability to communicate
2. Establish a system of communication for both the nurse and patient before transport
3. Use alternative methods when available and feasible (writing, behavioral)
4. Have family members, friends, and translators assist in explaining the transport process to the patient

5. Use communication techniques based on the patient's age
6. Consider allowing family member or translator to accompany patient during transport
7. Learn key words or use a reference for important words and phrases of a foreign language

During Transport
1. Allow patient to use aids when possible (e.g., hearing aids)
2. Reduce distractions and stress (use headphones and music)
3. Maintain eye contact and physical contact,

Table 13-1 Nursing Diagnoses, Interventions, and Evaluative Criteria for Specific Patient Populations (Elderly Patient, Pregnant Patient, and the Patient with a Communication Problem)

Diagnosis	Interventions	Evaluative Criteria
Ineffective thermoregulation related to the age of the patient and the need to take the patient out of a controlled environment for resuscitation transport.	Keep the patient covered during transport. Administer warm fluids for fluid. Administer warm humidified oxygen. Monitor the patient for signs and symptoms of hypothermia including altered mental status and shivering.	Patient will state feeling comfortable. Patient's temperature will remain within normal limits.
High risk for injury related to seizures from eclampsia during transport.	Check blood pressure frequently. Administer medications as prescribed (magnesium sulfate, diazepam). Turn patient on side to protect airway. Have suction available and working. Establish an airway as needed. Administer high-flow O_2. Assess fetal status (heart tone and movement). Have calcium gluconate available for potential magnesium sulfate toxicity.	The potential for seizure activity will be recognized. The patient's seizure activity will cease with treatment. The patient's airway will be protected. The patient's risk of injury from toxicity will be decreased through appropriate preparation.
Impaired communication related to the patient's inability to speak or understand English.	Identify methods that may be used to communicate with patient during transport. Use a reference manual or learn important phrases that may be used during transport. Identify resource people. Learn important words and phrases for languages that may be encountered in one's service area.	The patient will be able to communicate with the nurse. The patient will be comfortable during the transport process.

if permitted by the patient, to decrease anxiety
4. Give simple explanations during transport
5. Always assume that the patient understands what is going on
6. Allow the patient time to respond

SUMMARY

The care and transport of patients who are elderly, pregnant, or have a communication problem require an understanding of the aging process, the physiological changes related to pregnancy, and the impact that alterations in the communication process may have on patients. The nurse needs to plan care for these patients based on these additional care challenges. Table 13-1 contains a summary of the care of these patients using nursing diagnoses. The case study at the end of this chapter offers a further example of the care and transport of the pregnant patient.

CASE STUDY

Case Scenario

A 23-year-old pregnant woman was involved in a motor vehicle crash before arrival of the nurse and physician transport team. The life squad related that the patient had been without vital signs for 5 minutes. Cardiopulmonary resuscitation was in progress. Transport time to the closest facility was 15 minutes by air and 45 minutes by ground.

History obtained from the patient's husband indicated that the patient was 9 months' pregnant. Inspection of her abdomen showed the fundus to be above her diaphragm. Because of the transport distance, the physician elected to perform a perimortem cesarean section to enhance both the mother and infant's chances of survival.

An abdominal incision was made, and a fe-male infant was immediately delivered. The child's size indicated that she was full term.

Transport Care and Interventions

Resuscitation was continued for the mother with no changes noted after the delivery. The mother was transported by ground to the closest facility where she eventually died.

Initially the infant had a pulse rate of 50 with no spontaneous respirations. Cardiopulmonary resuscitation was initiated, and the baby was intubated with a 2.5 uncuffed tube. Epinephrine and atropine were given through the endotracheal tube. The infant was flown to the neonatal unit.

The neonatal team assumed resuscitation upon the infant's arrival. An umbilical catheter was inserted, and fluid resuscitation in addition to pharmacological resuscitation was initiated. Despite aggressive resuscitation, the baby died about 1 hour after delivery. Unbeknownst to the nurse and physician, the child had sustained a skull fracture from the impact of the motor vehicle crash.

Discussion

The incidence of trauma occurring during pregnancy is estimated to be between 6% to 7%. In a study done by Drost, Rosemurgy, Sherman, Scott, & Williams (1990), 64% of pregnant women who were traumatically injured sustained blunt trauma from motor vehicle crashes. One of the common complications of blunt trauma is abruptio placenta (Figure 13-6) and uterine rupture.

When a pregnant women has sustained a life-threatening injury, a perimortem cesarean section may be considered to potentially save both the mother and the child's life. Delivery of the child facilitates maternal blood flow. Indications for a perimortem cesarean section include a fetal gestation age of 24 to 26 weeks and older and the amount of time the mother has been without vital signs. Delivery should occur within 9 minutes of the cessation of maternal

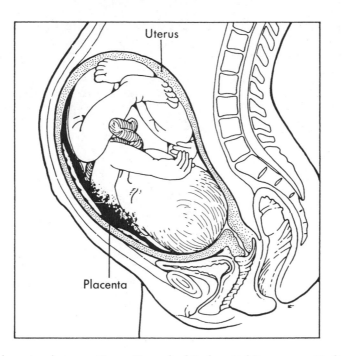

Fig. 13-6   Abruptio placenta. (From *Manual of Prehospital Emergency Medicine* by R.H. Miller & J.K. Wilson, 1992, St. Louis, Mosby.)

vital signs to ensure the greatest possibility of fetal survival (Strong & Lowe, 1989). About 15% of infants delivered by perimortem cesarean section survive and are healthy.

The procedure is performed by making a midline abdominal incision. Once the location of the infant has been identified in the uterine cavity, the child's head is lifted out of the uterus and delivered. The child's airway should be cleared and the rest of the body delivered (Strong & Lowe, 1989).

Even though this is a rare problem to be encountered in the field, being prepared to perform this procedure may be the only chance both the mother and infant may have for survival. Anticipating this potential problem, as well as having the appropriate equipment, may mean the difference between life and death for mother and child.

REFERENCES

Burns, J, & Bayley, E. (1992). Elderly in E. Bayley & S. Turcke (Eds.), *A comprehensive curriculum for trauma nursing* (pp. 467-478). Boston: Jones & Bartlett.

Cardona, V., Hurn, P., Mason, P., Scanlon-Schilpp, A., Veise-Berry, S. (1988). *Trauma nursing: From resuscitation through rehabilitation*. Philadelphia: W.B. Saunders.

Champion, H., Copes, W., Buyer, D., Flanagan, M., Bain, L., & Sacco, W. (1989). Major trauma in geriatric patients. *American Journal of Public Health, 79*(9),1278-1281.

Dandan, I. (1992). Trauma in the elderly. *Topics in Emergency medicine, 14*(3),39-46.

Drost, T., Rosemurgy, A., Sherman, H., Scott, L., & Williams, K. (1990). Major trauma in pregnant women: Maternal/fetal outcome. *Journal of Trauma, 31*(5),574-578.

Elliott, J., Spii, T., & Balazs, K. (1992). Maternal transport of patients with advanced cervical dilatation: To fly or not to fly? *Obstetrics and Gynecology, 79*(3),380-382.

Henninger, B. (1992). Obstetric. In E. Bayley & S. Turcke (eds.), *Trauma nursing* (pp. 455-466). Boston: Jones & Bartlett.

Henry, M., & Stapleton, E. (1992). *EMT prehospital care.* Philadelphia: W.B. Saunders.

Janing, J. (1992). Tarnishing the golden years. *The Journal of Emergency Services, 24*(9), 40-43, 58.

Judd, R. (1991). EMS strategies and the elderly. *Journal of Emergency Services, 23*(2), 29, 54.

Kauder, D., & Schwab, W. (1991). Trauma in the elderly. *Journal of Emergency Services, 23*(2), 22-26.

Manley, L. (1993). Trauma in pregnancy. In J. Neff & P. Kidd (Eds.), *Trauma nursing: Art and science* (pp. 499-525). St. Louis: Mosby.

Miller, R., & Wilson, J. (1992). *Manual of prehospital care.* St. Louis: Mosby.

Nelson, M. (1988). The high-risk obstetrical patient. *Air medical crew national standard curriculum.* Pasadena, CA: Association of Air Medical Services.

Newman, R. (1993). Trauma and the elderly. In J. Neff & P. Kidd (Eds.), *Trauma nursing: Art and science* (pp. 555-588). St. Louis: Mosby.

Poulton, T., Gutierrez, P. (1992). Fetal monitoring during air medical transport. *Journal of Air Medical Transport, 11*(11-12), 13-17.

Riley, T., Cleary, V. (1987). Field conditions affecting patient management. In V. Cleary, P. Wilson, & G. Super (Eds.), *Prehospital care* (pp. 88-89). Rockville, MD: Aspen Publications.

Rhodes, J. (1990). Double trouble: Trauma for two. *Emergency Medical Services, 10,* 29-31.

Sherman, H., Scott, L., Rosemurgy, A. (1990). Changes affecting the initial evaluation and care of the pregnant trauma victim. *Journal of Emergency Medicine, 8,* 575-582.

Skidmore-Roth, L. (1993). *Mosby's nursing drug reference.* St. Louis: Mosby.

Skinner, G. (1991). Obstetric emergencies. In G. Lee (Ed.). *Flight nursing: Principles and practice* (pp. 498-538). St. Louis: Mosby.

Strong, T., & Lowe, R. (1989). Perimortem cesarean section. *American Journal of Emergency Medicine, 7*(5), 489-494.

Thompson, J., McFarland, G., Hirsch, J., Tucker, S., & Bowers, A. (1993). *Mosby's manual of clinical nursing* (2nd ed.). St. Louis: Mosby.

PART THREE

Issues in Prehospital Nursing

CHAPTER 14

Challenges in Prehospital Nursing

OBJECTIVES

1. Describe the use of continuous quality improvement in the practice of prehospital nursing care
2. Discuss the legal and ethical challenges faced by the nurse in the prehospital care environment
3. Identify the sources of stress in the prehospital care environment
4. Discuss methods of stress management
5. Describe critical incident stress management

COMPETENCIES

1. Identify a continuous quality improvement project for prehospital nursing
2. Develop a policy that describes when to cease resuscitation in the field
3. Employ methods to manage individual stress in the prehospital care environment

The practice of nursing in the prehospital care environment involves not only being educated, skilled, and competent in caring for patients in various circumstances but also being prepared to face challenges that may not be encountered in hospital nursing practice. Some of these challenges include developing methods to continuously improve professional care skills, making legal and ethical decisions, and managing the stress that is a common component of prehospital nursing care.

The purpose of this chapter is to describe and discuss the implications of three particular challenges that nurses may face when caring for the patient in the prehospital environment. These include continuous quality improvement (CQI) and quality management (QM), ethical and legal issues, and stress management.

CONTINUOUS QUALITY IMPROVEMENT AND QUALITY MANAGEMENT IN PREHOSPITAL NURSING CARE

Quality assurance is a familiar concept among all business and industries. Since its introduction into hospital nursing practice by the Joint Commission of Accreditation of Healthcare Organizations (JCAHO) in the late 1970s, quality assurance has been an important part of each hospital's plan of care (O'Leary & O'Leary, 1992). Quality assurance has been described as the sum of all activities that are undertaken to provide confidence that the products or services available maintain the standard of excellence established for those particular products or services (Polsky, 1992).

Measuring quality assurance requires the de-

337

velopment of a plan to meet standards of care, which has been accomplished through chart audits and case reviews (Butler, 1992). Quality assurance identifies when care did not meet a particular standard, but it does not address the reasons why or what may be done to improve.

During the past decade the problems with using only a quality assurance program to assess the quality of care have come under scrutiny. Limitations to the use of quality assurance include its narrow definition of quality care, its focus on only one group of care providers, and its failure to account for the effects of the interactions of all those involved in a patient's care (Fanucci, Hammill, Johannson, Leggett, & Smith, 1993). Because of the limitations of quality assurance and the observation that patient care does not occur within a vacuum, the process of CQI and QM is now being advocated by industries and JCAHO for use in hospitals (O'Leary & O'Leary, 1992).

CQI examines not only the quality of care that is being provided but also what can be done to improve the care. Quality improvement involves the process of patient care, allows input from all involved to establish norms and find ways to maintain these norms, and speaks of a commitment to improvement (Resource Document, 1992).

CQI as used in health-care is based on Deming's theory of continuous quality improvement derived from studies of Japanese management in industries after World War II. The ideas integral to CQI include the following (Fanucci, Hammill, Johannson, Leggett, & Smith, 1993; O'Leary & O'Leary, 1992; Southard & Eastes, 1993):

1. The need for CQI to be developed and maintained internally
2. The need for each institution to have a statement of its philosophy, mission, and purpose, and for all to be committed to this institutional statement
3. The need for CQI to be practiced throughout the entire organization

4. The philosophy that the quality of care can always be improved
5. The need for each organization to create a climate of creativity
6. The need for leadership skills to be taught and developed
7. The importance of CQI being organized around patient care not around the organization itself
8. The encouragement of education and self-improvement.
9. The need of CQI to be action oriented

Use of CQI/QM in Prehospital Care

Because CQI is still essentially in its infancy in hospital nursing practice, its use outside of the hospital is still developing. The American College of Emergency Physicians, the National Association of Emergency Physicians, the National Flight Nurses Association, and the Association of Air Medical Services have produced documents that address the use of QM and CQI in the prehospital setting (Balazs, 1993; Polsky, 1992; Swor, 1993).

One major problem faced by nurses and caregivers who practice in this environment is the lack of standardization and specific guidelines for care. Even though the Department of Transportation established a curriculum outline in 1973 that has been periodically reevaluated to describe practice in the prehospital care environment, each state, county, city, and, at times, individual organizations have adapted and applied these guidelines as needed. Multiple systems are involved in the provision of prehospital care, including referral systems, dispatch systems, types of vehicles used for transport, types of equipment used by individual care providers, protocols used, and the variety of patients transported (Swor, 1992). The complexities of these systems pose a unique challenge to quality management.

Methods that may be used to monitor or measure CQI include prospective, concurrent, and retrospective evaluations (Johnson, 1992).

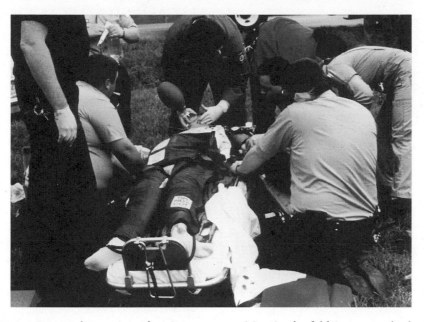

Fig. 14-1   Direct observation of patient care provision in the field is one method of employing continuous quality improvement in prehospital nursing practice.

Examples of prospective evaluation are personnel education and training records, continuing education records, skills evaluation, and preceptor apprenticeships. Concurrent evaluation may occur through direct observation of skill performance (Figure 14-1). Retrospective evaluation includes chart review, critique of specific cases, and chart audits with specific criteria.

Specific indicators for care need to be developed, and these indicators must be measurable and objective (Southard and Eastes, 1993). The indicators may be either sentinel events or rate based. Sentinel events are events that are serious enough to warrant specific review, for example, patients who die within 24 hours of transport or the discovery of an esophageal intubation. Rate-based indicators are less high risk and may be reviewed with other data, for example, activation times of the transport team. Box 14-1 contains examples of some indicators

that are used by the National Flight Nurses Association and the Association of Air Medical Services.

The key issues in the use of QM/CQI in the practice of nursing in the prehospital setting are the need to establish some mutually agreed upon standards of care for patient transport including the qualifications and education for those nurses providing that care, the development of methods to evaluate the care provided, provision of feedback about what is found, and the need to recognize that change may be necessary to provide the optimum level of care each patient may require (Davis & Billitier, 1993; Kallsen, 1993). Continuous quality management must involve the entire organization or systems involved in the organization, empower individuals to make change, and include commitment and support from management to be successful and make a difference in patient care.

Box 14-1

**ASSOCIATION OF AIR MEDICAL
SERVICES/NATIONAL FLIGHT
NURSES ASSOCIATION QUALITY
ASSURANCE RESOURCE
DOCUMENT INDICATORS**

Medical

1. Airway
   a. Appropriateness of intubation by air medical personnel
   b. Success rate of intubation attempts
   c. Documentation of endotracheal tube placement
   d. Appropriate size of endotracheal tube

Operational

2. Timeliness of care
   a. Scene times on the ground less than 20 minutes
   b. Bedside time preparation less than 30 minutes
3. Safety
   a. All patients secured to aircraft stretcher with two or more straps
   b. Flight following completed and documented by communications personnel every 15 minutes on radio
   c. Weekly fuel samples of on-site fueling reservoirs meet minimum quality-control standards
   d. Documentation of safety training of all air medical personnel
   e. Documentation of geographically appropriate survival training

Note. From *AAMS/NFNA QA Resource Document Indicators* by K. Balazs, 1993, Pasadena, CA: Association of Air Medical Services.

LEGAL AND ETHICAL CHALLENGES

The legal and ethical challenges of providing care in the prehospital care environment are probably some of the most interesting but potentially difficult situations that caregivers may face. Some of the legal and ethical issues that caregivers may confront include patients who refuse care, patients who refuse to be transported, questions raised related to cardiopulmonary resuscitation, personnel safety in the patient care situation, and social and psychiatric situations.

Although some legal and ethical issues are interrelated, many ethical problems are not governed by laws. Laws vary from state to state and may not reflect ethical behavior. Ethical analysis should provide a framework for the determination of moral duty, obligation, and conduct (Adams, 1993).

Refusal of Treatment and to be Transported

One of the most common legal problems confronted by the prehospital nurse is a patient's refusal to be treated or transported. When a patient refuses to be treated or transported, the caregiver needs to determine if the patient is competent to refuse services. Patients should be able to demonstrate the ability to understand their options related to their care and the consequences of the actions that they may choose (Sucov, Verdile, Garettson, & Paris, 1992). In addition, the patient must be an adult (over the age of 18, an emancipated minor, a minor who is married, or a member of the military) or the parent/legal guardian of a minor. If the patient is competent, the patient's wishes need to be respected or the caregiver runs the risk of being charged with assault and battery. This can be a difficult situation, particularly if the patient's family, referring hospital personnel, or individuals at the scene of the response believe the patient should be transported. It is advisable to contact medical direction for assistance and to document the patient's decision-making ability carefully.

Patients with an intracranial injury, intoxicated by alcohol or drugs, suffering from a metabolic disorder (hyperglycemia, hypoglycemia, hypernatremia, hypothermia, hypothermia, and so forth) or mentally ill may not be capable of making a competent decision (Adams, 1993). It is important that whichever decision is made, that it be made carefully and with respect for the patient.

Two studies found that there are potential hazardous consequences related to refusal of treatment or transport whether the refusal comes from the patient, the patient's family, or the EMS provider (Sucov, Verdile, Garrettson, & Paris, 1992; Zachariah, Bryan, Pepe, & Griffin, 1992). In the study by Zachariah, Bryan, Pepe, and Griffin (1992), 15 patients who were not transported because of denial or mutual agreement and were able to be contacted were found by the researchers to have medical problems ranging from peritonitis to pneumonia that eventually needed hospitalization or other medical care. Sucov, Verdile, Garrettson, and Paris (1992) noted that when patients refused transport, it was difficult to follow-up to ensure that there were no complications related to their refusal to be treated or transported. Both studies agreed that the problem of refusal requires preestablished protocols, medical direction involvement, and a method of quality management that provides for patient follow-up to identify potential problems that may result from lack of treatment or transport. Figures 14-2 and 14-3 offer examples of forms that may be used to document refusal of care.

Other Legal Considerations

Two other legal considerations that may concern the nurse in prehospital practice include confidentiality and documentation. The patient's privacy needs to be respected. Careful use of descriptions that may identify the patient

during radio communications or casual conversations helps to ensure patient privacy (Frew, 1990). The clash between patient privacy and caregiver safety is always a potential. This issue has been debated intensely during the past 12 years because of the spread of the human immunodeficiency virus (HIV) in the general population. In some states prehospital caregivers may have access to a patient's HIV status if they are exposed to an infectious individual and provide documentation. However, in some areas of the country this information is not accessible. In addition, other potentially dangerous diseases may be encountered such as hepatitis B virus, which may cause serious illness in prehospital care providers if they are exposed. (Refer to Chapter 11 for a discussion of infectious diseases in the prehospital care environment.)

Finally, documentation is equally important in the prehospital care environment as in the hospital environment, yet it can be more challenging. Time constraints, lighting, and vehicle movement are only a few of the things that may interfere with the ability to complete a patient record. Currently, research is in progress to use computer technology for documentation, including the use of an electric pen and screen device, as well as voice-activated documentation (Trofino, 1993). Figure 14-3 offers an example of a nursing record that is used for both ground and air patient transport.

Ethical Considerations

According to Raffin (1992) the goals of critical care are to save the salvageable, restore health, relieve suffering, and when there is no hope, not to interfere with allowing the patient to die a peaceful and dignified death. As prehospital caregivers, nurses are educated and trained to sustain the lives of patients in the process of dying. This may be accomplished through the use of life-support devices such as mechanical ventilators, balloon pumps, or left

AGAINST MEDICAL ADVICE

RELEASE

_____
RUN REPORT NUMBER

I, _____ , acknowledge that on
　　Name

_____　　_____　　/　　_____　　/　　_____
Date　　　　　EMT-II/Paramedic (circle one)　　Cert #　　　　Service Provider Agency

explained my condition to me and advised me of some of the
potential risks and/or complications which could or would arise
from refusal of medical care. I have also been advised that other
unknown risks and/or complications are possible. Being aware that
there are known and unknown potential risks and/or complications,
it is still my desire to refuse the advised medical care.

I do hereby release _____ ,
　　　　　　　　　　　Service Provider Agency

its agents, employees, base hospital, base hospital physician(s)
and mobile intensive care nurse(s) from all liability resulting
from any adverse medical condition(s) caused by my refusal of the
recommended medical care.

_____　　_____am/pm
Signature of Patient/Parent/Legal Guardian　　Date

_____　　_____
First Witness　　　　　　　　　　　Second Witness

If witness acted as translator, check here [ ]

Name of Translator_____

REFUSAL TO SIGN RELEASE

On _____ , _____ did:
　　Date　　　　　　Patient/Responsible Party

[ ] refuse advised medical care.

[ ] refuse to sign the above RELEASE.

_____　　_____
First Witness　　　　　　　　　　　Second Witness

RISK OF REFUSING MEDICAL CARE

In addition to various unknown risks and/or complications, some of
the potential risks and/or complications are:

_____

_____

S-SV EMS Agency Form 850B　　　　　　　　　　　　　　September 27, 1991

Fig. 14-2　　Example of document illustrating refusal for care.

PATIENTS REFUSING CARE
MICN DOCUMENTATION FORM

DATE	TIME	EMT NAME	EMS RESPONSE FORM NUMBER

COMPLAINT

VITAL SIGNS: _____ _____ _____ _____   Yes [ ]   No [ ]
             BP   PULSE   RESP.   AGE   (If Minor: Parent/Legal Guardian Present?)

YES NO   YES NO

[ ] [ ] DRUGS/ALCOHOL/UNDER THE INFLUENCE   [ ] [ ] OD

[ ] [ ] VERBALIZED SUICIDE   [ ] [ ] THREATENED SOMEONE ELSE

[ ] [ ] GRAVELY ILL   [ ] [ ] POSSIBLE ACTIVE BLEEDING

[ ] [ ] CONFUSED/UNABLE TO MAKE CLEAR JUDGEMENT   [ ] [ ] LOC ALTERED IN ANY WAY

IF THE ANSWER TO ANY OF THE ABOVE IS YES, DO NOT RELEASE THE PATIENT WITHOUT FURTHER ACTION OR INVESTIGATION. SEE "PATIENT REFUSING CARE" POLICY FOR ACTION RECOMMENDATIONS.

IF THE ANSWERS TO ALL OF THE ABOVE ARE NO, PROCEED.

YES NO

[ ] [ ] ALERT-ORIENTED

       [ ] Name   [ ] Day/Year   [ ] Where he/she lives   [ ] Where he/she is: why?   [ ] What happened

What specific steps have been taken to inform the patient of the consequences of not receiving care? _____
_____

YES NO

[ ] [ ] Does patient understand the risk of no medical care?

[ ] [ ] Is the patient willing to see a physician on his/her own?

[ ] [ ] Has the patient signed an "Against Medical Advice Statement"?

[ ] [ ] AMA witnessed?

[ ] [ ] Refuse to sign AMA is documented on AMA?

OUTCOME:

AGENCY CALLED_____ BADGE NUMBER_____

              _____ BADGE NUMBER_____

HOLD PLACED 5170_____ 5150_____ MINOR PLACED IN PROTECTIVE CUSTODY _____

ELDER PLACED ON ADULT PROTECTIVE SERVICES_____ PATIENT HAS OTHER TRANSPORTATION TO HOSPITAL _____

PATIENT RELEASED ON OWN_____ BASE RN/MICN _____ PHYSICIAN CALLED _____

Fig. 14-3   Example of document illustrating refusal for care.

ventricular assist devices; fluid resuscitation; administration of blood; drug administration; and transport to the most appropriate place for additional medical care such as an organ transplant (Raffin, 1992). However, the transport process is incredibly frightening to patients not only because of the illness or injury that the patient has suffered but also because of the potential of facing death and the need to leave family and friends or other support systems. Critical care and transport may not be in the best interest of the patient, particularly when the patient's goals are different from the caregiver's goals. The way these decisions are made are evaluated in the process of biomedical/ethical decision making.

The principles of biomedical ethics are beneficence, nonmaleficence, autonomy, and justice (Raffin, 1992). Beneficence involves looking at the benefits of care decisions made in relation to the good they bring to the patient. Sometimes these actions are performed to offer the greatest good for the patient without consideration of the best interests of the patient (Ulrich & Blazing, 1991), for example, a protocol that calls for CPR to be initiated on all patients no matter what the cause of the arrest.

Nonmaleficence is the principle of doing no harm. Autonomy involves patients' choice about the type of care they may want. As previously discussed, sometimes the patient's ability to make decisions is impaired. When a patient is incapacitated due to illness or injury, the patient's family or the health caregivers may need to make decisions (Dworkin, 1993).

Finally the principle of justice involves fair allocation of resources for patient care. Justice or fairness also entails the rendering of emergency care without regard to race, color, national origin, worthiness, or patient behaviors (e.g., drug abuse) (Ulrich & Blazing, 1991).

Raffin (1992) recommends that four key principles be considered when making ethical decisions related to the critically ill or injured patient. These include the following:

1. Establishing the authority for decision making (patient, family, judicial system)
2. Establishing effective communication with the patient and the patient's family
3. Determining early the quality of the patient's life and the patient's desires as related to quality of life
4. Recognizing the patient's rights and autonomy

In general, prehospital care providers have the duty to provide patient care by being educated and skilled in their work and being sure that the equipment they use is functioning. However, the duty to provide care does not require prehospital caregivers to put themselves at risk (Adams, 1993). Safety is always of the utmost priority.

It can be very difficult to make ethical decisions in field situations. Prehospital caregivers lack prior relationships with the patient and the patient's family, generally are not aware initially of what the patient's and family's wishes are for care, and many times do not have access to all the information in the patient's medical records (Jecker, 1992).

Ethical decision making by nurses does not occur in a vacuum. Nurses needs to reflect on their personal values related to death, quality of life, and technology and the maintenance of life. Preplanning for potential ethical issues can decrease the anxiety and stress that may accompany that decision-making process. Case discussion, protocols, and identification of available resources are examples of methods that may employed.

Decisions Concerning Resuscitation

Both society and trauma resuscitators will accept that the patient who has a fatal injury will die with dignity, not being subject to extensive and expensive resurrection techniques" (Mattox, 1993, p. 735).

One of the most difficult decisions that the nurse must make in prehospital care practice involves the initiation or cessation of cardiopulmonary resuscitation. The survival rate for out-of-hospital cardiac arrests as the result of trauma varies from 1.4% to 3.2% (Wright, Dronen, Combs, & Storer, 1989). Kellermann, Staves, and Hackman (1988) found that only 1.6% of the patients who sustained out-of-hospital cardiac arrest (n = 240) survived to hospital discharge. Two were discharged home neurologically intact and two to nursing homes with severe neurological deficits. Out-of-hospital cardiac arrest carries a low survival rate.

Nurses practicing in the prehospital care environment will encounter patients in four different categories of cardiopulmonary arrest (Johnson & Maggione, 1993): (1) patients with advanced directives or do-not-resuscitate orders (DNR), (2) patients without advanced directives but are expected to die, (3) patients who die unexpectedly but have a poor prognosis (traumatic arrests), and (4) patients who experience sudden death but may survive with immediate and appropriate interventions.

Currently the recognized guidelines for indications not to perform CPR from the American Heart Association are refusal by a competent person, presence of DNR orders, patients who are decapitated, and patients with rigor mortis, tissue decomposition, and extreme lividity (Jecker, 1992). Even with these guidelines, CPR is not initiated by prehospital care providers because of other factors. In a study done by Johnson and Maggione (1993), 68% of the emergency medical technicians surveyed indicated that on one or more occasions they had been in a situation in which resuscitation was withheld. Reasons given for not resuscitating patients included the advanced age of the patient, presence of a terminal illness, and uncertainty of downtime.

Many states, counties, hospitals, and Emergency Medical Service systems have initiated "portable" DNR orders that can be carried by the patient and honored outside of the hospital. The American College of Emergency Physi-cians offers guidelines for setting up "portable" DNR orders for EMS systems.

However, problems may still occur even with the use of DNR orders. Some of these problems include the following (Iserson, 1989; Jecker, 1992):

1. Less than 10% of the population with a terminal illness have DNR orders.
2. Advanced directives contain provisions that allow for patients to change their minds.
3. Discussing DNR status during patient resuscitation is difficult for both the family and prehospital caregivers.

Education of patients, families, and caregivers offers one solution to this difficult dilemma. As pointed out by Dworkin (1993, p. 217), ". . . making someone die in a way that others approve, but he or she believes a horrifying contradiction of his or her life, is a devastating, odious form of tyranny." Box 14-2 contains some recommendations for resolving and meeting this challenge. Figures 14-4 and 14-5 con-

---

Box 14-2

RECOMMENDATIONS FOR DEVELOPING GUIDELINES FOR CEASING RESUSCITATION

1. Evaluation of the futility of the resuscitation
   - Cause of the arrest
   - Amount of time patient has been down
2. Development of a consensus for a do-not-resuscitate protocol involving hospitals and prehospital care providers
3. Research of the outcome of out-of-hospital CPR to identify survivability and quality of life when patient has sustained out-of-hospital CPR

Note. From "Ceasing Futile Resuscitation in the Field: Ethical Considerations" by N. Jecker, 1993, *Archives of Internal Medicine, 152*(12), 30-35.

UNIVERSITY OF CINCINNATI HOSPITAL
UNIVERSITY AIR CARE NURSING

POLICY	Page 1 of 1

POLICY: Pronouncing Patients as Dead at other Hospitals

FILE: p-9-a	DATE ORIGINATED: 11/86
REVISED: 5/90	REVIEWED: 4/92

PREVIOUS REVIEWS/REVISIONS: 11/86-11/91

PRECAUTIONS:

RESPONSIBILITY: Flight Nurse and Flight Physician

EQUIPMENT:

Purpose:
To provide guidelines for the Flight Team when making the decision to pronounce a patient dead at an other hospital.

Procedure:

A.   When it has been decided that a patient is to be pronounced dead at an other hospital, this decision is to be made in collaboration with the nursing and medical staff at the referring institution.

B.   A flight record will be initiated by the flight crew and will document any care provided and patient outcome (s).

C.   If the referring agency requests it, a copy of the chart will be provided for them.

D.   Whenever there is a question as to whether a patient should be pronounced dead at an other facility, radio or telephone contact with the Faculty should be established.

Reviewed by: Renee' S. Holleran, Daniel Storer, David Thomson

T. Jane Swaim
T. Jane Swaim
Administrator & Chief Nursing Officer, Interim

Fig. 14-4   Protocol used as guideline for pronouncing patients dead and ceasing resuscitation in the prehospital environment.

POLICY: Pronouncing Patients Dead-Scene

FILE:p-10-a	DATE ORIGINATED: 11/86
REVISED: 5/90	REVIEWED: 4/92

PREVIOUS REVIEWS/REVISIONS: 11/86- 11/91

PRECAUTIONS:

RESPONSIBILITY:

EQUIPMENT:

Purpose:
To provide guidelines for the pronouncing dead of patients by the University Air Care Flight Physician at the scene of an accident, injury, or illness.

Procedure:

A.   Due to the presence of a physician on the University Air Care Team, a patient may be pronounced dead in the field in the following circumstances.
   1.   If in the judgement of the University Air Care Physician the patient is clinically dead with no chance of survival.
   2.   The requesting agency, rescue personnel, and family members _if and when present_ are comfortable with the decisions to terminate resuscitative efforts.
   3.   There are no medical-legal contraindications to pronouncing the patient dead in the field, such as in homicide or suicide cases.
B.   The following are specific situations that if present, would generally prohibit pronouncing a patient dead in the field:
   1.   Rescue personnel have been working diligently to save the victim's life and feel that the patient should be transported to a higher level of care.
   2.   Invasive surgical procedures such as chest tube insertion has been accomplished by the University Air Care Team.
   3.   Advanced skills for establishing an adequate airway such as endotracheal intubation and cricothyrotomy, may be necessary to determine the likelihood of survival for a patient. These procedures do not preclude pronouncing a patient dead in the field, but if accomplished, should cause the University Air Care Team to carefully consider all the factors associated with pronouncing a patient dead in the field.   *Continued.*

Fig. 14-5   Protocol used as guideline for pronouncing patients dead and ceasing resuscitation in the prehospital environment.

Continued.

```
┌─────────────────────────────────────────────────────────────────────┐
│  Pronouncing Patients Dead-Scene              Page 2 of 2             │
│  ═══════════════════════════════════════════════════════════════     │
│                                                                       │
│    4.    A patient may not at any time be pronounced dead in the      │
│          aircraft or on the helipad.                                  │
│    5.    In the event that a flight nurse is flying without a         │
│          physician, he/she cannot pronounce a patient dead.           │
│    6.    Whenever there is a question as to whether a patient         │
│          should be pronounced dead in the field, radio contact        │
│          with Emergency Medicine Faculty should be established.        │
│                                                                       │
│                                                                       │
│  Reviewed by:   Renee' S. Holleran, Daniel Storer, David Thomson      │
│                                                                       │
│                                                                       │
│  ──────────────────────────────────────────────────────────────────  │
│  T. Jane Swain                                                        │
│  Administrator & Chief Nursing Officer, Interim                       │
│                                                                       │
└─────────────────────────────────────────────────────────────────────┘
```

Fig. 14-5, cont'd   Protocol used as a guideline for pronouncing patients dead and ceasing resuscitation in the prehospital environment.

tain examples of protocols that are used as guidelines for pronouncing patients dead and ceasing resuscitation in the prehospital environment.

STRESS

Stress has been defined as the body's nonspecific response to any demand (Hardin, 1985). When a person cannot cope with the challenges of a particular situation, stress arises. A person's perception, competency, and support systems all contribute to the ability to manage stress.

In the practice of prehospital nursing, stress is a state of physical and psychological arousal (Mitchell, 1992). The nature of the work and the environments in which one practices always require that the nurse be prepared to respond and function appropriately.

Factors that contribute to an individual's re-

actions and ability to handle stress in a healthy or unhealthy manner include the following:

- Intensity of the stress
- Number of times the stress is encountered
- Amount exposure to the stress
- Perceived threat the stress may cause
- Perception of the stress
- Previous experience with the stress or similar stressors
- Presence of support systems

Sources of Stress

There are myriad of sources of stress in the prehospital care environment. Both the physical and psychological environment can produce stress. Box 14-3 contains examples of physical and psychological sources of stress in the prehospital care environment, and Figures 14-6 and 14-7 illustrate some of the situations that may be sources of stress in the prehospital care environment.

```
┌─────────────────────────────────────────────┐
│                  Box 14-3                     │
│         SOURCES OF PHYSICAL AND               │
│       PSYCHOLOGICAL STRESS IN THE             │
│           PREHOSPITAL CARE                    │
│              ENVIRONMENT                      │
│                                               │
│  Physical                                     │
│  1. Limited space in which to provide patient │
│     care                                      │
│  2. Lack of appropriate patient care equip-   │
│     ment                                      │
│  3. Malfunctioning patient care equipment     │
│  4. Malfunctioning transport vehicle          │
│  5. Ambient outdoor temperature (excessive    │
│     heat or cold)                             │
│  6. Noise, odors, and vibration               │
│  7. Illness or injury of the nurse            │
│  8. Significant exposures to infectious       │
│     diseases                                  │
│                                               │
│  Psychological                                │
│  1. Pediatric patients                        │
│  2. Death of the patient                      │
│  3. The patient's illness or injury           │
│  4. Family or relatives of the patient        │
│  5. Team member interactions                  │
└─────────────────────────────────────────────┘
```

Reactions to Stress

There are physical, emotional, and cognitive reactions to stress. These reactions may be acute, occurring during the time or immediately after the stressful incident. If the stress continues, these reactions may have long-term effects. Boxes 14-4 and 14-5 contain examples of acute and long-term reactions to stress (Mitchell, 1992).

Stress Management

The management of stress needs to be an integral part of the care provided for the prehospital nurse. The effects of long-term stress, particularly the traumatic stress encountered in the prehospital environment, may lead to deterio-

ration in job performance, personality changes, anxiety states, and depression (Mitchell, 1992).

Just as there are myriad stress sources, there are many ways that stress may be prevented and managed (Bell, 1991a; Bell, 1991b). General stress management includes identifying the source of the stress, assessing life priorities, finding and using support systems, and physical exercise. Box 14-6 provides an outline of methods that may be used to prevent and manage stress (Bell, 1991b; O'Rear, 1992b).

Critical Incident Stress Management

As previously discussed, stress is an inherent component of the practice of prehospital nursing. However, the nature of prehospital nursing also leaves one at risk of being exposed to critical incident stress (CIS). CIS has been described as a heightened state of physical, cognitive, behavioral, and emotional arousal (Mitchell, 1992). Examples of sources of critical incident stress are listed in Box 14-7. The effects of CIS include not only those already discussed but also a tendency to reexperience the trauma when confronted with similar patients or care situations, avoiding similiar care situations, flashbacks, and excessive startle reactions (Mitchell, 1992).

To prevent and cope with CIS, critical incident stress management (CISM) has been developed. The components of CISM include education, CIS teams, significant-other and family support, management support, peer support, and mutual aid from community stress-management programs (Mitchell, 1992). CISM teams are located throughout the world. The majority of these teams are composed of professionals from multiple disciplines, including EMS providers, nurses, physicians, and mental health workers.

Functions of a CISM team include stress management education and the provision of a defusing or a debriefing. A defusing is a short version of a debriefing that is held within a few hours after the critical incident. A defusing is composed of an introduction, discussion of the

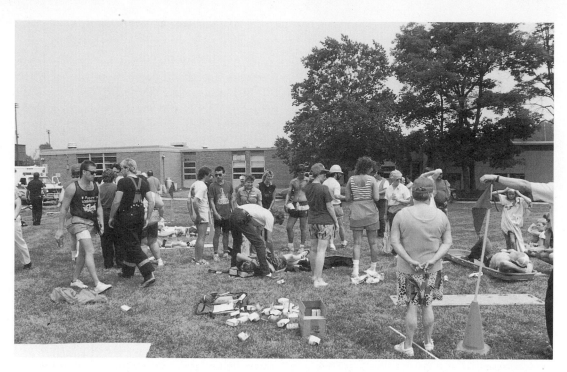

Fig. 14-6   A disaster response as an example of a source of stress in the prehospital care environment.

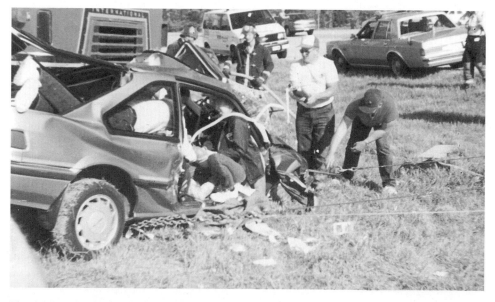

Fig. 14-7   Example of a patient entrapped for a long period of time as a source of stress in the prehospital care environment.

Box 14-4
EXAMPLES OF ACUTE REACTIONS TO STRESS

Physical	Emotional	Cognitive
Exhaustion	Nightmares	Confusion
Headaches	Inability to sleep	Inability to prioritize tasks
Nausea and vomiting	Fear	Loss of attention
Diarrhea	Guilt	Calculation problems
Sweating	Feelings of helplessness	Loss of concentration
Increased heart rate	Anger	Easily distracted
Difficulty breathing	Irritability	

Box 14-5
EXAMPLES OF LONG-TERM EFFECTS OF STRESS

Physical	Emotional	Cognitive
Headache	Setting inflexible rules	Anomia
Nausea and vomiting	Alterations in personal finances	Inability to make decisions
Chronic illness	Depression	Memory loss
		Hyperexcitability

---

incident, and a description of some of the reactions of those involved in the incident (Mitchell, 1992).

A debriefing is a formal process that generally occurs within 72 hours of the incident. Debriefings are conducted by CISM teams that are composed of mental health professionals and educated peer counselors. The debriefing is composed of seven phases, which are summarized in Box 14-8.

Stressors and critical incident stress are inherent realities in the practice of prehospital nursing. It is hoped that learning how to recognize, prevent, and manage stress will decrease the potentially devastating effects stress may have and

will help keep nurses practicing in the prehospital care environment.

CASE STUDIES

Legal Issue (Patient Refusal for Transport)
Scenario
The transport team was called to a community hospital to transport a victim of a motor vehicle crash. The patient was a 25-year-old man who was an unrestrained backseat passenger in a car that had been broadsided. The patient's parents, who were in the front seat, were killed on impact.

Box 14-6
STRESS MANAGEMENT

Physical Care

Participating in an exercise program
Using relaxation techniques (imagery, deep
breathing, and meditation)
Following an appropriate diet
Limiting or eliminating the use of tobacco
and alcohol

Emotional Care

Learning and using time-management tech-
niques
Acquiring problem-solving skills
Using humor
Spending time with people not involved in
the same work

Diversions

Allotting some private time each day
Writing a journal
Volunteering for work different from current
work (Figure 14-8)
Finding a hobby
Listening to music
Caring for a pet
Planning group activities away from work
(Figure 14-9)

Interpersonal Care

Spending time with family
Sharing feelings with others
Attending assertiveness training

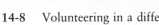

Fig. 14-8   Volunteering in a different environment than work, e.g., volunteering on a farm.

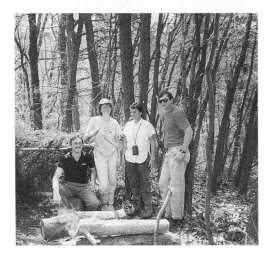

Fig. 14-9   A group outing—camping.

Upon arrival at the referring hospital, the patient was found to be awake and alert. His injuries included facial lacerations and no other obvious signs of injury. His skin was cool and clammy, and his blood pressure was 80 by palpation with a pulse rate of 90. The patient stated that he did not want to be transferred because he did not want to leave his parents.

The nurse and other team members conferred with the referring physician and nursing staff. Even though the patient was alert, his blood pressure and mechanism of injury suggested potential internal injuries. The patient was told that he would have to be transferred to a facility that could appropriately evaluate him. He was secured to a backboard and stretcher and transported.

Box 14-7

SOURCES OF CRITICAL INCIDENT STRESS

A fellow worker who has been taken hostage

Serious injury, illness, or death of a co-worker

Violent, threatening patients

Suicide or unexpected death of a co-worker

Loss of life of a patient after prolonged extrication or resuscitation

Caring for a patient who is a friend, relative, or co-worker

Incidents attracting extensive media attention

Any incidents where the sights, sounds, and odors are so distressing as to produce a high level of immediate or delayed emotional response

---

Note. From "Critical Incident Stress Debriefing" by N.A. Bell, 1991, *Emergency, 23*(9), 30-35, 58. "Comprehensive Traumatic Stress Management in the Emergency Department" by J. Mitchell, 1992, *Leadership and Management, 1*(8), 3-14. "Post-Traumatic Stress Disorder: When the Rescuer Becomes the Victim" by J.A. O'Rear, 1992, *Journal of Emergency Medical Services, 17*(1), 30-35.

Box 14-8

PHASES OF DEBRIEFING

Phase I	Introduction of group members, encouragement of active participation if members feel comfortable with it
Phase II	Each person is asked to discuss and describe their role in the incident. It is easy to initiate this phase by reconstructing the entire incident
Phase III	Participants are encouraged to discuss and describe their initial feelings after the incident
Phase IV	A discussion of which parts of the incident elicited the most physical and emotional response
Phase V	CISM asks the group what signs and symptoms of stress they may have experienced since the incident
Phase VI	Reentry phase, in which the team elicits any questions or comments about the process
Phase VII	Wrap-up session. Some groups provide refreshments and additional time to socialize

---

Note. From "Comprehensive Traumatic Stress Management in the Emergency Department" by J. Mitchell, 1992, *Leadership and Management, 1*(8), 3-14.

During transport, his blood pressure continued to decrease to about 60 by palpation. Fluid resuscitation was continued. The patient continued to voice his refusal to be transferred. Upon arrival at the receiving facility, the patient became confused, and despite three units of packed red blood cells, his blood pressure remained in the sixties and seventies. A peritoneal lavage revealed gross blood. The patient was taken to the operating room where a splenectomy was performed and the patient was eventually stabilized.

Discussion

When making the decision to transfer patients against their wishes, the nurse must take several factors into consideration. The first is the patient's ability or competency to make a decision. Even though this patient was awake and alert, his vital signs were unstable. The mechanism of injury was significant, and two other passengers had been killed in the same crash.

A follow-up visit was made to the patient by the transport nurse. Ironically the patient did not remember the entire transport incident. He stated that he initially had refused care because he was afraid that the caregivers were ignoring his parents, and he felt since he was awake and not hurting that all attention should have been focused on them. He thanked the nurse and other team members for their care and decision to move him for definitive care.

Ethical Issues (Pronouncing Patients Dead in the Field)

Scenario

A 60-year-old restrained male driver was struck by a tractor-trailer on the driver's side of the car. Upon the nurse and the transport team's arrival, the first responders were attempting to extricate the patient (Figure 14-7). Because the patient was having agonal respirations and had only a carotid pulse, the patient was intubated while still entrapped and intravenous access obtained. The patient remained entrapped for over 45 minutes.

About 20 minutes before the patient was removed from the car, he became pulseless. Cardiac compressions could not be given while the patient was entrapped. When cardiac compressions were attempted, the patient's sternum was found to be crushed and compressions were ineffective. In agreement with all those providing care for the patient, resuscitation was stopped and the patient pronounced dead at the scene of the crash.

Discussion

Ceasing resuscitation in the field can be a difficult decision. The nurse needs to take into account the mechanism of injury, initial vital signs and care, the amount of time it would take to transport the patient to definitive care, and the feelings of those who have been participating in the resuscitation. There are always problems to be considered related to futile resuscitation, which include safety of personnel and the fact that prolonged resuscitation can be emotionally difficult for all involved.

It is quite helpful to have preestablished protocols (see Figures 14-4 and 14-5) before these issue arise. It also important to discuss these decisions with others involved in the patient's care.

There is never a simple answer to this particular dilemma. Each case must be individually considered and reviewed. Anticipating these problems and having preexisting solutions may decrease the stress that is a part of this decision-making process.

REFERENCES

Adams, J. (1993). Ethical challenges in emergency medical services. *Prehospital and Disaster Medicine, 8*(2), 179-182.

Balazs, K. (1993). *AAMS/NFNA QA resource document indicators.* Pasadena, CA: Association of Air Medical Services.

Bell, N. (1991a). Critical incident stress debriefing. *Emergency, 9,* 30-35, 58.

Bell, N. (1991b). Exorcising stress. *Emergency, 23*(9), 36-39, 57.

Butler, S. (1992). Recording and using trauma data. In E. Bayley & S. Turke (Eds.). *Trauma nursing* (pp. 25-39). Boston: Jones & Bartlett.

Davis, E., & Billitier, J. (1993). The utilization of quality assurance methods in emergency medical services. *Prehospital and Disaster Medicine, 8*(2), 127-132.

Dworkin, R. (1993). *Life's dominion.* New York: Knopf Publishers.

Fanucci, D., Hammill, M., Johannson, P., Leggett, J., & Smith, M. (1993). Quantum leap into continuous quality improvement. *Nursing Management, 24*(6), 28-30.

Frew, S. (1990). Emergency medical services legal issues for the emergency physician. *Emergency Medicine Clinics of North America, 8*(1), 41-55.

Hardin, S. (1985). Chronic occupational distress in nursing. In J. McClosky & H. Grace. *Current issues in nursing.* (pp. 425-435). Boston: Blackwell Scientific Publications.

Iserson, K. (1989). Prehospital DNR orders. *Hastings Center Report, 12,* 17-19.

Jecker, N. (1992). Ceasing futile resuscitation in the field: Ethical considerations. *Archives of Internal Medicine, 152*(12), 3035.

Johnson, D., & Maggione, W. (1993). Resuscitation decision making by New Mexico Emergency Medical Technicians. *American Journal of Emergency Medicine, 11*(2), 139-142.

Johnson, J. (1992). Introduction to quality improvement. In S. Polsky (Ed.). *Continuous quality improvement* (pp.

1-19). Dallas: American College of Emergency Physicians.

Kallsen, G. (1993). Quality assurance in EMS. In R. Swor (Ed.). *Quality management in prehospital care* (pp. 3-13). St. Louis: Mosby.

Kellermann, A., Staves, D., & Hackman, B. (1988). In-hospital resuscitation following unsuccessful prehospital advanced cardiac life support. *Annals of Emergency Medicine, 17*(5), 589-594.

Mattox, K. (1993). "Ideal" posttraumatic parameters. *Journal of Trauma, 34*(5), 734-735.

Mitchell, J. (1992). Comprehensive traumatic stress management in the emergency department. *Leadership and Management, 1*(8), 3-14.

O'Leary, D., & O'Leary, M. (1992). From quality assurance to quality improvement. *Emergency Medicine Clinics of North America, 10*(3), 477-491.

O'Rear, J. (1992a). Posttraumatic stress disorder: When the rescuer becomes the victim. *Journal of Emergency Medical Services, 17*(1), 30-35.

O'Rear, J. (1992b). Preventing negative stress. *Journal of Emergency Medical Services, 17*(1), 36-39.

Polsky, S. (1992). *Continuous quality improvement in EMS.* Dallas: American College of Emergency Physicians.

Raffin, T. (1992). Perspectives on clinical medical ethics. In J. Hall, G. Schmidt, & L. Wood (Eds.). *Principles of critical care* (pp. 2185-2203). New York: McGraw-Hill.

Resource Document. (1992). Nursing care of the trauma patient.

Southard, P., & Eastes, L. (1993). Trauma quality management. In J. Neff & P. Kidd (Eds.). *Trauma nursing* (pp. 79-111). St. Louis: Mosby.

Sucov, A., Verdile, V., Garettson, D., & Paris, P. (1992). The outcome of patients refusing prehospital transportation. *Prehospital and Disaster Medicine, 7*(4), 365-371.

Swor, R. (1992). Quality assurance in EMS. *Emergency Medicine Clinics of North America, 10*(3), 597-610.

Swor, R. (1993). *Quality management in prehospital care.* St. Louis: Mosby.

Trofino, J. (1993). Voice-activated nursing documentation: On the cutting edge. *Nursing Management, 24*(7), 40-42.

Ulrich, S., & Blazing, M. (1991). Ethical dilemmas in emergency practice. *Topics in Emergency Medicine, 13*(3), 22-34.

Wright, S., Dronen, S., Combs, T., & Storer, D. (1989). Aeromedical transport of patients. *Annals of Emergency Medicine, 18*(8), 721-726.

Zachariah, B., Bryan, D., Pepe, P., & Griffin, M. (1992). Follow-up and outcome of patients who decline or are denied transport by EMS. *Prehospital and Disaster Medicine, 7*(4), 359-364.

CHAPTER 15

The Future of Prehospital Nursing

I have realized that the past and the future are real illusions, that they exist only in the present, which is what there is and all that there is.

WATTS, *1989*

Most people are curious about the future and what effect it may have on their lives. Nursing is no different. Societal, economic, and technological changes have created new roles for nursing outside of the walls of the hospital. Societal changes that affect prehospital care include the increase in the aging population, survival from chronic illnesses, and violence. With each passing year the cost of health care rises, and the number of those either uninsured or underinsured increases (Bradley, 1991). Will prehospital nursing be affordable and accessible to all or will cost prohibit its use? The question remains as to where these changes will lead the practice of prehospital nursing.

This chapter summarizes the current literature's predictions on the future of prehospital care from both inside and outside the discipline of nursing. In addition, some of the contributing authors to this text have contributed their prognostications. Looking to the future brings meaning to both the past and the present.

SOCIETAL CHANGES

In 1985 there were approximately 28.5 million people over the age of 65 (Patterson & Kim, 1991). It is estimated that there will be 35 million this age or older by the year 2000 (Patterson & Kim, 1991). Each year, more and more Americans survive the effects of heart disease and cancer. Chronic illness is not an un-

common problem any more. The care of the elderly and the treatment of chronic illnesses will continue into the future as new medicine, healing traditions, and technologies are developed.

Perhaps the most frightening societal change over the past 20 years is the increase in societal violence. Approximately 26 million Americans carry weapons such as guns and knives (Patterson & Kim, 1991). Both homicide and suicide have dramatically increased. About 25,000 Americans are killed by drunk drivers each year (Callahan, 1990; Patterson & Kim, 1991). Both prehospital and emergency department personnel have found themselves not only caring for the victims of violence, but also becoming victims during the course of providing patient care in some situations (Callahan, 1990; Gregory, 1992; Pane, Winiarski, & Salness, 1990; Patterson & Kim, 1991; Wagner, 1990; Wasserberger, Ordog, Kolodny, & Hardin, 1992).

Societal violence has greatly affected and will continue to impact those in the prehospital care environment. Scene safety, protective gear, and violence prevention education will become intricate parts of prehospital nursing practice.

ROLE OF NURSING IN PREHOSPITAL CARE

The first chapter of this book describes and discusses the history and some of the current roles of nursing in prehospital practice. Although there are accepted roles, a clear delineation of prehospital nursing's role has not been established. As pointed out by the study completed by Johnson, Childress, Herron, Boyko, Nowacki, Scanzello, and Lynch (1993), only six states have a certification for prehospital nursing. Other states require nurses either to have an EMT licensure or to take some type of challenging examination to practice in the prehospital care environment.

One of the most important future challenges prehospital nurses must face is to describe and define the role of nursing in prehospital care. Once this has been accomplished, a generic curriculum must be developed that describes the knowledge base, skills, experience, and additional course work necessary to practice in the prehospital care environment.

This will have to be a collaborative effort made not only by nurses but also by EMTs, paramedics, firefighters, and physicians. Some recent work has begun on this task through the establishment of an Emergency Services Committee by the Emergency Nurses Association and the collaborative development of the Certified Flight Nurse Examination with the Emergency Nurses Association and the National Flight Nurses Association.

One problem concerns the lack of a central authority in the Emergency Medical Services system in the United States. Nursing along with other EMS organizations have begun to address this issue through meetings and working together on mutual issues such as funding for services. Soon, the new assessment-based curriculum will be ready for use by prehospital care providers (Gregory, 1992). The foundations have been built, but the rest of the building has yet to be completed.

RESEARCH

Perhaps one of the most important tasks that must be accomplished now and continued in the future is the development of collaborative research ideas, protocols, and projects. Prehospital care research is needed to describe practice and demonstrate that what is done before and during transport makes a difference in patient care (Benson, 1992). Prehospital research will aid in the evaluation of current practice, will maintain interest in the profession, and will

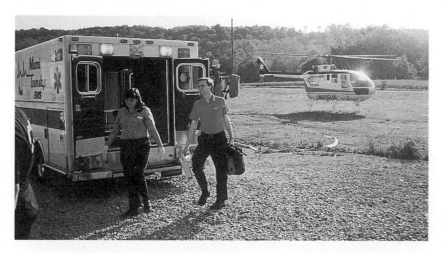

Fig. 15-1   Nurse in collaboration in the prehospital environment.

save lives and limit morbidity (Menegazzi, 1993).

Research challenges practitioners to take another look at the status quo. For example, current research related to the use of MAST pants (military antishock trousers) and fluid resuscitation has suggested that contemporary practices may be detrimental to certain types of patients (Kowalenko, Stern, Dronen, & Wang, 1992; Martin, Bickell, Pepe, Burch, & Mattox; Mattox, Bickell, & Pepe, 1989; Stern, Dronen, Birrer, & Wang, 1993). These studies have shown that the process of treating a hypotensive adult patient in the field requires a holistic approach and more collaborative evaluation.

Performing research in the prehospital care environment is not an easy charge. Several problems need to be addressed including identifying the type of research design that will work in the field, the problem with double blinding in the field, controlling for extraneous variables, defining a study sample, establishing inclusion and exclusion criteria, and minimizing selection biases (Menegazzi, 1993). Other problems that have been encountered are related to continued enthusiasm about a particular project, collection of data over a long period of time, failure to enroll the right patients, and lack of supplies and funding to do the research project (Menegazzi, 1993).

Collaborative research holds one of the keys to the future of prehospital care, as well as prehospital nursing practice. Discovering what we do and whether it makes a difference defines who we are and provides the framework for better patient care.

TECHNOLOGY

Equipment that was once limited to intensive care units, operating rooms, and emergency departments is now routinely used before and during transport. For example, end-tidal CO_2 monitoring can be used for monitoring tube placement, as well as for directing intracranial pressure management during transport (Sanders, 1989). Other examples of technological advances for field use include "heart-starters," which evaluate how long the patient has been in arrest based on the quality of the EKG wave detected. Depending on the length of time down, the machine will advise whether to shock the patient or begin CPR and drug management (Menegazzi, 1993). Needleless systems for drug and fluid administration will decrease the risk of disease exposure (Evans, Kramer, & Mistler, 1993).

Communications between the field and receiving facilities will change. Examples of this include the use of video cameras at the scene of the illness or injury directed back to the receiving facility. The teams at the receiving facility can then advise and direct care based on visual and verbal information. This also offers a method of implementing quality management in prehospital patient care.

Computers will be of particular use in the field and during transport. Laboratory, EKG, and physiological data may be rapidly transmitted during the transport process. Charting may involve the use of preprogrammed data screens (e.g., advanced cardiac life support), allowing for some narrative documentation as events occur.

THE FUTURE

As the future unfolds, so will the roles for prehospital nursing. Case management, implementation of research protocols, delivery of care in the field without transport, and the development and implementation of illness and injury prevention strategies are only some of the phenomena prehospital nurses may be a part of in the years to come. Prehospital nursing does have a collaborative role to play in the care of the patient before, during, and after transport. Continuing to discover, develop, and define this role through research and collaborative efforts will probably be the most important challenges prehospital nurses will face.

The future is a collective effort. You can't decide on the future alone, and you especially can't create it alone (Popcorn, 1991).

REFERENCES

Benson, K. (1992). What's at stake? *Emergency, 24*(12), 40-41.

Bradley, V. (1991). *Megatrends in emergency nursing.* Park Ridge, IL: Emergency Nurses Association.

Callahan, B. (1990). Armed America: Demands on the EMS system. *Emergency Medical Services, 11,* 24-26.

Evans, J., Kramer, A., & Mistler, A. (1993). Future trends in prehospital care. Personal communication.

Gregory, A. (1992). Playing prophet. *Emergency, 24*(12), 28-35.

Johnson, R., Childress, S., Herron, H., Boyko, S., Nowacki, J., Scanzello, N., & Lynch, M. (1993). Regulation of prehospital nursing practice: Where do we stand? Unpublished abstract.

Kowalenko, T., Stern, S., Dronen, S., & Wang, X. (1992). Improved outcome with hypotensive resuscitation of uncontrolled hemorrhagic shock in a swine model. *Journal of Trauma, 33*(3), 349-353.

Martin, R., Bickell, W., Pepe, P., Burch, J., & Mattox, K. (1992). Prospective evaluation of perioperative fluid resuscitation in hypotensive patients with penetrating truncal injury: A preliminary report. *Journal of Trauma, 33*(3), 354-362.

Mattox, K., Bickell, W., & Pepe, P. (1989). Prospective MAST study in 911 patients. *Journal of Trauma, 30*(8), 1104-1112.

Menegazzi, J. (1993). Pragmatic problems in prehospital research. *Prehospital and Disaster Medicine, 8*(1), S15-S19.

Pane, G., Winiarski, A., & Salness, K. (1990). Aggression directed toward emergency department staff at a university teaching hospital. *Annals of Emergency Medicine, 19*(3), 284-286.

Patterson, J., & Kim, P. (1991). *The day America told the truth.* New York: Prentice Hall Press.

Popcorn, F. (1991). *The Popcorn report.* New York: Harper Business.

Sanders, A. (1989). Capnometry in emergency medicine. *Annals of Emergency Medicine, 18*(12), 1287-1290.

Stern, S., Dronen, S., Birrer, P., & Wang, X. (1993). Effect of blood pressure on hemorrhage volume and survival in a near-fatal hemorrhage model incorporating vascular injury. *Annals of Emergency Medicine, 22*(2), 155-163.

Wagner, L. (1990). Hospitals feeling the trauma of violence. *Modern Healthcare, 5,* 23-28.

Wasserberger, J., Ordog, G., Kolodny, M., Hardin, E. (1992). Weapons in the emergency department. *Annals of Emergency Medicine, 21*(5), 656.

Watts, A. (1989). Time. In J. Winokur (Ed.). *Zen to go* (pp. 70-73). New York: New American Library.

Appendixes

State Emergency Medical Services Agencies

ALABAMA

The Office of Emergency Medical Services
Alabama Department of Health
434 Monroe Street
Montgomery, AL 36130-1701
205/242-5865

ALASKA

Emergency Medical Services
DHSS/Public Health
P. O. Box 110616
Juneau, AK 99811-0616
907/465-3027

ARIZONA

Office of Emergency Medical Services
Arizona Department of Health Services
100 W. Clarendon, Suite 300
Phoenix, AZ 85013
602/255-1170

ARKANSAS

Division of Emergency Medical Services
Arkansas Department of Health
4815 W. Markham Street, Slot 38
Little Rock, AR 72205-3867
501/661-2178

CALIFORNIA

Emergency Medical Services Authority
1930 Ninth Street, Suite 100
Sacramento, CA 95814
916/322-4336

COLORADO

Colorado Department of Health
EMS Division, EMSD-ADM-A3
4300 Cherry Creek Drive S.
Denver, CO 80222
303/692-2980

CONNECTICUT

Emergency Medical Services Office
Department of Health
150 Washington Street
Hartford, CT 06106
203/566-7336

DELAWARE

Emergency Medical Services
Capitol Square
Jesse S. Cooper Memorial Building
Dover, DE 19901
302/739-4710

DISTRICT OF COLUMBIA

Emergency Health and Medical Service
District of Columbia Commission of Public Health
1660 S Street N.W., Room 1223
Washington, DC 20036
202/673-6744

FLORIDA

Emergency Medical Services
Department of Health and Rehabilitation
1317 Winewood Blvd.
Tallahassee, FL 32399-0700
904/487-1911

GEORGIA
Emergency Medical Services
Georgia Department of Human Resources
878 Peachtree Street N.E., Room 207
Atlanta, GA 30309
404/894-6505

HAWAII
Emergency Medical Services
State Department of Health
3627 Kilauea Avenue, Room 102
Honolulu, HI 96816
808/735-5267

IDAHO
Emergency Medical Services Bureau
Department of Health and Welfare
450 W. State Street
Boise, ID 83720
208/334-5994

ILLINOIS
Division of Emergency Medical Services
Illinois Department of Public Health
525 W. Jefferson Street
Springfield, IL 62761
217/785-2080

INDIANA
Indiana EMS Commission
302 W. Washington, Room E-208
Indianapolis, IN 46204-2258
317/232-3980

IOWA
Emergency Medical Services
Iowa Department of Public Health
Lucas State Office Building
Des Moines, IA 50319-0075
515/281-3239

KANSAS
Board of Emergency Medical Services
109 S. W. Sixth Street
Topeka, KS 66603-3805
913/296-7296

KENTUCKY
Emergency Medical Services Branch
Department for Health Services
275 E. Main
Health Services Building
Frankfort, KY 40621
502/564-8965

LOUISIANA
Bureau of Emergency Medical Services
P. O. Box 94215, Bin 8
Baton Rouge, LA 70804
504/342-4881

MAINE
Maine Emergency Medical Services
16 Edison Drive
Augusta, ME 04347
207/289-3953

MARYLAND
Emergency Medical Services
MIEMSS
22 S. Greene Street
Baltimore, MD 21201
410/328-5074

MASSACHUSETTS
Office of Emergency Medical Services
Department of Public Health
150 Tremont Street, Second Floor
Boston, MA 02111
617/727-8338

MICHIGAN
Division of EMS
Michigan Department of Public Health
P. O. Box 30195
Lansing, MI 48909
517/335-9502

MINNESOTA
Emergency Medical Services
Minnesota Department of Health
P. O. Box 9441
Minneapolis, MN 55440
612/623-5484

MISSISSIPPI
Emergency Medical Services
State Department of Health
P. O. Box 1700
Jackson, MS 39215-1700
601/987-3880

MISSOURI
Bureau of Emergency Medical Services
Missouri Department of Health
P. O. Box 570
Jefferson City, MO 65102
314/751-6356

MONTANA
Emergency Medical Services
Department of Health/Environmental Science
Cogswell Building
Helena, MT 59620
406/444-3895

NEBRASKA
Division of Emergency Medical Services
301 Centennial Mall S., Third Floor
Box 95007
Lincoln, NE 68509-5007
402/471-2158

NEVADA
Emergency Medical Services Office
Nevada State Health Division
505 E. King Street, Suite 204
Carson City, NV 89710
701/687-3065

NEW HAMPSHIRE
Bureau of EMS
Health and Welfare Building
6 Hazen Drive
Concord, NH 03301-6527
603/271-4569

NEW JERSEY
Emergency Medical Services
State Department of Health
CN-364
Trenton, NJ 08625
609/292-6789

NEW MEXICO
Primary Care and EMS Bureau
Department of Health
P. O. Box 26110
Santa Fe, NM 87502-6110
505/827-2509

NEW YORK
Emergency Medical Services Program
Department of Health
74 State Street, Fourth Floor
Albany, NY 12207
518/474-0911

NORTH CAROLINA
Office of Emergency Medical Services
701 Barbour Drive (27603)
P. O. Box 29530
Raleigh, NC 27626-0530
919/733-2285

NORTH DAKOTA
Division of Emergency Health Services
Department of Health/Consolidated Labs
600 E. Boulevard Avenue
Bismarck, ND 58505-0200
701/224-2388

OHIO
Ohio Department of Highway Safety
Division of Emergency Medical Services
P. O. Box 7167
Columbus, OH 43266-0563
614/466-9447

OKLAHOMA
Emergency Medical Services
Department of Health, Special Health Services
1000 N.E. 10th, Room 1104
Oklahoma City, OK 73117-1299
405/271-4027

OREGON
Emergency Medical Services
State Health Division
P. O. Box 14450
Portland, OR 97214-0450
503/731-4011

PENNSYLVANIA
Division of Emergency Medical Services
Health and Welfare Building, Room 1033
P. O. Box 90
Harrisburg, PA 17108
717/787-8740

RHODE ISLAND
Emergency Medical Services Division
Department of Health, Room 404
3 Capitol Hill
Providence, RI 02908-5097
401/277-2401

SOUTH CAROLINA
Emergency Medical Services Division
Department of Health and Environmental Control
2600 Bull Street
Columbia, SC 29201
803/734-4905

SOUTH DAKOTA
Emergency Medical Services Program
Department of Health
118 W. Capitol Street
Pierre, SD 57501
605/773-3737

TENNESSEE
Division of Emergency Medical Services
Department of Health and Environment
287 Plus Park Blvd.
Nashville, TN 37247-0701
615/367-6278

TEXAS
Emergency Medical Services Division
Texas Department of Health
1100 W. 49th Street
Austin, TX 78756-3199
512/458-7550

UTAH
Bureau of Emergency Medical Services
Department of Health
P. O. Box 16990
Salt Lake City, UT 84116-0990
801/538-6435

VERMONT
Emergency Medical Services Division
Department of Health
Box 70
131 Main Street
Burlington, VT 05402
802/863-7310

VIRGINIA
Division of Emergency Medical Services
State Department of Health
1538 E. Parham Road
Richmond, VA 23228
804/371-3500

WASHINGTON
EMS and Trauma Systems
Department of Health
P. O. Box 47853
Olympia, WA 98504-7853
206/705-6700

WEST VIRGINIA
Emergency Medical Services
West Virginia Department of Health
1411 Virginia Street E., Second Floor
Charleston, WV 25301
304/558-3956

WISCONSIN
Emergency Medical Services
Division of Health
P. O. Box 309
Madison, WI 53701-0309
608/266-7743

WYOMING
Emergency Medical Services Program
State of Wyoming
Hathaway Building, Room 527
Cheyenne, WY 82002
307/777-7955

APPENDIX 2

Organizations and Associations

AMBULANCE MANUFACTURERS DIVISION (AMD)
National Truck Equipment Association
38705 Seven Mile Road, Suite 345
Livonia, MI 48152-1057
800/866-6832, 313/462-2108

AMERICAN ACADEMY OF ORTHOPAEDIC SURGEONS
Thomas C. Nelson
Executive Director
6300 N. River Road
Rosemont, IL 60018
708/823-7186

AMERICAN ACADEMY OF PEDIATRICS (AAP) COMMITTEE ON PEDIATRIC EMERGENCY CARE
James E. Strain
Executive Director
141 N.W. Point Blvd.
Elk Grove Village, IL 60009
708/228-5005

AMERICAN AMBULANCE ASSOCIATION (AAA)
David Nevins
Executive Vice President
3814 Auburn Blvd., Suite 70
Sacramento, CA 95821
916/483-3827

AMERICAN ASSOCIATION OF CRITICAL-CARE NURSES
Sarah J. Sanford, RN, MA, FAAN, CNAA
Chief Executive Officer
101 Columbia
Aliso Viejo, CA 92656-1491
800/899-AACN, 714/362-2000

AMERICAN COLLEGE OF EMERGENCY PHYSICIANS (ACEP)
Collin C. Rorrie, PhD
Executive Director
1125 Executive Circle
Irving, TX 75038
214/550-0911

AMERICAN COLLEGE OF HEALTHCARE EXECUTIVES (ACHE)
Thomas C. Dolan, PhD, FACHE
President
840 N. Lake Shore Drive
Chicago, IL 60611
312/943-0544

AMERICAN COLLEGE OF OSTEOPATHIC EMERGENCY PHYSICIANS
5200 S. Ellis
Chicago, IL 60615
312/947-4922

AMERICAN COLLEGE OF SURGEONS/ COMMITTEE ON TRAUMA
Director, Trauma Department
55 E. Erie Street
Chicago, IL 60611
312/664-4050

AMERICAN HEART ASSOCIATION (AHA)

Dudley H. Hafner
Executive Vice President
7272 Greenville Avenue
Dallas, TX 75231
214/373-6300

AMERICAN MEDICAL ASSOCIATION (AMA)

James S. Todd, MD
Executive Vice President
515 N. State Street
Chicago, IL 60610
312/464-5000

AMERICAN MEDICAL DIRECTORS ASSOCIATION (AMDA)

Lorraine Tamove
Executive Director
10480 Little Patuxent Parkway, Suite 760
Columbia, MD 21044
410/740-9743

AMERICAN NATIONAL RED CROSS

Robert Burnside
Director, Health and Safety
17th and D Streets N.W.
Washingtion, DC 20006
202/639-3557

AMERICAN PEDIATRIC SURGICAL ASSOCIATION COMMITTEE ON TRAUMA

University of Florida
Health Science Center
653 W. Eighth Street
Jacksonville, FL 33209-6511
904/549-3910

ASSOCIATED PUBLIC-SAFETY COMMUNICATIONS OFFICERS INC. (APCO)

Executive Director
2040 S. Ridgewood Avenue
South Daytona, FL 32119
904/322-2500

ASTM-COMMITTEE F30 ON EMS

Manager
1916 Race Street
Philadelphia, PA 19103
215/299-5521

CENTER FOR STUDIES IN HEALTH POLICY

1155 Connecticut Avenue N.W., Suite 400
Washington, DC 20036
202/659-3270

CITIZEN CPR FOUNDATION

Board of Directors
P. O. Box 911
Camel, IN 46032
317/575-0036

COMMISSION ON ACCREDITATION OF AIR-MEDICAL SERVICES (CAAMS)

Executive Director
P. O. Box 1305
Anderson, SC 29622
803/287-4177

COMMISSION ON ACCREDITATION OF AMBULANCE SERVICES (CAAS)

Executive Director
P. O. Box 619911
Dallas, TX 75261-9911
214/580-2829

DISASTER RESEARCH CENTER

Director
University of Delaware
Newark, DE 19716
302/831-6618

DOCTORS FOR DISASTER PREPAREDNESS

President
Box 272
2509 N. Campbell
Tucson, AZ 85716
602/325-2680

EMERGENCY MEDICAL SERVICE INSTITUTE
Executive Director
4240 Greensburg Pike
Pittsburgh, PA 15221
412/351-6604

EMERGENCY MEDICINE FOUNDATION
Executive Director
P. O. Box 619911
Dallas, TX 75261-9911
214/550-0911

EMERGENCY NURSES ASSOCIATION (ENA)
President
216 Higgins Road
Park Ridge, IL 60068
708/698-9400

EMS FOR CHILDREN
Division of Maternal, Infant, Child and Adolescent
Health
Maternal and Child Health Bureau
Health Resources and Services
Administration, Room 18-A 30
Parklawn Building
5600 Fishers Lake
Rockville, MD 20857
301/443-4026

INTERNATIONAL ASSOCIATION OF FIRE CHIEFS (IAFC)
Executive Director
4025 Fair Ridge Drive, Suite 300
Fairfax, VA 22038-2862
703/273-0911

INTERNATIONAL ASSOCIATION OF FIRE FIGHTERS (IAFF)
General President
1750 New York Avenue N.W., Third Floor
Washington, DC 20006
202/737-8484

INTERNATIONAL CRITICAL INCIDENT STRESS FOUNDATION
President
5018 Dorsey Hall Drive, Suite 104
Ellicott City, MD 21042
410/730-4311 (emergency, 410/313-2473)

INTERNATIONAL SOCIETY FOR BURN INJURIES
Secretary-Treasurer
325 Ninth Avenue
Surgery Department Za-16
Seattle, WA 98104
206/223-3140

INTERNATIONAL SOCIETY OF FIRE SERVICE INSTRUCTORS (ISFSI)
Chief Executive Officer
30 Main Street
Ashland, MA 01721
508/881-5800, 800/435-0005

JOINT COMMISSION ON ACCREDITATION OF HEALTHCARE ORGANIZATIONS
President
1 Renaissance Blvd.
Oakbrook Terrace, IL 60181
708/916-5600

NATIONAL ASSOCIATION FOR SEARCH AND RESCUE (NASAR)
Executive Director
11200 Waples Mill Road, Suite 300
Fairfax, VA 22030
703/352-1349

NATIONAL ASSOCIATION OF EMERGENCY MEDICAL TECHNICIANS (NAEMT)
President
9140 Ward Parkway
Kansas City, MO 64144
816/444-3500

**NATIONAL ASSOCIATION OF EMS
PHYSICIANS (NAEMSP)**
Executive Director, Executive National Resource
Center
230 McKee Place
Pittsburgh, PA 15213
412/578-3222, 800/228-3677

**NATIONAL ASSOCIATION OF STATE EMS
DIRECTORS (NASEMSD)**
President
1947 Camino Vida Roble, Suite 202
Carlsbad, CA 92008
619/431-7054

**NATIONAL COUNCIL OF STATE EMS
TRAINING COORDINATORS (NCSEMSTC)**
Chairperson
P. O. Box 11910, Iron Works Pike
Lexington, KY 40578
606/231-1923

**NATIONAL EMERGENCY NUMBER
ASSOCIATION (NENA)**
Executive Director
1500 W. Third Avenue, Suite 228
Columbus, OH 43212
800/332-3911

**NATIONAL EMS FOR CHILDREN RESOURCE
ALLIANCE (NERA)**
Project Director
1001 W. Carson Street, Suite S
Torrance, CA 90502
310/328-0720

**NATIONAL FLIGHT NURSES ASSOCIATION
(NFNA)**
President
6900 Grove Road
Thorofare, NJ 08086
609/384-6725

**NATIONAL FLIGHT PARAMEDICS
ASSOCIATION (NFPA)**
President
35 S. Raymond Avenue, Suite 205
Pasadena, CA 91105
818/405-9851

**NATIONAL HEAD INJURY FOUNDATION
INC.**
President
1776 Massachusetts Avenue N.W.
Suite 100
Washington, DC 20036
202/296-6643

**NATIONAL INSTITUTE FOR BURN
MEDICINE**
Director
909 E. Ann Street
Ann Arbor, MI 48104
313/769-9000

**NATIONAL INSTITUTE FOR URBAN SEARCH
AND RESCUE (NI/USR)**
President
P. O. Box 91648
Santa Barbara, CA 93190-1648
800/767-0093

NATIONAL REGISTRY OF EMTS (NREMT)
Executive Director
6610 Busch Blvd., P.O. Box 29233
Columbus, OH 43229
614/888-4484

NATIONAL RURAL HEALTH ASSOCIATION
Executive Director
301 E. Armour Blvd., Suite 420
Kansas City, MO 64111
816/756-3140

NATIONAL SAFETY COUNCIL
President
1121 Spring Lake Drive
Itasca, IL 60143-3201
708/285-1121

NATIONAL STUDY CENTER FOR TRAUMA AND EMS

Director
UMAB
22 S. Greene Street
Baltimore, MD 21201
410/328-5085

PROFESSIONAL AEROMEDICAL TRANSPORT ASSOCIATION

Executive Director
P. O. Box 7519
Alexandria, VA 22307
703/660-9200, 800/541-7517

RADIO EMERGENCY ASSOCIATION COMMUNICATION TEAM (REACT) INTERNATIONAL INC.

Office Manager
242 Cleveland
Wichita, KS 67214
316/263-2100

SOCIETY FOR ACADEMIC EMERGENCY MEDICINE (SAEM)

Executive Director
901 N. Washington Avenue
Lansing, MI 48906
517/485-5484

SOCIETY OF CRITICAL CARE MEDICINE

Executive Director
8101 E. Kaiser Blvd.
Anaheim, CA 92808-2214
714/282-6000

SOCIETY OF TRAUMA NURSES

President
P. O. Box 340278
Sacramento, CA 95834-0278
916/568-0617

UNDERSEA AND HYPERBARIC MEDICAL SOCIETY

Executive Director
9650 Rockville Pike
Bethesda, MD 20814
301/571-1818

WILDERNESS MEDICAL SOCIETY

President
P. O. Box 2463
Indianapolis, IN 46206
317/631-1745

WOMEN IN THE FIRE SERVICE

Executive Director
P. O. Box 5446
Madison, WI 53705
608/233-4768

GOVERNMENT AGENCIES

CENTERS FOR DISEASE CONTROL AND PREVENTION (CDC)

Director
1600 Clifton Road N.E.
Atlanta, GA 30333
404/639-3311

FEDERAL COMMUNICATIONS COMMISSION (FCC)

Public Service
1919 M Street N.W., Room 254
Washington, DC 20554
202/632-7000

FEDERAL EMERGENCY MANAGEMENT AGENCY

Director
16825 S. Seton Avenue
Emmitsburg, MD 21727
301/447-1185

NATIONAL HIGHWAY TRAFFIC SAFETY ADMINISTRATION (NHTSA)
Chief, EMS Division, NTS-42
400 Seventh Street S.W.
Washington, DC 20590-0001
800/424-9393, 202/366-5440

UNITED STATES FIRE ADMINISTRATION
EMS Program Manager
16825 S. Seton Avenue
Emmitsburg, MD 21727
301/447-1080, 301/447-1185

U. S. DEPARTMENT OF TRANSPORTATION
Emergency Medical Services Division
Chief
400 Seventh Street S.W.
Room 5119-H, NTS-42
Washington, DC 20590
202/366-5440

Index